a LANGE medical book

CURRENT CONSULT

CARDIOLOGY

Differential Diagnosis

A—Z   Dx and Tx

a LANGE medical book

CURRENT CONSULT

CARDIOLOGY

Edited by

Michael H. Crawford, MD
Professor of Medicine
Lucie Stern Chair in Cardiology
University of California, San Francisco
Chief of Clinical Cardiology
UCSF Medical Center
San Francisco, California

Komandoor Srivathson, MD
Assistant Professor of Medicine
Mayo Medical School
Rochester, Minnesota
Senior Associate Consultant
Mayo Clinic Arizona
Scottsdale, Arizona

Dana P. McGlothlin, MD
Assistant Professor of Medicine
University of California,
    San Francisco
San Francisco, California

Lange Medical Books/McGraw-Hill
Medical Publishing Division

New York   Chicago   San Francisco   Lisbon   London
Madrid   Mexico City   Milan   New Delhi   San Juan
Seoul   Singapore   Sydney   Toronto

Current Consult: Cardiology

ISBN: 0-07-144010-0

ISSN: 1557-3478

Notice

Medicine is an ever-changing science. As new research and clinical experience broaden our knowledge, changes in treatment and drug therapy are required. The authors and the publisher of this work have checked with sources believed to be reliable in their efforts to provide information that is complete and generally in accord with the standards accepted at the time of publication. However, in view of the possibility of human error or changes in medical sciences, neither the authors nor the publisher nor any other party who has been involved in the preparation or publication of this work warrants that the information contained herein is in every respect accurate or complete, and they disclaim all responsibility for any errors or omissions or for the results obtained from use of the information contained in this work. Readers are encouraged to confirm the information contained herein with other sources. For example and in particular, readers are advised to check the product information sheet included in the package of each drug they plan to administer to be certain that the information contained in this work is accurate and that changes have not been made in the recommended dose or in the contraindications for administration. This recommendation is of particular importance in connection with new or infrequently used drugs.

This book was set in Adobe Garamond by Pine Tree Composition, Inc.
The editors were Hilarie Surrena, Harriet Lebowitz, and Penny Linskey.
The production supervisor was Sherri Souffrance.
The text was designed by Eve Siegel.
The index was prepared by Kathrin Unger.

Quebecor Dubuque was printer and binder.

This book is printed on acid-free paper.

INTERNATIONAL EDITION ISBN: 0-07-110513-1
Copyright © 2006. Exclusive rights by The McGraw-Hill Companies, Inc. for manufacture and export. This book cannot be re-exported from the country to which it is consigned by McGraw-Hill. The International Edition is not available in North America.

Current Consult Cardiology: 2 Parts

Differential diagnosis for
cardiac-related symptoms and signs

Key diagnosis and treatment
information for over 175 diseases
and symptoms

CONTENTS: Alphabetical

CONTENTS: Topical

Guide to *Current Consult: Cardiology*

Current Consult: Cardiology is designed to provide rapid, efficient access to the exact information you need when you only have a few minutes to review a topic. It is a single-source reference for use in the clinical setting. The two parts of the book which are color-coded include:

- Differential Diagnosis: the GREEN PAGES
- A-Z Diagnosis and Treatment: the WHITE PAGES

The **DIFFERENTIAL DIAGNOSIS** section is a unique index and valuable feature that groups disease topics according to related signs, symptoms, and patient presentations. It offers differential diagnoses for patient evaluation, along with an immediate connection to the appropriate disorders.

A—Z DIAGNOSIS AND TREATMENT presents carefully selected information on cardiovascular topics in a convenient two-page format for each disorder. Perfect as a reference when a rapid review of practical points is needed, the WHITE PAGES are not only organized alphabetically, but are also accompanied by an additional Contents list that categorizes the topics by subject area; for example, ischemic heart disease, vascular disease and valvular heart disease groupings. Each disease entry in the A—Z section highlights:

- Key Features, including Essentials of Diagnosis
- Clinical Presentation and Differential Diagnosis
- Diagnostic Evaluation, including Imaging Studies
- Ongoing Management, including Complications and Prognosis
- Treatment, such as Medications, Therapeutic Procedures, and Surgery
- Resources, such as Practice Guidelines, References, and Web Sites

How to Use *Current Consult: Cardiology*
- If you know the diagnosis for which you need an immediate consult, go directly to that disorder in the WHITE PAGES, or
- If you are searching for a differential diagnosis for certain symptoms, signs, or patient presentations, consult the Differential Diagnosis section – the GREEN PAGES. After selecting the most likely diagnoses, go to the WHITE PAGES, A—Z Diagnosis and Treatment, to get complete diagnosis and treatment information.

We hope that *Current Consult: Cardiology* will be a useful and handy resource, providing the guidance that you need—when you need it—to enhance the care of your patients.

Michael H. Crawford, M.D.
San Francisco, California

Differential Diagnosis

Canon Waves in the Jugular Venous Pulse

More Common
- Atrioventricular nodal-His block

Less Common
- Nonparoxysmal junctional tachycardia
- Pacemaker syndrome
- Ventricular tachycardia

Chest Pain: at Rest, Transient

More Common
- Angina pectoris, unstable

Less Common
- Variant or Prinzmetal's angina

Chest Pain: Exertional, Transient

More Common
- Aortic stenosis
- Ischemic heart disease, chronic

Less Common
- Cardiac Syndrome X (microvascular angina pectoris)
- Coronary artery disease, symptomatic, non-revascularizable
- Hypertrophic cardiomyopathies
- Subclavian coronary artery steal syndrome

Chest Pain: Pleuritic

More Common
- Myocarditis
- Pericarditis, acute

Less Common
- Left ventricular free wall rupture, acute
- Myocardial infarction, acute ST-elevation
- Pulmonary embolism

Chest Pain: Prolonged

More Common
- Myocardial infarction, acute non-ST segment elevation
- Myocardial infarction, acute ST segment elevation

Less Common
- Myocarditis
- Pericarditis, acute

Continuous Murmur

More Common
- Patent ductus arteriosus

Less Common
- Aortic stenosis and regurgitation
- Periprosthetic valve leak
- Ventricular septal defect with aortic regurgitation

Cyanosis

More Common
- Cor pulmonale/right-heart failure
- Pulmonary embolism

Less Common
- Atrioventricular canal defects
- Eisenmenger's syndrome
- Epstein's anomaly
- Pulmonary atresia
- Tetralogy of Fallot
- Total anomalous pulmonary venous drainage
- Transposition of the great arteries
- Tricuspid atresia
- Truncus arteriosus

Dyspnea, at Rest

More Common
- Congestive heart failure
- Pulmonary edema

Less Common
- Aortic regurgitation, acute
- Cardiac tamponade
- High altitude pulmonary edema
- Mitral regurgitation, acute
- Pulmonary embolism

Dyspnea, on Exertion

More Common
- Aortic regurgitation, chronic
- Aortic stenosis
- Cardiomyopathy
- Congestive heart failure
- Cor pulmonale

- Hypertrophic cardiomyopathy
- Ischemic heart disease
- Mitral stenosis
- Mitral regurgitation
- Mixed valve diseases
- Pulmonary hypertension, primary

Less Common
- Heart disease in pregnancy
- High output heart failure
- Hyperthyroid heart disease
- Mitral valve prolapse
- Pulmonic stenosis
- Pulmonary embolism
- Tricuspid stenosis

Edema

More Common
- Congestive heart failure
- Cor pulmonale, right-heart failure
- Deep venous thrombosis
- Venous insufficiency

Less Common
- Carcinoid and the heart
- Hypothyroid heart disease
- Localized lymphedema
- Pericarditis, constrictive

Ejection Sound or Systolic Click

More Common
- Aortic stenosis
- Bicuspid aortic valve
- Mitral valve prolapse

Less Common
- Epstein's anomaly
- Pulmonary hypertension, primary
- Pulmonic stenosis

Elevated Blood Pressure

More Common
- Aortic regurgitation, chronic
- Cerebral vascular disease
- Hypertension, systemic
- Metabolic syndrome

Less Common
- Acromegaly
- Coarctation of the aorta

- Cocaine-induced cardiovascular disease
- Cushing's syndrome
- Hyperaldosteronism, primary
- Hyperparathyroidism
- Hypertension, gestational
- Hypertension, renovascular
- Pheochromocytoma

Elevated Jugular Venous Pulse

More Common
- Cardiac tamponade
- Congestive heart failure
- Cor pulmonale / right-heart failure

Less Common
- Carcinoid
- Cardiomyopathy, restrictive
- Eisenmenger's syndrome
- Myocardial infarction, right ventricular
- Pericarditis, constrictive
- Superior vena cava syndrome
- Tricuspid regurgitation
- Tricuspid stenosis

Enlarged Heart

More Common
- Aortic regurgitation, chronic
- Cardiomyopathy
- Congestive heart failure
- Mitral regurgitation, chronic
- Mixed valve disease
- Pericardial effusion

Less Common
- Athlete's heart
- Atrial septal defect
- Chagas' heart disease
- Eisenmenger's syndrome
- Left ventricular aneurysm

Fourth Heart Sound

More Common
- Aortic stenosis
- Hypertension
- Ischemic heart disease, chronic
- Myocardial infarction

Less Common
- Athletes' heart

- Cardiomyopathy, restrictive
- Epstein's anomaly
- Hemochromotosis
- Hypertrophic cardiomyopathies

Global or Focal Disturbance of Cerebral Function

More Common
- Atrial fibrillation
- Cardiogenic Shock
- Cerebral vascular disease
- Hypertensive emergencies

Less Common
- Cardiomyopathy, idiopathic dilated
- Digitalis toxicity
- Infective endocarditis
- Left ventricular aneurysm
- Mitral stenosis
- Patent foramen ovale / atrial septal aneurysm

Localized Reduced Blood Pressure or Pulse Amplitude

More Common
- Peripheral arterial atherosclerosis obliterans
- Thoracic aortic dissection

Less Common
- Aortic coarctation
- Aortic stenosis, supravalvular
- Takayasu's arteritis

Low Systemic Blood Pressure

More Common
- Cardiac tamponade
- Cardiogenic shock
- Congestive heart failure
- Orthostatic hypotension

Less Common
- Adrenal insufficiency
- Athlete's heart
- Hypotension complicating hemodialysis
- Hypothyroid heart disease

Murmur, Diastolic

More Common
- Aortic regurgitation
- Mitral stenosis

Less Common
- Periprosthetic valve leaks
- Pulmonic regurgitation
- Tricuspid stenosis
- Truncus arteriosus

Murmur, Holosystolic

More Common
- Mitral regurgitation, chronic
- Periprosthetic valve leaks
- Tricuspid regurgitation

Less Common
- Atrioventricular canal defects
- Ventricular septal defect
- Ventricular septal rupture, acute

Murmur, Systolic, Ejection (Crescendo, Decrescendo)

More Common
- Aortic stenosis
- Bicuspid aortic valve
- Mitral valve prolapse

Less Common
- Hyperthyroid heart disease
- Hypertrophic cardiomyopathy
- Pulmonic stenosis

Palpitation, Tachycardia

More Common
- Atrial flutter / fibrillation
- Atrioventricular nodal re-entrant tachycardia
- Atrioventricular reciprocating tachycardia
- Automatic (ectopic) atrial tachycardia
- Sinus tachycardia

Less Common
- Atriofascicular tachycardia
- Cocaine-induced cardiovascular disease
- Hyperthyroid heart disease
- Intra-atrial re-entrant tachycardia
- Multifocal atrial tachycardia

- Permanent form of functional reciprocating tachycardia
- Postural tachycardia syndrome
- Sinus node re-entry
- Ventricular tachycardia

Syncope

More Common
- Atrioventricular nodal-His block
- Neurocardiogenic
- Orthostatic hypotension

- Sinus bradycardia
- Sinus node dysfunction
- Ventricular tachycardia

Less Common
- Brugada syndrome
- Congenitally corrected transposition of the great arteries
- Carotid sinus hypersensitivity
- Effort syncope
- Long QT syndrome
- Hypertrophic cardiomyopathy
- Pacemaker malfunction

- Pulmonary emboli
- Tricyclic antidepressants

Wide Pulse Pressure

More Common
- Aortic regurgitation
- Hyperthyroid heart disease
- Peripheral arterial atherosclerosis obliterans

Less Common
- High output heart failure

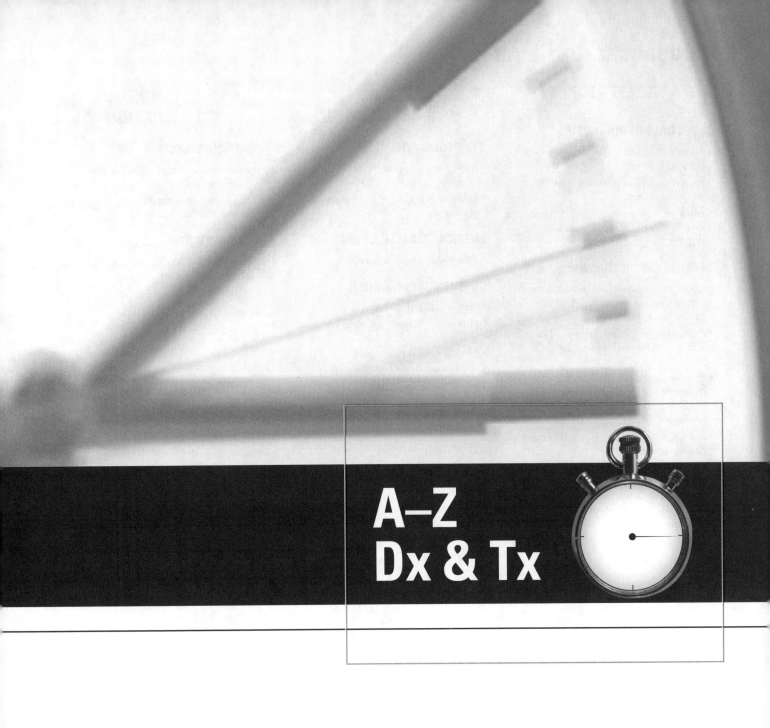

A–Z
Dx & Tx

Abdominal Aortic Aneurysm

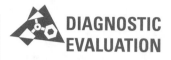 KEY FEATURES

ESSENTIALS OF DIAGNOSIS

- Dilatation of the infrarenal aorta (> 3 cm in diameter)
- Incidence increases with age and more common in men
- Most are asymptomatic until rupture; then 75% of patients die suddenly before reaching the hospital

GENERAL CONSIDERATIONS

- Up to 10% of men over age 65 have abdominal aortic aneurysm (AAA) by ultrasound screening
- Autopsy series discover ruptured AAA in 8 of 100,000 men and 3 of 100,000 women
- Pathologically, AAAs are characterized by loss of the media and fewer elastin fibers, but more collagen. Also, there are findings of inflammation of the aventitia
- After age, smoking is the most common risk factor for AAA
- Hypertension is associated with rupture, but not the development of AAA. Other traditional atherosclerotic risk factors are not associated with AAA

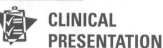 CLINICAL PRESENTATION

SYMPTOMS AND SIGNS

- Most are asymptomatic and found incidentally
- Back, abdominal, or flank pain can occur

PHYSICAL EXAM FINDINGS

- Pulsatile abdominal mass

DIFFERENTIAL DIAGNOSIS

- Tumor adjacent to aorta
- Pulsatile liver from tricuspid regurgitation
- Musculoskeletal back pain
- Acute abdomen (eg, pancreatitis)
- Aortic dissection
- Ureteric colic

DIAGNOSTIC EVALUATION

IMAGING STUDIES

- Abdominal ultrasound is the best initial screening test
- CT scanning is superior for identifying rupture in painful AAAs

DIAGNOSTIC PROCEDURES

- Angiography is often misleading and is not recommended

TREATMENT

CARDIOLOGY REFERRAL

- Suspicion of heart disease pre-procedure or surgery

HOSPITALIZATION CRITERIA

- Painful AAA
- Ruptured AAA
- Planned surgery

MEDICATIONS

AAA < 5.5 cm
- Watchful waiting
- Stop smoking
- Treat hypertension

AAA > 5.5 cm
- Repair unless risk is prohibitive

THERAPEUTIC PROCEDURES

- Endovascular repair with a percutaneous graft-stent combination is experimental but may be life-saving in nonsurgical candidates

SURGERY

- Surgical replacement with a synthetic graft

MONITORING

- ECG monitoring in hospital
- Blood pressure in hospital

DIET AND ACTIVITY

- Restrict activity if rupture suspected; exercise stress testing contraindicated

ONGOING MANAGEMENT

HOSPITAL DISCHARGE CRITERIA

- After successful procedure or surgery

FOLLOW-UP

- If < 5.5 cm, reevaluate in 3 months, then 6 months, and, if stable, yearly

COMPLICATIONS

- Rupture
- Embolization distally may cause limb ischemia
- Fistula into the gastrointestinal tract, especially after aortic surgery
- Fistula into the inferior vena cava

PROGNOSIS

- Fifty percent of patients in the 4–5.5 cm aneurysm range can expect to need surgery due to expansion > 5.5 cm in 5 years
- The 30-day surgical mortality rate for aneurysm resection is 6%
- The outcome for ruptured aneurysms is poor:
  - 75% die before reaching the hospital
  - 50% do not survive surgery
  - The 30-day mortality rate for the remainder is 40%

PREVENTION

- Smoking cessation
- Control hypertension

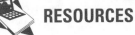

RESOURCES

PRACTICE GUIDELINES

- There is no proven benefit in operating on aneurysms < 5.5 cm in diameter that are asymptomatic
- The standard treatment is resection and replacement with a Dacron graft. The safety and durability of endovascular grafts is not known, but being studied

REFERENCES

- Jones KG et al: Interleukin-6 (IL-6) and the prognosis of abdominal aortic aneurysms. Circulation 2001;103:2260.
- Lederle FA et al: Immediate repair compared with surveillance of small abdominal aortic aneurysms. N Engl J Med 2002;346:1437.
- The UK Small Aneurysm Trial Participants: long-term outcomes of immediate repair compared with surveillance of small abdominal aortic aneurysms. N Engl J Med 2002;346:1445.

INFORMATION FOR PATIENTS

- www.drpen.com/441.9

WEB SITE

- www.emedicine.com/med/topic3443.htm

Acromegaly and the Heart

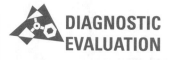 KEY FEATURES

ESSENTIALS OF DIAGNOSIS

- Elevated somatomedin C
- Inability to suppress growth hormone to < 2 ng/mL during glucose tolerance test
- Pituitary adenoma found on MRI
- Biventricular hypertrophy with systolic and diastolic dysfunction
- Hypertension, diabetes, and premature coronary artery disease

GENERAL CONSIDERATIONS

- Acromegaly is caused by excessive growth hormone secretion from a pituitary adenoma
- It is characterized by excess bone growth, organ enlargement, and premature death due to cardiorespiratory complications
- Rarely other endocrine tumors can secrete growth hormone

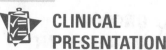 CLINICAL PRESENTATION

SYMPTOMS AND SIGNS

- Headache, bitemporal hemianopsia from tumor growth
- Impotence, galactorrhea or amenorrhea
- Diaphoresis, hoarseness, polyuria, polydipsia
- Carpal tunnel syndrome
- Symptoms of:
  - Heart failure, such as dyspnea
  - Coronary artery disease, such as chest pain

PHYSICAL EXAM FINDINGS

- Systemic hypertension
- Thick lips, macroglossia, bulbous nose, protrusive lower jaw
- Joint swelling, kyphosis
- Left ventricular lift
- Signs of congestive heart failure, such as pulmonary rales

DIFFERENTIAL DIAGNOSIS

- Other causes of cardiomyopathy and heart failure
- Other causes of hypertension
- Other causes of premature coronary artery disease

DIAGNOSTIC EVALUATION

LABORATORY TESTS

- Growth hormone, somatomedin C, and insulin-like growth factor levels
- Hyperglycemia, hypertriglyceridemia
- Hyperphosphatemia

ELECTROCARDIOGRAPHY

- Left ventricular hypertrophy
- Atrial and ventricular tachyarrhythmias

IMAGING STUDIES

- Chest x-ray: cardiomegaly
- Echocardiography: eccentric left ventricular hypertrophy, left atrial enlargement
- Doppler echocardiography: diastolic dysfunction

DIAGNOSTIC PROCEDURES

- Stress cardiac imaging or cardiac catheterization may be indicated to diagnose coronary artery disease

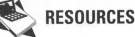

 TREATMENT

CARDIOLOGY REFERRAL

- Suspected cardiac disease
- Difficult to control hypertension

HOSPITALIZATION CRITERIA

- Heart failure
- Acute coronary syndromes
- Planned surgery

MEDICATIONS

- Pharmacologic therapy with somato-statin analogs, eg, octreotide 200–500 μg/day SC, or dopamine agonists, eg, bromocriptine 20–30 mg/day PO (start at 2.5 mg/day)
- Heart disease treated conventionally

THERAPEUTIC PROCEDURES

- Cardiac catheterization and angioplasty may be required

SURGERY

- Surgical removal of the pituitary tumor

MONITORING

- ECG monitoring in hospital as appropriate

DIET AND ACTIVITY

- Low-sodium, low-saturated-fat diet
- Activity restriction if heart disease present

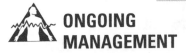 **ONGOING MANAGEMENT**

HOSPITAL DISCHARGE CRITERIA

- Resolution of problem
- Successful surgery

FOLLOW-UP

- Depends on condition

COMPLICATIONS

- Heart failure
- Acute coronary syndromes
- Tachyarrhythmias

PROGNOSIS

- Good with early recognition and treatment

RESOURCES

PRACTICE GUIDELINES

- Diastolic dysfunction due to hypertrophy is a major cause of death
- The coexistence of diabetes and hypertension contributes to hypertrophy and increases the risk of coronary artery disease

REFERENCE

- Colao A et al: Growth hormone and the heart. Clin Endocrinol (Oxf) 2001;54:137.

INFORMATION FOR PATIENTS

- www.nlm.nih.gov/medlineplus/ency/article/000321.htm

WEB SITE

- www.emedicine.com/med/topic27.htm

Adrenal Insufficiency and the Heart

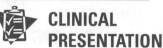 ## KEY FEATURES

ESSENTIALS OF DIAGNOSIS

- Inability to increase cortisol to > 20 mg/dL in response to synthetic adreno-corticotropic hormone (ACTH) during rapid ACTH stimulation testing
- Orthostatic hypotension, salt wasting, and hyperkalemia in primary adrenal insufficiency (Addison's disease)
- Hyponatremia in both primary and secondary (pituitary) adrenal insufficiency
- Elevated ACTH in Addison's disease

GENERAL CONSIDERATIONS

- Primary adrenal insufficiency (Addison's disease) is caused by destruction of the adrenal cortex usually by an autoimmune disease today (granulomatous diseases such as tuberculosis in the past)
- Secondary adrenal insufficiency is usually caused by withdrawal of steroids, which depress the hypothalamic pituitary adrenal axis, mainly affecting glucocorticoid production
- Incidence in the general population is <0.01%, but occurs more commonly in critically ill patients

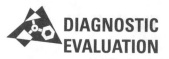 ## CLINICAL PRESENTATION

SYMPTOMS AND SIGNS

- Fatigue
- Anorexia, nausea, vomiting, abdominal pain
- Depressed mentation, coma

PHYSICAL EXAM FINDINGS

- Hyperpigmented skin if chronic, vitiligo
- Decreased pubic and axillary hair
- Dehydration
- Hypotension
- Fever

DIFFERENTIAL DIAGNOSIS

- Other causes of orthostatic hypotension
- Other causes of hypovolemic shock
- Other causes of hyperkalemia, hyponatremia, hypercalcemia, hypoglycemia, and acidosis

DIAGNOSTIC EVALUATION

LABORATORY TESTS

- Electrolytes and glucose show: hyponatremia, hyperkalemia, hypercalcemia, hypoglycemia, and acidosis
- CBC: anemia, lymphocytosis, and eosinophilia
- Serum cortisol < 25 mg/dL in critically ill patients

ELECTROCARDIOGRAPHY

- Sinus brady or tachycardia
- Nonspecific ST-T–wave changes
- Signs of hyperkalemia (peaked T waves)
- Short QT if hypercalcemic

IMAGING STUDIES

- Echocardiogram shows small cardiac chambers with normal function

DIAGNOSTIC PROCEDURES

- Rapid ACTH stimulation test causes cortisol to increase to ≥ 20 mg/dL in primary adrenal insufficiency

TREATMENT

CARDIOLOGY REFERRAL

- Significant cardiac arrhythmias

HOSPITALIZATION CRITERIA

- Suspected adrenal insufficiency

MEDICATIONS

- Hydrocortisone 100 IV every 6–8 hours acutely
- Saline and glucose IV
- Treatment of precipitating infection
- Long-term adrenal hormone replacement, such as hydrocortisone PO 20 mg in the morning and 10 mg in the evening, plus fludrocortisone 0.05–0.1 mg PO daily in primary adrenal insufficiency

MONITORING

- ECG in hospital as appropriate

DIET AND ACTIVITY

- High-sodium diet and fluids until condition is controlled by therapy
- Restricted activity until treatment is underway

ONGOING MANAGEMENT

HOSPITAL DISCHARGE CRITERIA

- Resolution of problem

FOLLOW-UP

- Frequent visits until stabilized
- Follow-up visit with any intercurrent illness or when subject to significant stress for the purpose of adjusting replacement doses

COMPLICATIONS

- Adrenal crisis
- Hypovolemic shock
- Death

PROGNOSIS

- Good, with treatment and appropriate medication dosage adjustments as necessary to avoid crisis

PREVENTION

- Judicious use of corticosteroids can prevent secondary adrenal insufficiency

RESOURCES

PRACTICE GUIDELINES

- The treatment of adrenal crisis can be lifesaving
- Patient's presentation may mimic an acute abdominal emergency; exploratory surgery can be lethal in this setting
- Adrenal crisis should be considered in anyone with unexplained hypovolemic shock

REFERENCE

- Zolga GP, Marik P: Endocrine and metabolic dysfunction syndromes in the critically ill. Crit Care Clin 2001;17:25.

INFORMATION FOR PATIENTS

- www.drpen.com/255.4

WEB SITES

- www.emedicine.com/med/topic42.htm
- www.emedicine.com/med/topic65.htm

AIDS and the Heart

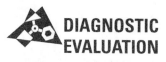 KEY FEATURES

ESSENTIALS OF DIAGNOSIS

- Pericardial effusion
- Lymphocytic myocarditis
- Dilated cardiomyopathy and left ventricular systolic dysfunction
- Myocardial Kaposi's sarcoma and non-Hodgkin's lymphoma
- Pulmonary hypertension secondary to multiple pulmonary infarctions, or primary pulmonary hypertension
- Accelerated atherosclerosis as a consequence of longer survival and the use of antiretroviral agents

GENERAL CONSIDERATIONS

- Most HIV-infected patients with cardiac abnormalities have acquired immune deficiency syndrome (AIDS)
- Pericardial effusion is the most common cardiac pathology (10–40% of patients) and is associated with a poor prognosis
- The cause of idiopathic myocarditis is uncertain, but may be due to direct myocardial infection by the HIV virus, autoimmune mechanisms, other viruses, or opportunistic infection
- Clinically important dilated cardiomyopathy is present in 1–3%
- Cardiac tumors such as Kaposi's sarcoma, intracavity growth, and obstruction should be considered
- Pulmonary hypertension is present in 0.5% of HIV-infected patients and is associated with poor survival
- Protease inhibitors that are a part of most HAART (highly active antiretroviral treatment) regimens are associated with metabolic abnormalities that lead to accelerated atherosclerosis and increased cardiovascular risk
- Prolonged QT interval and torsades de pointes have been described in one third of hospitalized patients with HIV infection, even without drug therapy

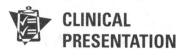 CLINICAL PRESENTATION

SYMPTOMS AND SIGNS

- Worsened fatigue
- Breathlessness/dyspnea
- Edema
- Chest pain

PHYSICAL EXAM FINDINGS

- Patients with significant pericardial disease:
  - Elevated jugular venous pressure
  - Muffled heart sounds or a pericardial friction rub
- Patients with a dilated cardiomyopathy
  - Elevated jugular venous pressure
  - Pulmonary rales
  - Displaced sustained apical impulse
  - Gallop rhythms
- Patients with pulmonary hypertension
  - Increased P_2
  - Right ventricular lift
  - Murmur of tricuspid regurgitation

DIFFERENTIAL DIAGNOSIS

- Idiopathic dilated cardiomyopathy
- Heart failure secondary to foscarnet used for cytomegalovirus infection
- Dilated cardiomyopathy secondary to interferon-alfa used to treat Kaposi's sarcoma
- Other causes of pericardial effusion

DIAGNOSTIC EVALUATION

LABORATORY TESTS

- HIV serology
- CD4 count
- Other tests based on the clinical situation

ELECTROCARDIOGRAPHY

- Low-voltage QRS and/or electrical alternans may suggest a pericardial effusion
- Rare patients may have PR depression and/or diffuse ST elevation with acute pericarditis
- Q waves in patients with prior myocardial infarction
- Prolonged QT interval

IMAGING STUDIES

- Chest x-ray:
  - Enlarged cardiac silhouette due to a pericardial effusion or cardiomegaly
- Echocardiogram (routine echo not indicated to screen for cardiovascular involvement):
  - Pericardial effusion
  - Cardiac chamber enlargement
  - Reduced ventricular function
- Stress testing:
  - May be indicated in patients with symptoms of myocardial ischemia or ventricular dysfunction

DIAGNOSTIC PROCEDURES

- Cardiac catheterization:
  - Coronary angiography may be indicated in patients presenting with signs or symptoms of myocardial ischemia or infarction

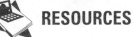

TREATMENT

CARDIOLOGY REFERRAL

- Unexplained dyspnea
- Chest pain
- Asymptomatic or symptomatic cardiomyopathy
- Prolonged QT interval

HOSPITALIZATION CRITERIA

- Decompensated heart failure
- Acute coronary syndrome
- Syncope
- Ventricular or atrial arrhythmias

MEDICATIONS

- Management of hyperlipidemia
- Management of heart failure similar to that for dilated cardiomyopathy
- Therapy for infections
- Chemotherapy for Kaposi's sarcoma and lymphoma
- Pulmonary vasodilator therapy for patients with symptomatic pulmonary hypertension

THERAPEUTIC PROCEDURES

- Percutaneous coronary intervention for coronary stenosis in selected patients
- Pericardiocentesis, pericardial window, biopsy as needed

SURGERY

- Coronary artery bypass surgery in selected patients
- Cardiac transplantation in selected patients

MONITORING

- ECG monitoring
- Fluid balance

DIET AND ACTIVITY

- Low-sodium diet for patients with heart failure
- Cardiac diet for patients with ischemic heart disease
- Restricted activity if heart failure or unstable coronary syndrome is present

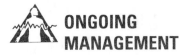
ONGOING MANAGEMENT

HOSPITAL DISCHARGE CRITERIA

- After appropriate treatment of pericardial disease, coronary artery disease, or heart failure

FOLLOW-UP

- Within 2 weeks of hospital discharge
- Follow-up exam every 3–4 months based on symptoms
- Echocardiography as indicated based on symptoms and exam findings

COMPLICATIONS

- Sudden death
- Progressive heart failure
- Future ischemic events

PROGNOSIS

- Poor prognosis in patients with a pericardial effusion (even if asymptomatic)
  - The effusion is rarely the cause of death, but is a marker of advanced HIV infection
- Poor prognosis in HIV-infected patients with pulmonary hypertension

PREVENTION

- Antibiotic prophylaxis

RESOURCES

PRACTICE GUIDELINES

- HIV-infected patients are often treated with therapies for their cardiovascular disease in much the same way as patients without HIV, including consideration of cardiac transplantation in patients with HIV and end-stage heart failure

REFERENCE

- Barbaro G: Cardiovascular manifestations of HIV infection. Circulation 2002;106:1420.

INFORMATION FOR PATIENTS

- http://www.nlm.nih.gov/medlineplus/aids.html
- http://www.nlm.nih.gov/medlineplus/cardiomyopathy.html
- http://www.nlm.nih.gov/medlineplus/pulmonaryhypertension.html

WEB SITES

- http://www.emedicine.com/med/topic289.htm
- http://www.emedicine.com/med/topic2946.htm

Angina Pectoris, Unstable

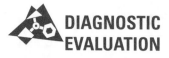 KEY FEATURES

ESSENTIALS OF DIAGNOSIS

- New or worsening symptoms (angina, pulmonary edema) or signs (ECG changes) of myocardial ischemia
- Absence or mild elevation of cardiac biomarkers (creatinine kinase and its MB fraction or troponin I or T) without prolonged ST-segment elevation on ECG
- Unstable angina and non–ST-elevation myocardial infarction (MI) are closely related in pathogenesis and clinical presentation and are often considered one entity

GENERAL CONSIDERATIONS

- Formerly called intermediate coronary syndrome
- Accounts for 40–50% of all admissions to coronary care units
- Imbalance between myocardial oxygen demand and supply
- May be triggered in stable patients by extrinsic factors such as anemia, thyrotoxicosis, arrhythmia, or hypotension
- Unstable plaque with fissure or rupture is the mechanism
- Thrombosis (luminal) and vasoconstriction are factors in causing ischemia

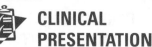 CLINICAL PRESENTATION

SYMPTOMS AND SIGNS

- Chest pain typically lasts 15–30 min
- Atypical locations include neck, jaw, arms, and epigastrium
- Dyspnea, fatigue, diaphoresis, feeling of indigestion, and desire to burp or defecate may be presenting symptoms or accompany other symptoms
- Symptoms occur at rest or provoked by minimal activity
- Chest tightness may be frequent or prolonged
- May follow an acute MI or coronary revascularization

PHYSICAL EXAM FINDINGS

- Physical finings are nonspecific
- S_3 or S_4 may be heard
- Ischemic mitral regurgitation may be detected
- Features of left heart failure may be seen
- Arrhythmias and conduction disturbances may occur
- Hypotension

DIFFERENTIAL DIAGNOSIS

- Stable angina pectoris
- Variant angina
- MI
- Aortic dissection
- Acute myopericarditis
- Acute pulmonary embolism
- Esophageal reflux
- Cholecystitis
- Peptic ulcer disease
- Cervical radiculopathy
- Costochondritis
- Pneumothorax

DIAGNOSTIC EVALUATION

LABORATORY TESTS

- Elevated biomarkers (creatinine kinase and its MB fraction or troponin I or T) identify high-risk patients
- CBC, basal metabolic panel

ELECTROCARDIOGRAPHY

- ECG may show ST depression
- Left bundle branch block may mask ischemic change
- Normal ECG does not exclude cardiac ischemia
- ST depression identifies high-risk patients

IMAGING STUDIES

- Echocardiogram if heart failure symptoms predominate
- Chest x-ray

DIAGNOSTIC PROCEDURES

- Coronary angiography in high-risk patients
- Nuclear stress test or stress echocardiogram in low-risk patients with normal ECG and cardiac biomarkers
- Additional tests depend on differential diagnosis
- CT of chest if pulmonary embolism or dissection is suspected

---

TREATMENT

CARDIOLOGY REFERRAL

- High-risk patients with abnormal ECG or elevated cardiac biomarkers
- Low-risk patients may be observed in chest pain units with cardiology follow-up the next day

HOSPITALIZATION CRITERIA

- Prior coronary disease or revascularization
- Abnormal ECG or cardiac biomarkers
- Abnormal resting nuclear study during chest pain
- Abnormal echocardiogram

MEDICATIONS

- Hospitalization with ECG monitoring, bed rest, oxygen
- Elimination of hypertension, dysrhythmias, anemia, heart failure, thyrotoxicosis
- Aspirin 162 mg/day
- Nitrates for pain—IV 20–30 μg/min
- Heparin, either unfractionated or low molecular weight, eg, enoxaparin 1 mg/kg subcutaneously every 12 hours
- Beta blockers for continued pain, eg, metoprolol 25 mg PO bid
- Calcium channel blockers when beta blockers are contraindicated or pain is refractory, eg, amlodipidine 5 mg/day PO
- Clopidogrel for patients who cannot take aspirin or for use before angioplasty in high-risk patients (300 mg PO × 1, then 75 mg/day PO)
- Platelet glycoprotein IIb/IIIa inhibitors for high-risk patients, especially if percutaneous revascularization planned, eg, eptifibatide 180 μg/kg IV bolus, followed by 2 mg/min IV infusion (1 mg/min/kg if creatinine > 2 mg/dL) for up to 72 hours

THERAPEUTIC PROCEDURES

- Percutaneous coronary intervention early for high-risk patients
- Intra-aortic balloon pump counterpulsation

SURGERY

- Coronary artery bypass surgery for high-risk patients

MONITORING

- Holter monitoring
- Telemetry

DIET AND ACTIVITY

- Cardiac low-fat diet
- Gradual exercise in rehabilitation unit

ONGOING MANAGEMENT

HOSPITAL DISCHARGE CRITERIA

- Lack of symptoms after 24 hours with a negative stress test
- Post-revascularization after an appropriate period of observation
- Precipitating causes under control

FOLLOW-UP

- Outpatient evaluation 2 weeks after discharge
- Revascularized patients: medications for secondary prevention such as aspirin, beta blocker, angiotensin-converting enzyme inhibitor, statin
- Nonrevascularized patients: secondary prevention therapy plus a noninvasive stress test 3–6 weeks after discharge

COMPLICATIONS

- During hospitalization: refractory chest pain, ST-elevation myocardial infarction, hemodynamic instability, heart failure, and arrhythmias, including life-threatening ventricular arrhythmias
- After discharge: recurrence of ischemia either secondary to failed medical therapy or complication of revascularization, such as in-stent thrombosis, restenosis, or occluded graft

PROGNOSIS

- Advanced treatment strategies have led to substantial improvement in prognosis
- Refractory angina, MI, and death at 23%, 12%, and 1.7%, respectively, at 1 week are improved by aspirin and heparin to 10.7%, 1.6%, and 0% within first week
- Combination of early invasive strategy, IIb/IIIa inhibitor, heparin, and aspirin have reduced the 6-month mortality rate to 3.3% in TACTICS-TIMI 18 trial

PREVENTION

- **A**: Antiplatelet therapy (aspirin, 81 mg/day and clopidogrel, 75 mg/day)
- **B**: Beta blockers, blood pressure control
- **C**: Cholesterol-modifying medication (statins)
- **D**: Dietary management
- **E**: Exercise and weight control

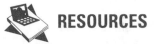

RESOURCES

PRACTICE GUIDELINES

- Bertrand ME, Simoons ML, Fox KA et al: Management of acute coronary syndromes: acute coronary syndrome without persistent ST segment elevation: recommendations of the Task Force of the European Society of Cardiology. Eur Heart J 2000;21:1406.
- Braunwald E, Antman EM, Beasley JW: ACC/AHA 2002 guideline update for the management of patients with unstable angina and non-ST-segment elevation myocardial infarction–summary article: a report of the American College of Cardiology/American Heart Association Task Force on Practice Guidelines. J Am Coll Cardiol 2002;40:1366.

REFERENCES

- TACTICS-TIMI 18 investigators: Comparison of early invasive and conservative strategies in patients with unstable coronary syndromes treated with the glycoprotein IIb/IIIa inhibitor tirofiban. N Engl J Med 2001;344: 1879.

WEB SITE

- www.acc.org

Ankylosing Spondylitis and the Heart

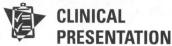 KEY FEATURES

ESSENTIALS OF DIAGNOSIS

- Characteristic lumbar spine and sacroiliac arthritis; positive HLA-B27 assay
- Aortic root sclerosis and dilation, leaflet thickening, and subaortic bump on echocardiography
- Aortic regurgitation

GENERAL CONSIDERATIONS

- Ankylosing spondylitis is an inflammatory disease that mainly affects the vertebral and sacroiliac joints
- Less frequently, it affects other organs, including the heart
- Its incidence is 1 per 2,000 people and occurs predominantly in white males < 40 years old
- Cardiac involvement usually follows articular manifestations by 1–2 decades
- The most common cardiovascular manifestations are:
  - Aortitis with or without aortic valve regurgitation
  - Conduction disturbances
  - Mitral regurgitation
  - Myocardial dysfunction
  - Pericardial disease
- Aortitis usually occurs in the proximal ascending aorta, frequently involving the sinuses of Valsalva and resulting in dilatation and thickening of the aortic root and annulus; the resulting leaflet retraction leads to mild to moderate aortic regurgitation
- Extension of this process into the anterior mitral valve leaflet may result in mitral regurgitation
- Extension of aortic fibrosis into the basal septum may interfere with the conduction system

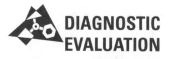 CLINICAL PRESENTATION

SYMPTOMS AND SIGNS

- Usually asymptomatic
- Dyspnea can occur
- Syncope can occur

PHYSICAL EXAM FINDINGS

- Typical decrescendo diastolic murmur of aortic regurgitation
- Pansystolic murmur of mitral regurgitation
- Bradycardia

DIFFERENTIAL DIAGNOSIS

- Other causes of aortic valve disease
- Other connective tissue diseases

DIAGNOSTIC EVALUATION

LABORATORY TESTS

- Positive test result for histocompatibility antigen HLA-B27

ELECTROCARDIOGRAPHY

- High-degree atrioventricular (AV) block can occur

IMAGING STUDIES

- Echocardiography findings:
  - Thickened, dilated aortic root with characteristic extension into the proximal anterior mitral leaflet (subaortic bump)
- Doppler echocardiography findings:
  - Color-flow Doppler evidence of aortic and mitral regurgitation

TREATMENT

CARDIOLOGY REFERRAL

- Cardiac symptoms
- Significant heart murmur

HOSPITALIZATION CRITERIA

- Heart failure
- Pericarditis
- Syncope
- High-degree AV block with bradycardia

MEDICATIONS

- Specific anti-inflammatory pharmacotherapy
- Antibiotic prophylaxis for endocarditis
- Vasodilators for severe aortic regurgitation

THERAPEUTIC PROCEDURES

- Pacemaker

SURGERY

- Rarely valve replacement

MONITORING

- ECG monitoring in hospital as appropriate

DIET AND ACTIVITY

- Diet and activity guidelines as appropriate for the cardiac condition

ONGOING MANAGEMENT

HOSPITAL DISCHARGE CRITERIA

- Resolution of problem
- Successful pacemaker placement
- Successful surgery

FOLLOW-UP

- As appropriate for specific cardiac problem

COMPLICATIONS

- Endocarditis
- Heart failure
- Pericardial tamponade
- Syncope

PROGNOSIS

- Overall prognosis is good; most patients have mild cardiovascular disease that does not require surgery

PREVENTION

- Antibiotic prophylaxis for endocarditis

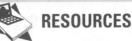

RESOURCES

PRACTICE GUIDELINES

- Management would follow recommendations for the specific cardiac problem

REFERENCES

- Jimenez-Balderas FJ et al: Two-dimensional echo Doppler findings in juvenile and adult onset ankylosing spondylitis with long-term disease. Angiology 2001;52:543.
- Roldan CA et al: Aortic root disease and valve disease associated with ankylosing spondylitis. J Am Coll Cardiol 1998;32:1397.

INFORMATION FOR PATIENTS

- www.drpen.com/720.0

WEB SITE

- www.emedicine.com/med/topic 2700.htm

Aortic Regurgitation, Acute

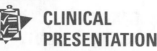 KEY FEATURES

ESSENTIALS OF DIAGNOSIS

- Usually due to aortic dissection, endocarditis, or trauma
- Sudden, severe dyspnea, orthopnea, and weakness
- Signs of pulmonary edema
- Soft S_1 and short decrescendo aortic murmur
- Characteristic Doppler echocardiographic findings:
  - Confirm aortic regurgitation (color jet)
  - Estimate its severity (short pressure half-time)
  - Estimate left ventricular pressure (premature closure of mitral valve, diastolic mitral regurgitation)

GENERAL CONSIDERATIONS

- Sudden, severe aortic regurgitation does not allow time for the left ventricle to adapt
- The acute volume load on a relatively noncompliant left ventricle leads to immediate and marked increases in filling pressures, which:
  - Are transmitted to the lungs
  - Result in acute pulmonary edema
- Since left ventricular diastolic volume is initially normal, total stroke volume does not increase and forward stoke volume decreases, resulting in:
  - Sympathetic stimulation
  - Peripheral vasoconstriction
  - Worsening of aortic regurgitation
- Acute aortic regurgitation is usually due to:
  - Leaflet abnormalities that cause sudden disruption or prolapse such as infective endocarditis
  - Other vasculitides or trauma
  - Occasionally, sudden root dilatation, as occurs with aortic dissection
  - Ruptured sinus of Valsalva aneurysm—most common congenital cause

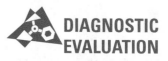 CLINICAL PRESENTATION

SYMPTOMS AND SIGNS

- Sudden, severe dyspnea, orthopnea, and weakness
- Rapid progression to hemodynamic collapse

PHYSICAL EXAM FINDINGS

- Normal pulse pressure
- Possible hypotension
- Pulmonary rales
- Normal left ventricular impulse
- Auscultation findings:
  - Soft S_1 due to premature closure of the mitral valve
  - S_3
  - Short high-pitched aortic diastolic murmur
- Absent pulses if due to aortic dissection

DIFFERENTIAL DIAGNOSIS

- Other causes of acute pulmonary edema
- Aorto-left ventricular fistula due to endocarditis

DIAGNOSTIC EVALUATION

LABORATORY TESTS

- CBC: Elevated white blood cell count and positive blood cultures if due to endocarditis
- Specific tests for various vasculitides may be helpful, such as antinuclear antibodies

ELECTROCARDIOGRAPHY

- Sinus tachycardia
- Atrioventricular nodal disease if cause is infective endocarditis

IMAGING STUDIES

- Chest x-rays to detect:
  - Wide mediastium if aortic dissection
  - Pulmonary edema
  - Broken ribs if due to trauma
- Echocardiography to detect:
  - Structural abnormalities of the valve or aortic root
  - Early closure of the mitral valve
- Transesophageal echo better if endocarditis or aortic dissection considered
- Doppler echocardiography—color flow identification of the leak:
  - If severe, a truncated continuous-wave Doppler signal of aortic regurgitation is found, since pressure between the aorta and the left ventricle equilibrate rapidly; this results in a short pressure half-time by continuous-wave Doppler of the jet
  - There may be diastolic mitral regurgitation
- MRI or CT scan useful to assess for dissection
- Magnetic resonance angiography can demonstrate aortic regurgitation

DIAGNOSTIC PROCEDURES

- Cardiac catheterization to demonstrate:
  - Elevated left ventricular diastolic, left atrial, pulmonary artery and right heart pressures in severe cases
  - There may be equilibration during diastole of left ventricle and ascending aorta pressures
- Aortography demonstrates aortic valve leak

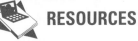

TREATMENT

CARDIOLOGY REFERRAL

- Severe acute aortic regurgitation
- Moderate acute aortic regurgitation with symptoms or signs of decompensation or left heart failure
- Suspicion of aortic dissection or endocarditis

HOSPITALIZATION CRITERIA

- Heart failure
- Severe aortic regurgitation
- Suspected endocarditis
- Suspected aortic dissection

MEDICATIONS

- Sodium nitroprusside 0.3–10 μg/kg/min IV to support patient until surgery
- Dobutamine 2–10 μg/kg/min if nitroprusside causes hypotension
- Appropriate antibiotics for endocarditis for 7–10 days before surgery if possible

THERAPEUTIC PROCEDURES

- Ascending aortic aneurysm may be treatable by a percutaneous stent graft

SURGERY

- Severe acute aortic regurgitation almost always requires urgent surgical correction or valve replacement
- Ascending aortic dissection almost always requires urgent surgical correction
- Endocarditis and severe aortic regurgitation almost always require urgent surgical correction
- Moderate acute aortic regurgitation often requires surgery during first 3 months

MONITORING

- Full ECG and hemodynamic monitoring for acute, severe aortic regurgitation
- Oxygen saturation monitoring

DIET AND ACTIVITY

- Low-sodium diet
- Bed rest until stabilized

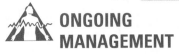

ONGOING MANAGEMENT

HOSPITAL DISCHARGE CRITERIA

- Resolution of symptoms with moderate aortic regurgitation
- Recovery from surgery with severe aortic regurgitation

FOLLOW-UP

- Three months after hospitalization; then 6 months (two times), then yearly

COMPLICATIONS

- Cardiogenic shock
- Serious arrhythmias
- Critical organ damage with dissection (heart, brain, kidneys)
- Septic emboli with endocarditis

PROGNOSIS

- Excellent if patient survives acute illness and surgery because left ventricle is usually normal

PREVENTION

- Endocarditis prophylaxis
- Hypertension control to prevent aortic dissection

RESOURCES

PRACTICE GUIDELINES

- Early surgical intervention is generally recommended

REFERENCES

- Movsowitz HD, Levine RA, Hilgenberg AD et al: Transesophageal echocardiographic description of the mechanisms of aortic regurgitation in acute type A aortic dissection: implications for aortic valve repair. J Am Coll Cardiol 2000;36:884.
- Murashita T, Kunihara T, Shiiya N et al: Is preservation of the aortic valve different between acute and chronic type A aortic dissections? Eur J Cardiothorac Surg 2001;20:967.
- Shah RP, Ding ZP, Ng AS et al: A ten-year review of ruptured sinus of Valsalva: clinicopathological and echo-Doppler features. Singapore Med J 2001;42:473.
- Song JK, Jeong YH, Kang DH et al: Echocardiographic and clinical characteristics of aortic regurgitation because of systemic vasculitis. J Am Soc Echocardiogr 2003;16:850.

INFORMATION FOR PATIENTS

- www.drpen.com/424.1

WEB SITE

- www.emedicine.com/med/topic156.htm

Aortic Regurgitation, Chronic

 KEY FEATURES

ESSENTIALS OF DIAGNOSIS

- After a long asymptomatic period, presentation with heart failure, arrhythmias or angina
- Wide pulse pressure with associated peripheral signs
- Diastolic decrescendo murmur at left sternal border
- Left ventricular (LV) dilation and hypertrophy with preserved function
- Diagnosis confirmed and severity estimated by Doppler echocardiography or aortography

GENERAL CONSIDERATIONS

- Caused by diseases of the valve leaflets or aortic root (dilatation), or both
- Root diseases: Marfan syndrome, cystic medial necrosis, aortic dissection, syphilis, and connective tissue diseases such as ankylosing spondylitis
- Leaflet diseases: rheumatic endocarditis, congenital and connective tissue diseases such as rheumatoid arthritis
- Causes a volume load on LV, which, if progressive, eventually leads to LV dysfunction

CLINICAL PRESENTATION

SYMPTOMS AND SIGNS

- Most remain asymptomatic for years
- Palpitation: arrhythmias or awareness of forceful heartbeat
- Angina pectoris, mechanism: low diastolic pressure plus LV hypertrophy
- Dyspnea and fatigue when LV dysfunction supervenes
- Congestive heart failure symptoms: orthopnea and edema

PHYSICAL EXAM FINDINGS

- Bounding peripheral pulses with wide pulse pressure
- Enlarged apical impulse
- Auscultation: LV gallops, high-pitched decrescendo murmur at the right second (aortic area) or left third intercostal space, systolic ejection murmur, occasional apical diastolic rumble (Austin Flint murmur)

DIFFERENTIAL DIAGNOSIS

- Pulmonic regurgitation associated with high pulmonary pressures (Graham Steell murmur)
- Patent ductus arteriosus
- Mitral stenosis mimicking an Austin Flint murmur
- Arteriovenous malformation with wide pulse pressure
- Arteriovenous fistula near heart with continuous murmur
- Left anterior descending coronary artery stenosis

DIAGNOSTIC EVALUATION

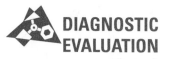

LABORATORY TESTS

- Tests pertinent to potential causes, such as:
  - Antinuclear antibody test for connective tissue disease
  - Fluorescent treponemal antibody absorption test

ELECTROCARDIOGRAPHY

- LV hypertrophy
- Left atrial enlargement
- Ventricular arrhythmias (ectopic beats)

IMAGING STUDIES

- Chest x-ray: cardiomegaly, aortic dilatation, pulmonary vascular congestion
- Echocardiography: LV and left atrial enlargement, eccentric ventricular hypertrophy
- Doppler echocardiography; severity can be assessed by:
  - Width of color flow jet at its origin relative to LV outflow tract diameter
  - Calculated regurgitant fraction from pulsed-wave Doppler comparison of LV outflow to mitral valve inflow
  - Regurgitant pressure half-time by continuous-wave Doppler
  - More severe aortic regurgitation showing a larger, denser jet and backward diastolic flow in the descending aorta
- Magnetic resonance and angiography
- Radionuclide angiography can assess the effect on LV size and performance

DIAGNOSTIC PROCEDURES

- Aortic root angiography
  - Penetration of the contrast and its persistence in LV are related to severity
  - Comparison of cardiac output and LV output can estimate regurgitant volume
- Cardiac catheterization can define hemodynamic burden and assess coronary artery patency pre-surgery

TREATMENT

CARDIOLOGY REFERRAL

- Symptoms
- Moderate to severe aortic regurgitation suspected or documented
- Evidence of LV enlargement or dysfunction

HOSPITALIZATION CRITERIA

- Heart failure and moderate to severe aortic regurgitation
- Syncope and moderate to severe aortic regurgitation
- Significant arrhythmias
- Unstable angina pectoris

MEDICATIONS

- Appropriate pharmacologic therapy of hypertension; avoid markedly lowering heart rate because it increases diastolic regurgitant time
- Antibiotic prophylaxis for infective endocarditis
- In asymptomatic patients with moderate to severe aortic regurgitation, chronic vasodilator therapy may delay onset of symptoms, occurrence of LV dysfunction, and need for valve surgery. eg, amlopidine 5 mg/day

SURGERY

- With moderate to severe aortic regurgitation and symptoms or LV dysfunction, valve replacement surgery is preferred

MONITORING

- ECG monitoring in hospital

DIET AND ACTIVITY

- Low-salt and low-calorie diet
- Avoidance of heavy isometric exercise and competitive sports

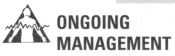

ONGOING MANAGEMENT

HOSPITAL DISCHARGE CRITERIA

- Resolution of symptoms and signs causing admission
- Recovery from successful surgery

FOLLOW-UP

- Mild aortic regurgitation: visit and echocardiography every 2–3 years
- Moderate aortic regurgitation: visit and echocardiography every year
- Severe aortic regurgitation: visit and echocardiography every 6 months

COMPLICATIONS

- Heart failure
- Serious ventricular arrhythmias
- Infective endocarditis
- Sudden death

PROGNOSIS

- Asymptomatic patients may remain stable for years
- Rate of progression to surgery about 4% per year
- Symptoms are a major determinant of outcome
- LV function after surgery may continue to improve for 2 years

PREVENTION

- Treatment of underlying causal diseases

RESOURCES

PRACTICE GUIDELINES

- Echocardiography indicated:
  - Confirm presence and severity of aortic regurgitation.
  - Assess cause of aortic regurgitation
  - Assess LV size and function
  - New or changing symptoms

  Enlarging aortic root seen on chest x-ray
- Aortic valve replacement indicated:
  - Chronic, severe aortic regurgitation with symptoms
  - Chronic, severe aortic regurgitation with LV ejection fraction < 0.50
  - Chronic, severe aortic regurgitation with progressive LV dilatation to severe degrees (end-diastolic dimension > 70 mm)

REFERENCES

- Bonow RO, Carbello B, de Leon AC Jr et al: ACC/AHA guidelines for the management of patients with valvular heart disease: executive summary. A report of the American College of Cardiology/American Heart Association Task Force on Practice Guidelines (Committee on Management of Patients with Valvular Heart Disease). Circulation 1998;98:1949.
- St John Sutton M: Predictors of long-term survival after valve replacement for chronic aortic regurgitation. Eur Heart J 2001;22:808.
- Willett DL, Hall SA, Jessen ME et al: Assessment of aortic regurgitation by transesophageal color Doppler imaging of the vena contracta: validation against an intraoperative aortic flow probe. J Am Coll Cardiol 2001;37:1450.

INFORMATION FOR PATIENTS

- www.drpen.com/424.1

WEB SITE

- www.emedicine.com/med/ CARDIOLOGY.htm

Aortic Stenosis

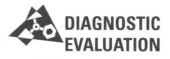 KEY FEATURES

ESSENTIALS OF DIAGNOSIS

- Angina pectoris
- Dyspnea (left ventricular [LV] heart failure)
- Effort syncope
- Systolic ejection murmur radiating to the carotid arteries
- Carotid upstroke delayed in reaching its peak and reduced in amplitude (parvus et tardus)
- Echocardiography shows thickened, immobile aortic valve leaflets
- Doppler echocardiography quantifies increased transvalvular pressure gradient and reduced valve area

GENERAL CONSIDERATIONS

- Definition/description:
  - Narrowing of the aortic valve orifice due to failure of the aortic leaflets to open fully
- Etiology/risk factors:
  - Aortic valve degeneration leads to valve leaflet thickening and calcification and has same risk factor profile as atherosclerosis
  - Rheumatic fever is less frequently a cause in the developed world and almost always occurs with mitral valve disease
- Demographics:
  - More common in men
  - Rheumatic aortic stenosis usually clinically manifests in middle age
  - Degenerative aortic stenosis is a disease of the elderly

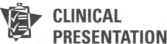 CLINICAL PRESENTATION

SYMPTOMS AND SIGNS

- Angina pectoris
- Effort syncope
- Dyspnea

PHYSICAL EXAM FINDINGS

- Harsh, medium-pitched, midsystolic murmur heard best in the aortic area, usually grade II–IV and may be heard at the apex
- Low-amplitude, delayed carotid artery upstroke (pulsus parvus et tardus), occasionally with a palpable shutter
- Soft second heart sound, occasionally with reversed splitting in severe cases
- Fourth heart sound
- Increased amplitude and duration of apical impulse
- Possible signs of congestive heart failure

DIFFERENTIAL DIAGNOSIS

- Discrete subvalvular aortic stenosis
- Supravalvular aortic stenosis
- Hypertrophic obstructive cardiomyopathy
- Pulmonic stenosis
- Ventricular septal defect

DIAGNOSTIC EVALUATION

LABORATORY TESTS

- Occasionally hemolytic anemia seen in severe cases
- Patients with a history of bleeding may exhibit reduced factor VIII and von Willebrand factor antigen levels
- Natriuretic peptide levels often elevated in symptomatic patients

ELECTROCARDIOGRAPHY

- LV hypertrophy, left atrial enlargement

IMAGING STUDIES

- Chest x-ray:
  - Normal heart size with LV prominence
  - Occasionally a dilated ascending aorta
  - Occasionally aortic valve calcification in severe cases
- Echocardiography:
  - Thickened aortic valve with reduced leaflet mobility
  - Concentric LV hypertrophy
  - Left atrial enlargement
- Doppler echocardiography
  - Valve area can be estimated by the continuity of flow equation from a measure of peak velocity through the valve and an estimate of stroke volume from the LV outflow tract
- Transesophageal echocardiography—the valve orifice can be imaged and measured if there is a question about the severity of stenosis

DIAGNOSTIC PROCEDURES

- Cardiac catheterization
  - Usually not required to make the diagnosis or determine severity, but always done before surgery or if patient's symptoms may be due to coronary artery disease
  - Aortic valve pressure gradient and stroke volume are measured and valve area calculated from the Gorlin formula
  - Coronary arteriography is done to define any disease because stress testing can be dangerous in patients with severe aortic stenosis

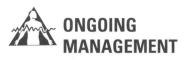

TREATMENT

CARDIOLOGY REFERRAL

- Symptomatic aortic stenosis

HOSPITALIZATION CRITERIA

- Unstable angina
- Congestive heart failure
- Hypotension
- Significant ventricular arrhythmias or nonexertional syncope

MEDICATIONS

- Endocarditis prophylaxis
- Cholesterol-lowering therapy if appropriate
- For severe heart failure, nitroprusside IV 0.3–5.0 µg/kg/min, given carefully; avoid oral vasodilators

THERAPEUTIC PROCEDURES

- Percutaneous balloon aortic valvuloplasty in patients with severe aortic stenosis who are not currently surgical candidates

SURGERY

- Indications:
  - Severe aortic stenosis
  - Symptoms or need for another cardiac operation
- Aortic valve is replaced with either the patient's pulmonic valve (with a pulmonic heterograft) or a prosthetic valve (biological or mechanical)
- Evidence is emerging that a heavily calcified valve or one that is progressing rapidly should be replaced even in an asymptomatic patient
- A reduced ejection fraction is not an exclusion criterion
- Age increases the risk of surgery, but is not an exclusion criterion

MONITORING

- Blood pressure
- ECG monitoring for admitted patients

DIET AND ACTIVITY

- Low-sodium, low-fat diet
- Mild-moderate stenosis: moderate, non-competitive exercise
- Severe stenosis: mild exercise only

ONGOING MANAGEMENT

HOSPITAL DISCHARGE CRITERIA

- Resolution of symptoms and a decision not to operate
- After successful surgery

FOLLOW-UP

- Mild stenosis: once every 1–2 years
- Moderate: every year
- Severe every 6 months
- Patients with changing symptoms: every 3 months until stable
- Echocardiograms should be done on every visit or every other visit, depending on the clinical situation

COMPLICATIONS

- Sudden death occurs with aortic stenosis, but rarely is the presenting manifestation
- Infectious endocarditis can occur
- Acute myocardial infarction may occur in the presence of normal coronary arteries due to increased myocardial oxygen demand from the pressure load on the left ventricle
- Cholesterol emboli may occur and cause brain or vision deficits

PROGNOSIS

- With appropriately timed surgery, prognosis is very good
- Bioprosthetic and autograft valves do not require anticoagulation in the aortic position, reducing the risk of bleeding complications
- Patients with symptoms and severe stenosis who do not have surgery rarely survive more than a few years

PREVENTION

- Antibiotic prophylaxis for infectious endocarditis
- Possibly cholesterol-lowering therapy to retard progression of degenerative aortic stenosis
- Rheumatic fever antibiotic prophylaxis in appropriate patients

RESOURCES

PRACTICE GUIDELINES

- Indications for echocardiography: diagnosis of aortic stenosis; assessment of severity; assessment of LV function; reassessment with change in symptoms or signs; yearly reevaluation of asymptomatic patients with severe aortic stenosis, every 2 years with moderate and every 5 years with mild stenosis
- Indications for valve replacement: symptomatic severe aortic stenosis; moderate to severe aortic stenosis undergoing other cardiac surgery; asymptomatic severe aortic stenosis and LV dysfunction

REFERENCES

- Aikawa K, Otto CM: Timing of surgery in aortic stenosis. Prog Cardiovasc Dis 2001;43:477.
- Khot U, Novaro G, Popovic Z et al: Nitroprusside in critically ill patients with left ventricular dysfunction and aortic stenosis. N Engl J Med 2003;348:1756.
- Palta S, Pai AM, Gill KS et al: New insights into the progression of aortic stenosis: implications for secondary prevention. Circulation 2000;101:2497.
- Qi W, Mathisen P, Kjekshus J et al: Natriuretic peptides in patients with aortic stenosis. Am Heart J 2001;142:725.
- Rosenhek R, Binder T, Porenta G et al: Predictors of outcome in severe, asymptomatic aortic stenosis. N Engl J Med 2000;343:611.
- Vincentelli A, Susen S, Le Tourneau T et al: Acquired von Willebrand syndrome in aortic stenosis. N Engl J Med 2003;349:343.

INFORMATION FOR PATIENTS

- www.drpen.com/hd424.1

WEB SITE

- www.emedicine.com/med/CARDIOLOGY.htm

Aortic Stenosis, Low-Gradient, Low-Output

 KEY FEATURES

ESSENTIALS OF DIAGNOSIS

- Severe aortic stenosis by valve area estimation (<1.0 cm^2)
- Low transvalvular gradient (mean < 40 mm Hg)
- Depressed left ventricular function (LVEF < 0.40)
- Transvalvular gradient—not aortic valve area—increases with dobutamine infusion

GENERAL CONSIDERATIONS

- About 5% of patients with significant aortic stenosis have low left ventricular (LV) ejection fraction and low transvalvular gradients
  - These patients have increased mortality rate with or without surgery
- Depressed LV function often improves after successful surgery in patients with severe aortic stenosis, but may not improve if associated with prior myocardial infarction or marked fibrosis
- Some patients with a small, calculated aortic valve area and low-gradient, low-output stenosis may have a cardiomyopathy and mild aortic stenosis, and not severe aortic stenosis
- Because of inaccuracies in the formulas for calculating aortic stenosis under low-output conditions or the inability of the weak LV to fully open thickened aortic valve leaflets, severe aortic stenosis is suggested
- If LV contractile reserve can be demonstrated and severe aortic stenosis is documented, then surgery is more often successful

 CLINICAL PRESENTATION

SYMPTOMS AND SIGNS

- Dyspnea is the predominant symptom
- Angina occurs in about 50% of patients with severe aortic stenosis
- Syncope is unusual

PHYSICAL EXAM FINDINGS

- Weak carotid pulse with slow upstroke (pulsus parvus et tardus)
- Enlarged LV impulse
- S_3 more common than S_4
- Systolic murmur may be unimpressive (grade I–II)
- Signs of heart failure may be present:
  - Pulmonary rales
  - Edema

DIFFERENTIAL DIAGNOSIS

- Mild to moderate aortic stenosis with LV dysfunction (valve area increases with dobutamine)
- Overestimation of stenosis severity because of failure to account for pressure recovery by Doppler echocardiography
- Technical errors in calculating aortic valve area and measuring valve gradient by Doppler echocardiography (eg, failure to account for a subvalvular gradient and inaccurate LV outflow tract measurement, resulting in underestimate)

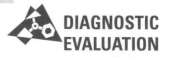 **DIAGNOSTIC EVALUATION**

LABORATORY TESTS

- Elevated brain natriuretic peptide

ELECTROCARDIOGRAPHY

- LV and left atrial hypertrophy

IMAGING STUDIES

- Chest x-ray:
  - Enlarged LV
  - Signs of pulmonary congestion
  - Aortic valve calcifications
- Echocardiography:
  - Hypertrophied or enlarged LV with reduced ejection fraction (< 0.40)
  - Enlarged left atrium
  - Thickened aortic valve leaflets with reduced mobility
- Doppler echocardiography:
  - Low transvalvular gradient (< 40 mm Hg mean)
  - Calculated valve area by continuity equation < 1.0 cm^2
  - Evidence of elevated LA pressure and pulmonary pressure

DIAGNOSTIC PROCEDURES

- Dobutamine stress echocardiography can identify patients with cardiomyopathy, low gradients, but not critical stenosis
  - With noncritical aortic stenosis, valve area increases with dobutamine
  - With critical stenosis, cardiac output rises, but valve area remains fixed
  - With end-stage cardiomyopathy, LV performance does not improve with dobutamine
- Cardiac catheterization is often needed to assess valve area at rest and with dobutamine because invasive pressure measurements are less influenced by pressure recovery
- Coronary angiography is frequently useful

TREATMENT

CARDIOLOGY REFERRAL

- Symptoms and suspected aortic stenosis
- Heart failure and suspected aortic stenosis
- Significant arrhythmias and suspected aortic stenosis

HOSPITALIZATION CRITERIA

- Symptoms and aortic stenosis
- Heart failure and aortic stenosis
- Significant arrhythmias and aortic stenosis

MEDICATIONS

- Patients shown to have reduced LV function and nonsevere aortic stenosis should be treated appropriately for heart failure
- Angiotensin-converting enzyme inhibitors are recommended in this situation

THERAPEUTIC PROCEDURES

- In patients thought to have too high a risk for surgery, percutaneous valvuloplasty can be considered

SURGERY

- Aortic valve replacement is the treatment of choice for severe aortic stenosis with symptoms and adequate LV contractile reserve

MONITORING

- ECG in hospital as appropriate

DIET AND ACTIVITY

- Low-sodium diet
- Restricted activity

ONGOING MANAGEMENT

HOSPITAL DISCHARGE CRITERIA

- Resolution of symptoms
- Successful surgery

FOLLOW-UP

- Medically treated patients should be seen every 3–6 months
- Postsurgical patients are seen at 3 months, then every 6 months

COMPLICATIONS

- Heart failure
- Sudden death
- Endocarditis

PROGNOSIS

- Patients with contractile reserve have a good prognosis with surgery
- Patients with inoperable condition have a poor prognosis

PREVENTION

- Preventive measures for atherosclerosis

RESOURCES

PRACTICE GUIDELINES

- Aortic valve replacement is indicated in almost all patients with severe symptomatic aortic stenosis with the possible exception of patients with low-gradient, low-output aortic stenosis with no evidence of contractile reserve or with severe coronary artery disease that cannot be revascularized
- Although operative mortality rate is high in patients with low gradient, low output aortic syndrome, if they survive surgery, outcome is likely improved

REFERENCES

- Monin J et al: Low-gradient aortic stenosis: operative risk stratification and predictors for long-term outcome: a multicenter study using dobutamine stress hemodynamics. Circulation 2003;108:319.
- Nishimura R et al: Low-output, low-gradient aortic stenosis in patients with depressed left ventricular systolic function: the clinical utility of the dobutamine challenge in the catheterization laboratory. Circulation 2002;106:809.
- Pereira J et al: Survival after aortic valve replacement for severe aortic stenosis with low transvalvular gradients and severe left ventricular dysfunction. J Am Coll Cardiol 2002;39:1356.

INFORMATION FOR PATIENTS

- www.drpen.com/hd424.1

WEB SITE

- www.emedicine.com/med/CARDIOLOGY.htm

Aortic Stenosis, Subvalvular

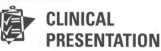 KEY FEATURES

ESSENTIALS OF DIAGNOSIS

- With no other congenital heart abnormalities, it is usually asymptomatic
- Low-pitched systolic ejection murmur is heard at the left sternal border radiating to the neck
- Two-dimensional echocardiography defines the anatomy of the obstruction
- Doppler echocardiography estimates the pressure gradient

GENERAL CONSIDERATIONS

- Subvalvular aortic stenosis accounts for 10–20% of fixed left ventricular outflow lesions in children
- Is more common in males by 2–3:1
- Associated congenital heart lesions are common, such as:
  – Ventricular septal defect
  – Patent ductus arteriosus
  – Coarctation of the aorta and bicuspid aortic valve
- Subvalvular aortic stenosis is rare at birth and is progressive even after surgical correction, suggesting that it maybe an acquired disorder
- The pathology ranges from a thin discrete membrane, to a fibromuscular ring, to a tunnel-like narrowing of the left ventricular outflow tract
- Most stenoses are membranes or ridges 5–15 mm below the aortic valve
- Aortic valve thickening and associated aortic regurgitation are common and may persist after membrane removal

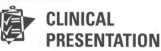 CLINICAL PRESENTATION

SYMPTOMS AND SIGNS

- Most patients are asymptomatic or have symptoms related to associated congenital heart disease
- When present, symptoms are similar to those of valvular aortic stenosis:
  – Dyspnea
  – Chest pain
  – Syncope
  – Palpitation

PHYSICAL EXAM FINDINGS

- A left ventricular lift and precordial thrill may be present
- Auscultation:
  – A fourth heart sound may be present
  – There is a low-pitched systolic ejection murmur best heard in the left third or fourth parasternal space
  – An early diastolic high-pitched murmur of aortic regurgitation is common

DIFFERENTIAL DIAGNOSIS

- Valvular aortic stenosis
- Supravalvular aortic stenosis
- Hypertrophic cardiomyopathy

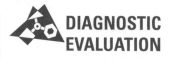 DIAGNOSTIC EVALUATION

ELECTROCARDIOGRAPHY

- Left ventricular hypertrophy is common

IMAGING STUDIES

- M-mode echocardiography shows coarse fluttering of the aortic valve and early systolic closure
- Two-dimensional echo defines the anatomy of the subvalvular obstruction
- If surgery is contemplated, transesophageal echo better defines the lesion for planning surgery
- Doppler echocardiography is used:
  – To estimate the pressure gradient across the lesion
  – If there is a ventricular septal defect, more than one obstructive lesion (eg, aortic valve stenosis or a tunnel-like left ventricle outflow tract), the estimated pressure gradient may not be reliable
  – For assessing other lesions

DIAGNOSTIC PROCEDURES

- Cardiac catheterization is best for distinguishing the hemodynamic contributions of multiple lesions

TREATMENT

CARDIOLOGY REFERRAL

- Suspected subvalvular aortic stenosis
- Symptoms of heart failure, angina, or rhythm disturbances

HOSPITALIZATION CRITERIA

- Heart failure
- Tachyarrhythmias/syncope
- Unstable angina

MEDICATIONS

- Endocarditis prophylaxis

THERAPEUTIC PROCEDURES

- Balloon angioplasty can be used on thin membranous lesions with good results
- Thicker membranes, rings, or tunnels usually require surgery

SURGERY

- Complete resection is treatment of choice for discrete subaortic stenosis
- Aortoventriculoplasty with or without aortic root and valve replacement is used for tunnel-like lesions

MONITORING

- ECG monitoring
- Hemodynamic monitoring

DIET AND ACTIVITY

- Low-sodium diet
- Moderate noncompetitive exercise if asymptomatic

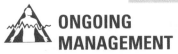

ONGOING MANAGEMENT

HOSPITAL DISCHARGE CRITERIA

- Resolution of symptoms
- Correction of lesion

FOLLOW-UP

- Yearly surveillance with a visit and periodic echocardiograms (every 1–3 years) for asymptomatic patients
- Because recurrences after surgery are common, routine surveillance is required usually at yearly intervals in asymptomatic patients

COMPLICATIONS

- Aortic regurgitation
- Infective endocarditis
- Heart failure
- Angina pectoris
- Arrhythmias, syncope, sudden death

PROGNOSIS

- The progression of subaortic stenosis is more rapid in children than in adults
- Survival after surgical correction is excellent and is related to residual obstruction and progression
- Postsurgical progression is common and is related to:
  – Initial gradient > 50 mm Hg
  – Tunnel-like lesions
  – Incomplete resection
  – Younger age at surgery

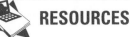

RESOURCES

PRACTICE GUIDELINES

- Intervention should be considered in children when the peak gradient is > 30 mm Hg, and > 50 mm Hg in adults
- Intervention is indicated for symptomatic patients with severe obstruction.

REFERENCES

- Gersony WM: Natural history of discrete subaortic stenosis: management implications. J Am Coll Cardiol 2001;38:843.
- Oliver JM, Gonzalez A, Gallego P et al: Discrete subaortic stenosis in the adult: increased prevalence and slow rate of progression of the obstruction and aortic stenosis. J Am Coll Cardiol 2001;38:835.

INFORMATION FOR PATIENTS

- www.drpen.com/hd424.1

WEB SITE

- www.emedicine.com/PED/topic2491.htm

Aortic Stenosis, Supravalvular

KEY FEATURES

ESSENTIALS OF DIAGNOSIS

- Phenotypic and molecular evidence of Williams syndrome
- Dyspnea on exertion and angina—common
- Elevated blood pressure in the right arm versus left arm
- Harsh systolic ejection murmur typical of valvular aortic stenosis
- Commonly associated are:
  - Aortic regurgitation
  - Peripheral pulmonary artery stenosis
  - Coarctation of the aorta
  - Mitral regurgitation
- Anatomy of the lesion and its severity defined by Doppler echocardiography

GENERAL CONSIDERATIONS

- Either localized or diffused narrowing of the ascending aorta beyond the sinuses of Valsalva
- Equal prevalence in both sexes
- Accounts for < 5% of fixed forms of congenital left ventricular outflow obstruction
- Three distinct presentations:
  - As a feature of Williams syndrome (deletion of elastin gene 7qll) with other abnormalities such as peripheral pulmonary artery stenosis, coarctation of the aorta, and stenoses of the origin of other arteries arising from the ascending aorta and arch
  - As an autosomal dominant familial form with associated peripheral pulmonary artery stenosis
  - As a sporadic form also with peripheral pulmonary artery stenosis, which is the most common form
- Three anatomic forms are recognized:
  - Discrete narrowing just above the ostia of the coronary arteries—the most common
  - A fibrous diaphragm just distal to the coronary ostia—the next most common
  - Diffused narrowing—least common
- Left main coronary artery obstruction may be present
- Premature coronary atherosclerosis develops

CLINICAL PRESENTATION

SYMPTOMS AND SIGNS

- Dyspnea on exertion
- Angina
- Symptoms usually develop in childhood

PHYSICAL EXAM FINDINGS

- Phenotypic features of Williams syndrome may be present
- Systolic blood pressure difference between the two arms, caused by preferential flow to the brachiocephalic vessels (higher pressure right arm)
- Systolic ejection murmur without an ejection sound
- Murmur of aortic regurgitation often present
- Murmur of mitral regurgitation may be present
- Systolic murmurs in the axillae representing peripheral pulmonary artery stenosis may be present
- Upper and lower extremity pulse differences due to coarctation of the aorta may be present

DIFFERENTIAL DIAGNOSIS

- Valvular aortic stenosis
- Subvalvular aortic stenosis
- Hypertrophic obstructive cardiomyopathy
- Left subclavian artery stenosis

DIAGNOSTIC EVALUATION

LABORATORY TESTS

- Molecular diagnosis of Williams syndrome

ELECTROCARDIOGRAPHY

- Left ventricular hypertrophy

IMAGING STUDIES

- Two-dimensional echocardiography demonstrates the supravalvular obstruction
- Continuous-wave Doppler identifies the pressure gradient
- Color-flow Doppler demonstrates the site of obstruction and ostial obstruction of the coronary arteries
- Chest x-ray may show:
  - Left ventricular enlargement
  - The three sign of aortic coarctation
  - Intercostal collaterals with coarctation

DIAGNOSTIC PROCEDURES

- Cardiac catheterization can detect the pressure gradient and identify patients who require surgery
- Angiography of the left and right sides can identify other vascular abnormalities

TREATMENT

CARDIOLOGY REFERRAL

- All patients with suspected supravalvular aortic stenosis should be referred to a cardiologist for evaluation

HOSPITALIZATION CRITERIA

- Angina
- Heart failure
- Need for surgery

MEDICATIONS

- Endocarditis prophylaxis
- Diuretics for heart failure
- Beta blockers for angina

THERAPEUTIC PROCEDURES

- Balloon angioplasty is not effective

SURGERY

- Resection of the aortic obstruction with patch aortoplasty or ascending aorta replacement is the preferred treatment
- Surgical correction of other anomalies should be done at the same time if indicated and feasible

MONITORING

- ECG monitoring in the hospital

DIET AND ACTIVITY

- Low-salt, low-fat diet
- General fitness exercise, but no strenuous or competitive activities

ONGOING MANAGEMENT

HOSPITAL DISCHARGE CRITERIA

- Resolution of symptoms
- Successful recovery from surgery

FOLLOW-UP

- Two weeks and 3 months postoperatively
- Every 6 months for stable patients

COMPLICATIONS

- Sudden cardiac death
- Endocarditis
- Heart failure
- Aortic regurgitation

PROGNOSIS

- Survival after repair is excellent
- Overall medical survival is influenced by the severity of other anomalies
- Aortic stenosis and coronary atherosclerosis are progressive, but the anomalies of other vessels are constant

PREVENTION

- Genetic counseling

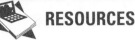

RESOURCES

PRACTICE GUIDELINES

- With symptoms, left ventricular dysfunction or a significant gradient at catheterization (peak > 50 mm Hg) surgery should be considered

REFERENCES

- Eronen M et al: Cardiovascular manifestations in 75 patients with Williams syndrome. J Med Genet 2002;39:554.

INFORMATION FOR PATIENTS

- www.drpen.com/hd424.1

WEB SITE

- www.emedicine.com/PED/topic2178.htm

Athlete's Heart

 ## KEY FEATURES

ESSENTIALS OF DIAGNOSIS

- History of athletic training and performance
- Enhanced exercise ability (maximum oxygen uptake > 40 mL/kg/min)
- Resting bradycardia
- Increased left ventricular mass noted on echocardiography

GENERAL CONSIDERATIONS

- The basic cardiac response to exercise training is myocardial hypertrophy, which may or may not involve chamber enlargement, depending on the type of training
- Pure isotonic (endurance) training results in the most chamber enlargement
- Pure isometric (strength) training results in the greatest degree of left ventricular wall thickening
- Exercise training also results in increased resting parasympathetic tone, resulting in resting bradycardia and other phenomena such as Mobitz I second degree atrioventricular (AV) block
- Left ventricular systolic and diastolic function is normal in the athlete's heart even if hypertrophy is marked
- The challenge for the clinician is distinguishing cardiac disease from normal cardiac adaptation to exercise training, especially in the former athlete whose cardiac effects of training may persist

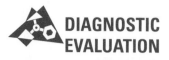 ## CLINICAL PRESENTATION

SYMPTOMS AND SIGNS

- Well-trained athletes are usually asymptomatic, but may have symptoms that are suggestive of cardiac disease (eg, chest pain or dyspnea) for other reasons, such as respiratory infection
- Excessive isotonic training occasionally leads to orthostatic dizziness and, rarely, syncope
- The hallmark of the athlete is an ability to perform exercise at a high level

PHYSICAL EXAM FINDINGS

- Slow pulse rate at rest
- Enlarged apical impulse
- S_3 or S_4 sounds

DIFFERENTIAL DIAGNOSIS

- Pathologic left ventricular volume increase (ie, dilated cardiomyopathy)
- Pathologic left ventricular hypertrophy, especially hypertrophic cardiomyopathy
- Pathologic bradycardia
- Coronary artery disease

DIAGNOSTIC EVALUATION

LABORATORY TESTS

- Creatinine kinase may be elevated after vigorous prolonged exercise

ELECTROCARDIOGRAPHY

- Sinus bradycardia, Mobitz I second-degree AV block, wandering atrial pacemaker
- Signs of left or right ventricular or atrial hypertrophy
- Myocardial infarction patterns due to chamber hypertrophy

IMAGING STUDIES

- Chest x-ray: may show cardiomegaly
- Echocardiography: may show chamber enlargement or hypertrophy with normal systolic and diastolic function
  - Hypertrophic cardiomyopathy is usually easily distinguished from the athlete's heart because 98% of athletes have left ventricular posterior wall thickness ≤ 12 mm, with a range up to 16 mm

DIAGNOSTIC PROCEDURES

- If doubt about athletic training exists, a cardiopulmonary exercise test can be done
  - Athletes characteristically have a maximum oxygen consumption > 40 mL/kg/min

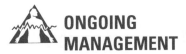

 TREATMENT

CARDIOLOGY REFERRAL

- Symptomatic bradycardia
- Cardiac symptoms in an athlete
- Marked left ventricular hypertrophy (posterior wall > 12 mm)

HOSPITALIZATION CRITERIA

- Suspicion of acute myocardial infarction

MEDICATIONS

- Orthostatic hypotension occasionally requires aldosterone agonists such as fludrocortisone 0.1–1.0 mg/day PO

THERAPEUTIC PROCEDURES

- For symptomatic bradycardia with orthostatic intolerance, reduce or stop isotonic training
- Cessation of training during viral illnesses reduces the incidence of myocarditis

SURGERY

- Athletes do well with surgery for other conditions

MONITORING

- ECG monitoring in hospital as appropriate

DIET AND ACTIVITY

- High-salt diet and increased fluids may help orthostatic symptoms

ONGOING MANAGEMENT

HOSPITAL DISCHARGE CRITERIA

- Resolution of myocardial ischemia

FOLLOW-UP

- Predicated by diagnosis

COMPLICATIONS

- Injury due to orthostatic intolerance

PROGNOSIS

- Excellent; athleticism may increase life span

PREVENTION

- Preventing injuries from athletic activities is critical

RESOURCES

PRACTICE GUIDELINES

- Since athletic training, activity, and competitions are stressful to the heart, individuals with cardiac disease need to be given reasonable guidelines for participation
- Athletes should be given preparticipation evaluations every 1–2 years

REFERENCES

- Pellicca A et al: Clinical significance of abnormal electrocadiographic patterns in trained athletes. Circulation 2000;102:278.
- Pellicca A et al: Remodeling of left ventricular hypertrophy in elite athletes after long term deconditioning. Circulation 2002;105:944.
- Pfisher GC et al: Preparticipation cardiovascular screening for U.S. collegiate student athletes. JAMA 2000;283:1597.

INFORMATION FOR PATIENTS

- www.nlm.nih.gov/medlineplus/ exerciseandphysicalfitness.htm

WEB SITE

- www.americanheart.org/presenter. jhtml?identifier=3004574

Atrial Fibrillation

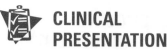

KEY FEATURES

ESSENTIALS OF DIAGNOSIS

- Irregularly irregular ventricular rhythm usually at rates > 100 beats/min
- Absence of P waves on the electrocardiogram (ECG)

GENERAL CONSIDERATIONS

- The most common chronic arrhythmia
- Present in 4% of the population > 60 years with a significantly higher percentage after the eighth decade
- Both paroxysmal and permanent forms of atrial fibrillation increase the risk of stroke
- In nonrheumatic heart disease patients, 15–20% of strokes are due to atrial fibrillation
- Common causes include:
  - Hypertensive heart disease
  - Systolic dysfunction of any cause
  - Mitral valve disease
  - Cardiac surgery
  - Hyperthyroidism
  - Idiopathic (lone atrial fibrillation)
- Atrial fibrillation associated with Wolff-Parkinson-White syndrome may lead to very rapid ventricular rates and be life threatening
- QRS complex is usually narrow (< 100 ms) but may be wide (> 120 ms) if there is aberrant conduction or preexisting bundle branch block
- Long, short cycle length fluctuations are common
- Faster ventricular rates may minimize cycle length fluctuation
- Regular ventricular rhythm in the presence of atrial fibrillation should raise suspicion of complete heart block
- Other causes of rapid regular ventricular rate include atrial flutter, junctional rhythm and ventricular tachycardia

CLINICAL PRESENTATION

SYMPTOMS AND SIGNS

- Palpitations, chest pain, and shortness of breath
- Symptoms of precipitating or associated conditions may mask symptoms of atrial fibrillation
- Alternatively, atrial fibrillation may produce symptoms in otherwise asymptomatic conditions
- Syncope is uncommon
- Atrial fibrillation may be an incidental finding in some patients (asymptomatic)

PHYSICAL EXAM FINDINGS

- Variable S_1, occasional S_3, and absent S_4
- Absence of *a* waves in the jugular venous pulse
- Pulse deficit (difference between the auscultated or palpated apical heart rate and palpated rate at the wrist) is common particularly at fast heart rates
- Irregularly irregular pulse
- Signs of precipitating conditions like thyrotoxicosis, rheumatic mitral stenosis and heart failure

DIFFERENTIAL DIAGNOSIS

- Multifocal atrial tachycardia
- Atrial flutter with variable atrioventricular (AV) block
- Sinus rhythm with consecutive premature atrial contractions

DIAGNOSTIC EVALUATION

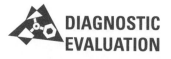

LABORATORY TESTS

- CBC, basal metabolic panel
- Thyroid function (serum thyroid-stimulating hormone)
- Arterial blood gas analysis to assess for hypoxemia

ELECTROCARDIOGRAPHY

- ECG to confirm atrial fibrillation (findings include fibrillatory wave, absence of p wave and varying R-R intervals)
- Holter monitoring for assessment of frequency of intermittent episodes, ventricular rate control on medication, or evaluation of syncope

IMAGING STUDIES

- Echocardiogram to evaluate for valvular heart disease, left ventricular function, and left atrial size
- Transesophageal echocardiogram to evaluate left atrial appendage thrombus if foregoing 3 weeks anticoagulation before cardioversion or evaluating source of systemic emboli
- Evaluation of pericardial disease with echocardiogram or chest CT
- Contrast CT pulmonary vein angiogram before planned left atrial ablation

DIAGNOSTIC PROCEDURES

- Atrial electrogram analysis of patients with a permanent dual-chamber pacemaker to detect atrial fibrillation

TREATMENT

CARDIOLOGY REFERRAL

- For rhythm control in a nonemergent setting due to symptomatic atrial fibrillation
- When rate control is suboptimal despite multiple medications to decide on AV nodal ablation and insertion of a pacemaker
- Initiation of antiarrhythmic medication
- Atrial fibrillation ablation being considered

HOSPITALIZATION CRITERIA

- Atrial fibrillation with chest pain
- Hemodynamic compromise
- Heart failure or positive biomarkers for myocardial injury
- Rapid ventricular response at rest or thyrotoxicosis

MEDICATIONS

- Ventricular rate control with beta blockers, calcium channel blockers, and digoxin alone or in combination
- Choice of antiarrhythmic therapy depends on left ventricular function (avoid class IC in ischemic heart disease or ibutilide and class IC in severe left ventricular dysfunction)
- Acute IV esmolol or diltiazem for rate control
- Cardioversion with countershock in unstable patients
- Elective cardioversion with countershock or antiarrhythmic agents (IV ibutilide, procainamide, amiodarone; or oral propafenone 600 mg or flecainide 300 mg as single dose) once left atrial thrombus has been excluded by transesophageal echocardiography or patient has received adequate anticoagulation for 3–4 weeks
- Anticoagulation for 4 weeks in postcardioversion patients
- Chronic anticoagulation in all patients except lone atrial fibrillation (age < 60 years and no structural heart disease) unless serious contraindication (in which case give at least aspirin)
- Rate control with anticoagulation is equivalent to rhythm control with antiarrhythmic agents regarding death and cardiovascular morbidity in asymptomatic elderly patients

THERAPEUTIC PROCEDURES

- Ablate and pace (AV nodal ablation with permanent pacemaker insertion) to control heart rate
- Left atrial substrate modification or focal ablation in suitable patients
- Wolff-Parkinson-White syndrome (WPW) ablation

SURGERY

- Maze procedure to prevent atrial fibrillation
- Ligation or amputation of left atrial appendage to prevent clot formation
- Surgical procedures usually done in combination with other necessary heart surgery, such as mitral valve replacement

MONITORING

- ECG monitoring in hospital

DIET AND ACTIVITY

- No specific restriction although this may be individualized

ONGOING MANAGEMENT

HOSPITAL DISCHARGE CRITERIA

- Rhythm control and patient asymptomatic
- Adequate ventricular rate control
- Symptoms under control

FOLLOW-UP

- INR monitoring if on warfarin therapy
- If rate control path is chosen in a symptomatic patient, adequacy of rate control to be assessed in 4–6 weeks with Holter monitoring
- Post-Maze or ablation patient usually requires symptom-guided and routine follow-up to evaluate success

COMPLICATIONS

- Stroke
- Systemic emboli
- Tachycardia cardiomyopathy
- Sudden death in WPW (R-R cycle length during atrial fibrillation < 250 ms)

PROGNOSIS

- Patients experience higher mortality than age-matched controls in sinus rhythm

PREVENTION

- Control of hypertension
- Timely management of valvular heart disease
- Appropriate management of congestive heart failure (CHF)

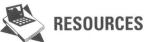

RESOURCES

PRACTICE GUIDELINES

- Indications for anticoagulation: warfarin for all patients except lone atrial fibrillation, aspirin as an alternative in low-risk patients or with contraindication to warfarin therapy
- Indication for cardioversion: hemodynamic instability, unacceptable symptoms; myocardial infarction, CHF or asymptomatic hypotension not responding to pharmacologic intervention

REFERENCES

- Prystowsky EN: Management of atrial fibrillation: Therapeutic options and clinical decisions. Am J Cardiol 2000;85:3D.
- Rockson SG, Albers GW: Comparing the guidelines: anticoagulation therapy to optimize stroke prevention in patients with atrial fibrillation. J Am Coll Cardiol 2004;43:929.

INFORMATION FOR PATIENTS

- www.drpen.com/427.31
- www.nlm.nih.gov/medlineplus/arrhythmia.html

WEB SITE

- www.acc.org

Atrial Flutter

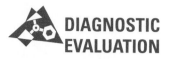 KEY FEATURES

ESSENTIALS OF DIAGNOSIS

- Regular ventricular rate of 75–150 bpm
- Irregular ventricular response secondary to variable atrioventricular (AV) block, usually induced by medication
- Prominent neck vein pulsations of about 300/min
- Flutter waves ("saw-tooth" in lead II) on ECG of 250–340/min

GENERAL CONSIDERATIONS

- Usually associated with organic heart disease more often than atrial fibrillation
- Typical atrial rate is 300 bpm, but 1:1 ventricular conduction is rare
- Ventricular rate is dependent on AV nodal conduction
- If flutter is suspected but not clearly seen on surface ECG, vagal maneuvers or IV adenosine can help unmask flutter waves
- Up to 33% of patients may experience atrial flutter after bypass surgery
- Cavotricuspid isthmus-dependent counterclockwise rotation (negative flutter waves in ECG lead II and positive in V1) is the most common
- Isthmus-dependent, clockwise flutter also occurs (positive waves in lead II)
- Non–isthmus-dependent atypical variety is uncommon

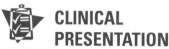 CLINICAL PRESENTATION

SYMPTOMS AND SIGNS

- Dizziness
- Palpitations
- Angina
- Dyspnea
- Weakness
- Fatigue
- Occasionally syncope
- Many of the symptoms are heart rate dependent

PHYSICAL EXAM FINDINGS

- Prominent neck vein pulsations of about 300 bpm
- Variable S_1 intensity

DIFFERENTIAL DIAGNOSIS

- Atrial tachycardia
- Paroxysmal supraventricular tachycardia

DIAGNOSTIC EVALUATION

LABORATORY TESTS

- Thyroid-stimulating hormone
- Basic metabolic panel
- Cardiac biomarkers depending on clinical situation

ELECTROCARDIOGRAPHY

- ECG to document rhythm
- Holter monitoring to detect rhythm disturbance
- Event recorder to detect infrequent episodes

IMAGING STUDIES

- Transthoracic echocardiogram to detect structural heart disease
- Depending on precipitating causes, chest x-ray or CT scan of the chest

DIAGNOSTIC PROCEDURES

- Occasionally in those with pacemakers, interrogation of the device may reveal the atrial flutter episodes

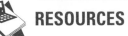

Atrial Flutter

TREATMENT

CARDIOLOGY REFERRAL

- All atrial flutter patients should be referred for cardiology evaluation because the condition is curable

HOSPITALIZATION CRITERIA

- All symptomatic patients should be hospitalized

MEDICATIONS

- Chronic anticoagulation with warfarin for stroke prevention
- Restoration of sinus rhythm with electrical cardioversion or overdrive pacing
- Chemical cardioversion with IV ibutilide 1 mg over 10 minutes; may be repeated
- Flecainide 300 mg or propafenone 600 mg orally as single dose to restore sinus rhythm (used in patients with structurally normal hearts)
- Rate control with beta blockers, calcium channel blockers, or digoxin either individually or in combination

THERAPEUTIC PROCEDURES

- Radiofrequency ablation is curative in 90%

SURGERY

- Rarely, pacemaker implantation followed by AV nodal ablation, especially with concurrent atrial fibrillation

MONITORING

- ECG monitoring in hospital

DIET AND ACTIVITY

- Dependent on comorbidity
- No special restrictions
- General healthy life style recommended

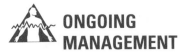

ONGOING MANAGEMENT

HOSPITAL DISCHARGE CRITERIA

- Resumption of sinus rhythm or symptom control (with rate control)
- Adequate anticoagulation

FOLLOW-UP

- Holter monitoring to evaluate the success of ablation 4 weeks after hospital discharge
- Subsequent follow-up depending on recurrence of symptoms

COMPLICATIONS

- Embolic events
- Rare complications of ablation such as cardiac perforation

PROGNOSIS

- Dependent on comorbid conditions
- Transition to atrial fibrillation not uncommon

PREVENTION

- Treatment of hypertension

RESOURCES

PRACTICE GUIDELINES

- Indication for anticoagulation: Manage antithrombotic therapy for patients with atrial flutter as for those with atrial fibrillation
- Catheter ablation is more effective in reducing the recurrence rate from 93% to 5% when used as first-line therapy

REFERENCES

- Blomstrom-Lundqvist C, Scheinman MM, Aliot EM et al: ACC/AHA/ESC guidelines for the management of patients with supraventricular arrhythmias—executive summary. A report of the American college of cardiology/American Heart Association Task Force on Practice Guidelines and the European Society of Cardiology Committee for Practice Guidelines (writing committee to develop guidelines for the management of patients with supraventricular arrhythmias) developed in collaboration with NASPE-Heart Rhythm Society. J Am Coll Cardiol 2003;42:1493.
- Cosio FG et al: Radiofrequency ablation of atrial flutter. J Cardiovasc Electrophysiol 1996;7:60.

INFORMATION FOR PATIENTS

- www.nlm.nih.gov/medlineplus/ arrhythmia.html

WEB SITE

- www.acc.org

Atrial Septal Defect (ASD)

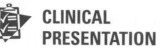

KEY FEATURES

ESSENTIALS OF DIAGNOSIS

- Widely fixed split S_2
- Midsystolic murmur
- Diastolic flow rumble at the lower left sternal border if the shunt is large
- Incomplete right bundle branch block (RBBB) with vertical QRS axis (ostium secundum ASD) and superior axis (ostium primum ASD) on ECG
- Prominent pulmonary arteries and right ventricular (RV) enlargement
- RV dilatation, increased pulmonary artery flow velocity, and left-to-right atrial shunt by Doppler echocardiography
- Oxygen step-up within the right atrium; right-sided catheter can pass into the left atrium across the defect

GENERAL CONSIDERATIONS

- Most common congenital lesion in adults (after bicuspid aortic valve)
- Classification is according to location
- Secundum ASD (most common) is a defect involving the septum secundum in the region of the fossa ovalis
- Primum ASD (also called atrioventricular [AV] canal defect) involves the ostium primum in the lower portion of the atrial septum
- Sinus venosus ASD is a defect in the upper septum near the entrance of the superior vena cava into the right atrium
- ASD is often asymptomatic until adulthood
- The pathophysiologic consequences depend on the quantity of blood shunted from the systemic to pulmonary circulation

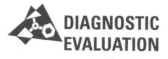

CLINICAL PRESENTATION

SYMPTOMS AND SIGNS

- Usually no symptoms in the young adult with an ASD and normal pulmonary artery pressures unless the defect is very large
- Symptoms more common in the fourth or fifth decade
- Dyspnea
- Diminished exercise tolerance
- Atrial arrhythmia increases with age and may be the most common presenting symptom in patients over 50
- Signs and symptoms of RV failure due to pulmonary hypertension or long-standing volume overload

PHYSICAL EXAM FINDINGS

- Prominent RV impulse
- Palpable pulmonary artery
- Systolic ejection murmur that does not vary with respiration
- Wide, fixed split S_2
- Right-sided diastolic flow rumble
- Right-sided S_3 gallop
- Holosystolic murmur of mitral regurgitation with ostium primum ASD
- With pulmonary hypertension, the P_2 is usually increased and a diastolic murmur of pulmonic insufficiency may be audible (Graham Steele murmur)
- Signs of RV failure with elevated jugular venous pressure and venous congestion in late stages
- Cyanosis in patients with Eisenmenger physiology

DIFFERENTIAL DIAGNOSIS

- Other causes of exertional dyspnea, of atrial arrhythmias, of RV failure, and of a midsystolic murmur (eg, pulmonic stenosis)
- The wide fixed split S_2 can be mimicked by complete RBBB, pericardial knock, and a late systolic click
- Other causes of pulmonary hypertension

DIAGNOSTIC EVALUATION

ELECTROCARDIOGRAPHY

- Incomplete RBBB in 90% of cases
- Right axis deviation with ostium secundum and sinus venosus ASDs
- First-degree AV block, complete RBBB, and left anterior fascicular block with superior and leftward axis with primum ASDs
- Ectopic atrial rhythm with superior P-wave axis occasionally with sinus venosus ASD
- RV hypertrophy
- Notch on the R wave ("crochetage" pattern) in the inferior leads
- Atrial arrhythmias (especially atrial fibrillation)

IMAGING STUDIES

- Chest radiograph: prominent main and branch pulmonary arteries, a small aortic knob, RV enlargement, an enlarged right atrium, and increased lung markings
- Transthoracic echocardiography (preferred initial imaging modality): right heart chamber enlargement and increased pulmonary artery flow velocity
  - Doppler findings of pulmonary hypertension may be present with or without reduced RV function
  - Left-to-right atrial shunt may be visualized with color-flow Doppler
  - Injection of IV agitated saline contrast may demonstrate bubbles within the left atrium, a result of interatrial right-to-left shunting

DIAGNOSTIC PROCEDURES

- Transesophageal echocardiography is the optimal method for evaluating the size and location of the defect venous return
- Cardiac catheterization is not necessary for a diagnosis, but may be necessary to accurately quantitate the shunt and measure the pulmonary vascular resistance

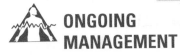

 TREATMENT

CARDIOLOGY REFERRAL

- Any newly diagnosed patient with ASD
- Any patient with a known uncorrected ASD who experiences reduced exercise tolerance, atrial arrhythmias, an embolic event, or signs and symptoms of RV failure, volume overload, or pulmonary hypertension

HOSPITALIZATION CRITERIA

- Severe right heart failure not responding to oral diuretics
- Embolic event
- Syncope (rare)

MEDICATIONS

- Associated arrhythmias may require treatment
- If signs of right heart failure are present, diuretics may be used
- If pulmonary hypertension develops, pulmonary vasodilator therapy may be considered

THERAPEUTIC PROCEDURES

- ASD closure is recommended for a left-to-right shunt > 1.5:1.0
- Smaller shunts can be closed if paradoxical systemic embolization cannot be controlled by other means, such as anticoagulation
- Small ostium secundum defects with adequate membranous tissue rims can be closed with a percutaneously delivered mechanical closure device

SURGERY

- Pulmonary hypertension and older age increase surgical risk
  - Surgery is relatively contraindicated with pulmonary vascular resistance > 10–15 U/m^2

MONITORING

- ECG monitoring in hospital

DIET AND ACTIVITY

- Low-sodium diet for patients with right heart failure
- Activity recommendations depend on size of ASD

ONGOING MANAGEMENT

HOSPITAL DISCHARGE CRITERIA

- Compensated right heart failure
- After recovery from ASD closure

FOLLOW-UP

- Minimal follow-up for pediatric postsurgical patients
- Older postsurgical patients with congestive heart failure or pulmonary hypertension should be followed up for evidence of progressive pulmonary hypertension or arrhythmia

COMPLICATIONS

- Complications of an undetected lesion include atrial arrhythmias, paradoxical embolization, cerebral abscess, pulmonary hypertension (Eisenmenger's syndrome in severe, late cases), and RV failure
- Device embolization or malposition
- Device thrombosis and embolism
- Atrial arrhythmias, especially after surgical repair

PROGNOSIS

- Excellent prognosis for patients with small ASDs or whose defect was closed early in life
- Survival rates less than expected, although the prognosis is still good, in patients whose ASD is closed in the third or fourth decade
- Poor prognosis in patients with severe fixed pulmonary stenosis who are not candidates for ASD closure

PREVENTION

- Early closure of ASDs with a large shunt is recommended to prevent pulmonary vascular disease and right heart failure

RESOURCES

PRACTICE GUIDELINES

- There are no systematic data defining the threshold value for Qp/Qs for repair of an ASD
- The American Heart Association recommended a threshold Qp/Qs of 1.5:1, but these guidelines specifically exclude patients > 21 years
- The Canadian Cardiac Society recommended a threshold Qp/Qs of > 2:1, or > 1.5:1 for patients with reversible pulmonary hypertension

REFERENCES

- Attie F, Rosas M, Granados N et al: Surgical treatment for secundum atrial septal defects in patients > 40 years old. J Am Coll Cardiol 2001; 38:2035.
- Hung J et al: Closure of patent foramen ovale for paradoxical emboli: intermediate term risk of recurrent neurological events following transcatheter device placement. J Am Coll Cardiol 2000;35:1311.
- Therrien J, Dore A, Gersony W et al: CCS Consensus Conference 2001 update: recommendations for the management of adults with congenital heart disease. Part I. Can J Cardiol 2001; 17:940.

INFORMATION FOR PATIENTS

- http://www.americanheart.org/presenter.jhtml?identifier=11065

WEB SITES

- http://www.emedicine.com/ped/topic1686.htm
- http://www.emedicine.com/ped/topic2493.htm
- http://www.emedicine.com/ped/topic171.htm

Atrial Tachycardia, Automatic (Ectopic)

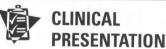 **KEY FEATURES**

ESSENTIALS OF DIAGNOSIS

- Heart rate 100–180 bpm
- P waves different from sinus P waves
- Initiated by an ectopic beat
- Gradual increase in heart rate during an episode

GENERAL CONSIDERATIONS

- Episodes may be brief and self-terminating or chronic and persistent
- Structural heart disease is common, particularly coronary artery disease (including acute myocardial infarction), valvular heart disease, and cardiomyopathy
- Concomitant atrial flutter or fibrillation is not uncommon
- Continuous tachycardia may cause tachycardia cardiomyopathy, mostly in children
- May be associated with digoxin toxicity

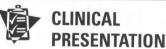 **CLINICAL PRESENTATION**

SYMPTOMS AND SIGNS

- Palpitations
- Dyspnea
- Dizziness
- Chest pain

PHYSICAL EXAM FINDINGS

- Tachycardia
- If the tachycardia is incessant, features of cardiomyopathy may be noted

DIFFERENTIAL DIAGNOSIS

- Reentrant atrial tachycardia
- Atypical AV nodal reentrant tachycardia
- AV reentrant tachycardia with slowly conducting pathway

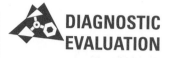 **DIAGNOSTIC EVALUATION**

LABORATORY TESTS

- CBC, basal metabolic panel
- Cardiac biomarkers
- If the patient has features of congestive heart failure, measurement of brain natriuretic peptide

ELECTROCARDIOGRAPHY

- ECG to define rhythm disturbance
- Holter monitoring to document frequency and duration of episodes
- Measurement of serum digoxin level if appropriate

IMAGING STUDIES

- Echocardiogram to exclude structural heart disease

DIAGNOSTIC PROCEDURES

- Electrophysiology study to determine mechanism of rhythm disturbance

TREATMENT

CARDIOLOGY REFERRAL

- All patients require cardiology assessment followed by electrophysiology referral as suggested by cardiologist

HOSPITALIZATION CRITERIA

- Patients with sustained or symptomatic arrhythmia

MEDICATIONS

- Sotalol is the best choice, followed by flecainide
- Propafenone and amiodarone are alternative choices
- Beta blockers are effective to slow the ventricular rate
- Digoxin is uniformly ineffective
- Type IA antiarrhythmic drugs are uniformly ineffective

THERAPEUTIC PROCEDURES

- Radiofrequency ablation
  - Electroanatomic or non-contact mapping may be required
- AV nodal ablation followed by pacemaker insertion if the arrhythmia focus could not be ablated

SURGERY

- Surgical excision or open cryoablation are not performed owing to advances in catheter ablation

MONITORING

- Patients managed by pharmacotherapy need ECG monitoring for effectiveness and assessment of side effects

DIET AND ACTIVITY

- No specific change other than healthy life style

ONGOING MANAGEMENT

HOSPITAL DISCHARGE CRITERIA

- After the arrhythmia is controlled or the ventricular rate is acceptable
- Twenty-four hours after ablation

FOLLOW-UP

- Patients on pharmacotherapy may require follow-up every 3–6 months

COMPLICATIONS

- Cardiomyopathy

PROGNOSIS

- Depends on underlying structural heart disease
  - If there is no structural heart disease, prognosis is good
  - If there is underlying heart disease and the cardiomyopathy is tachycardic in origin, then prognosis is better because left ventricular function improves with successful control of arrhythmia

PREVENTION

- Patients with digoxin-mediated arrhythmia may have been prevented by giving a smaller dose and careful monitoring

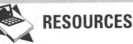

RESOURCES

PRACTICE GUIDELINES

- Indications for ablation: drug refractory or incessant atrial tachycardia, tachycardia-induced cardiomyopathy

REFERENCES

- Morady F: Catheter ablation of supraventricular arrhythmias: state of the art. J Cardiovasc Electrophysiol 2004;15:124.

INFORMATION FOR PATIENTS

- www.drpen.com/427

WEB SITES

- www.hrsonline.org
- www.acc.org

Atriofascicular Tachycardia (Mahaim Tachycardia)

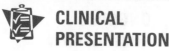

KEY FEATURES

ESSENTIALS OF DIAGNOSIS

- Wide QRS tachycardia (left bundle branch block and superior-axis morphology)
- Diagnosis confirmed at electrophysiologic study
- Progressive decrease in atrioventricular (AV) conduction through the pathway (anterograde decremental conduction)
- Coexistence with AV nodal reentrant tachycardia and other accessory pathways

GENERAL CONSIDERATIONS

- These pathways do not conduct retrogradely
- Antidromic tachycardia is the most common clinical tachycardia
- Minimal preexcitation during sinus rhythm
- More preexcitation during right atrial than lateral coronary sinus pacing (differential pacing)
- Earliest ventricular activation during tachycardia occurs at the right ventricular apex
- Atriofascicular pathways course along the right atrial free wall at the level of the tricuspid annulus and insert distally into right bundle branch
- Fasciculoventricular pathways give rise to fixed preexcitation and serve as bystanders during reentrant tachycardia
- Retrograde right bundle branch block prolongs the tachycardia cycle length
- Intermittent retrograde right bundle branch block causes long, short fluctuating cycle length of the tachycardia
- Mahaim pathway potentials and mechanical compression with the ablation catheter leading to loss of conduction are successful sites for ablation

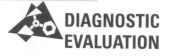

CLINICAL PRESENTATION

SYMPTOMS AND SIGNS

- Palpitations
- Presyncope
- Syncope

PHYSICAL EXAM FINDINGS

- When associated with congenital heart disease (Ebstein's anomaly), features of tricuspid regurgitation may be present

DIFFERENTIAL DIAGNOSIS

- Ventricular tachycardia
- Supraventricular tachycardia with aberrancy

DIAGNOSTIC EVALUATION

LABORATORY TESTS

- CBC, basic metabolic panel

ELECTROCARDIOGRAPHY

- During sinus rhythm, ECG may appear normal because of negligible preexcitation
- During tachycardia, ECG may resemble ventricular tachycardia
  - If the patient has structurally normal heart, Mahaim tachycardia should be in the differential diagnosis
- Holter monitoring to document rhythm disturbances

IMAGING STUDIES

- Echocardiogram if there is an associated murmur to identify Ebstein's anomaly

DIAGNOSTIC PROCEDURES

- Electrophysiologic study to confirm mechanism of tachyarrhythmias and establish diagnosis

TREATMENT

CARDIOLOGY REFERRAL

- All patients with an episode of symptomatic supraventricular tachycardia should be referred to a cardiologist

HOSPITALIZATION CRITERIA

- Symptomatic tachycardia, particularly syncope
- When ventricular tachycardia cannot be excluded

THERAPEUTIC PROCEDURES

- Radiofrequency (RF) ablation of the pathway

SURGERY

- Rarely required

MONITORING

- ECG monitoring in the hospital

DIET AND ACTIVITY

- No specific restrictions
- General healthy life style

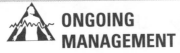

ONGOING MANAGEMENT

HOSPITAL DISCHARGE CRITERIA

- Twenty-four hours after RF ablation

FOLLOW-UP

- Four weeks after initial ablation
- Long-term follow-up with primary care physician

COMPLICATIONS

- Sudden death is rare

PROGNOSIS

- Once ablated, generally approaches normal life expectancy

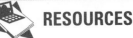

RESOURCES

PRACTICE GUIDELINES

- Wide QRS tachycardia in structurally normal heart; include this disorder in the differential diagnosis
- In Ebstein's anomaly with appropriate morphology of the tachycardia, consider this condition

REFERENCES

- Aliot E et al: Mahaim tachycardias. Eur Heart J 1998;19:E25.
- Pinski SL. The right ventricular tachycardias. J Electrocardiol 2000;33(Suppl):103.

INFORMATION FOR PATIENTS

- www.nlm.nih.gov/medlineplus/arrhythmia.html

WEB SITE

- www.hrsonline.org

Atrioventricular Canal Defects

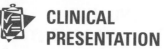 KEY FEATURES

ESSENTIALS OF DIAGNOSIS

- Infant with congestive heart failure
- Physical findings include primum atrial septal defect (ASD) plus mitral regurgitation
- Cardiac imaging shows a common atrioventricular (AV) valve annulus, one or more abnormal AV valves, and defects at the atrial or the ventricular level that can be detected in utero

GENERAL CONSIDERATIONS

- Also called endocardial cushion defect
- AV canal defect is a spectrum of lesions associated with maldevelopment of the AV septum and adjoining AV valves
- A partial AV canal defect has a cleft mitral valve along with a defect in the inferior portion of the AV septum
- Complete AV canal defect is a complex combination of :
  - An ASD
  - A nonrestrictive ventricular septal defect
  - Complex morphology of a common AV valve
- The condition is associated with other congenital anomalies such as:
  - Patent ductus arteriosus
  - Tetralogy of Fallot
  - Double-outlet right ventricle
  - Transposition of the great arteries
  - Unroofed coronary sinus with left superior vena cava
  - Asplenia or polysplenia syndromes
- Very common in Down's syndrome (approximately 20%)
- Large defects are usually repaired in the first 3–6 months of life

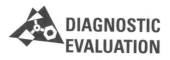 CLINICAL PRESENTATION

SYMPTOMS AND SIGNS

- Complete AV canal defects:
  - Presentation under age 1 year with a history of frequent respiratory infections and poor weight gain
  - Heart failure in infancy common
- Partial AV canal defects:
  - Presentation may be later, with dyspnea and signs and symptoms of right ventricular (RV) failure due to right-sided volume overload
- Patients with persistent complete AV canal defects > age 2 years invariably develop pulmonary vascular disease and possibly Eisenmenger syndrome

PHYSICAL EXAM FINDINGS

- Findings similar to patients with ASDs but may include the following:
  - Holosystolic apical murmur of mitral regurgitation
  - Holosystolic lower left sternal border murmur of interventricular communication

DIFFERENTIAL DIAGNOSIS

- Secundum ASD with mitral regurgitation due to rheumatic disease or prolapse
- Ventricular septal defect
- Other causes of heart failure

DIAGNOSTIC EVALUATION

ELECTROCARDIOGRAPH

- First-degree AV block
- Complete right bundle branch block
- Left anterior fascicular block
- RV hypertrophy

IMAGING STUDIES

- Chest x-ray:
  - Right atrial and ventricular cardiomegaly
  - Prominent right ventricular outflow tract
  - Increased pulmonary vascular markings
- Echocardiographic features of a *partial* AV canal defect:
  - Right atrial and ventricular enlargement
  - Increased pulmonary artery flow velocity
  - A defect in the inferior portion of the interatrial septum immediately adjacent to the AV valves, either of which may be deformed and incompetent
  - The mitral valve is often cleft and sometimes has a double orifice
  - Doppler findings of pulmonary hypertension may be present with or without RV dysfunction
- Echocardiographic features of a *complete* AV canal defect in addition to the ostium primum ASD:
  - A ventricular septal defect in the posterior basal inlet portion of the ventricular septum
  - A common AV valve orifice
- Echoardiography may reveal additional cardiovascular lesions, such as tetralogy of Fallot, double-outlet right ventricle, coarctation of the aorta, LV hypoplasia, and transposition of the great arteries

DIAGNOSTIC PROCEDURES

- Selective LV angiocardiography using contrast reveals:
  - Pathognomonic "gooseneck" deformity, which is due to elongation of the LV outflow tract
  - Inlet ventricular septal defect

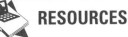

 TREATMENT

CARDIOLOGY REFERRAL

- Patients with complete AV canal defects are invariably diagnosed early in life and referred to a cardiologist
- Patients with partial AV canal defects diagnosed later in life should be referred to a cardiologist familiar with congenital heart disease

HOSPITALIZATION CRITERIA

- Heart failure

MEDICATIONS

- Appropriate treatment for heart failure
- Endocarditis prophylaxis

THERAPEUTIC PROCEDURES

- Pulmonary artery banding may be advised before surgical repair in patients with intractable heart failure and failure to thrive

SURGERY

- The surgery involves patch closure of the ASD and ventricular septal defect along with reconstruction of the mitral and tricuspid valves

MONITORING

- ECG monitoring in hospital

DIET AND ACTIVITY

- Normal activity and diet for patients who have had complete surgical repair without a residual shunt or significant valvular insufficiency
- Low-sodium diet for patients with significant valve regurgitation or heart failure
- Restricted activity for patients with uncorrected defects and fixed pulmonary vascular disease

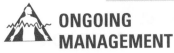 **ONGOING MANAGEMENT**

HOSPITAL DISCHARGE CRITERIA

- To be determined by the surgical team

FOLLOW-UP

- Every 6–12 months for patients without significant hemodynamic abnormalities
- Every 6 months or less for patients with residual AV valve regurgitation, to examine for symptoms and signs of heart failure

COMPLICATIONS

- Residual AV valve regurgitation (common) or stenosis (rare) may require re-operation
- Rarely, surgery can damage the AV node and/or the bundle of His, requiring permanent pacemaker insertion
- Supraventricular arrhythmias

PROGNOSIS

- Without surgical intervention:
  - Most patients die by age 2 or 3 years
  - Survivors usually develop Eisenmenger physiology and typically die in late childhood or young adulthood
- Survival after surgical repair:
  - Approximately 80% for the first year
  - 75% at 10 years
  - 65% at 20 years
- Postoperative complications and pulmonary hypertension are risk factors for higher mortality rate
- Reoperation for AV valve regurgitation or stenosis may be required in approximately 10% within the first year and 15% after 15–20 years

PREVENTION

- Operative repair should be considered before age 6 months to prevent obstructive pulmonary vascular disease and right heart failure

RESOURCES

PRACTICE GUIDELINES

- Patients with or without Down's syndrome have similar survival rate after surgical repair, and all should be referred for early surgical repair
- Endocarditis prophylaxis should be continued even after surgery

REFERENCE

- Boening A et al: Long-term results after surgical correction of atrioventricular septal defects. Eur J Cardiothorac Surg 2002;22:167.

INFORMATION FOR PATIENTS

- www.nlm.nih.gov/medlineplus/congenitalheartdisease.html
- www.heartcenteronline.com/myheartdr/common/articles.cfm?ARTID=426

WEB SITES

- http://www.emedicine.com/ped/topic2775.htm
- http://www.emedicine.com/ped/topic2498.htm

Atrioventricular Nodal-His Block

 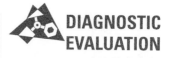

KEY FEATURES

ESSENTIALS OF DIAGNOSIS

- First degree: prolonged PR interval > 0.20 second
- Second degree, type I (Mobitz): progressive increase in PR interval, then failure of AV conduction and absent QRS complex
- Second degree, type II (Mobitz): abrupt failure of AV conduction without prior increase in PR intervals
- High degree: AV conduction ratio > 3:1
- Complete or third degree: independent atrial and ventricular rhythms, with failure of AV conduction despite temporal opportunity for it to occur

GENERAL CONSIDERATIONS

- Common causes: degenerative process, ischemia, calcific aortic valve disease, AV node ablative procedures, medications, infections (aortic valve endocarditis), aortic valve surgery, and infiltrative diseases like amyloidosis
- Escape rhythm originating from cells of the atrionodal area has a faster depolarization rate (45–60/min) and responds to autonomic modulation
- Escape rhythm from the nodal-His area has a slower rate (about 40 bpm) and generally does not respond to autonomic influence

CLINICAL PRESENTATION

SYMPTOMS AND SIGNS

- Syncope, lightheadedness, confusion
- Effort intolerance and exercise-related shortness of breath
- Rarely, bradycardia-mediated prolongation of QT interval may precipitate polymorphic ventricular tachycardia and cardiac arrest

PHYSICAL EXAM FINDINGS

- Clinical signs of complete AV block: cannon a waves in the jugular venous pulse and variable S_1 intensity
- Significant increase of systolic and pulse blood pressure due to large stroke volume secondary to bradycardia
- Rales in the chest and palpable liver if venous pressures are elevated due to bradycardia

DIFFERENTIAL DIAGNOSIS

- Causes of Mobitz I and first-degree AV block: increased vagal tone; drugs that prolong AV conduction such as beta blockers, digoxin, and calcium channel blockers
- Causes of Mobitz II and third-degree AV block: degenerative conduction system disease (Lev disease and Lenègre syndrome)
- Acute myocardial infarction: inferior myocardial infarction causes complete heart block at the AV node; anterior myocardial infarction causes heart block distal to it
- Other causes: acute myocarditis (viral, Lyme disease), digoxin toxicity, congenital heart blocks

DIAGNOSTIC EVALUATION

LABORATORY TESTS

- Electrolytes measurement particularly for hyperkalemia
- Thyroid-stimulating hormone

ELECTROCARDIOGRAPHY

- ECG with rhythm strip to document rhythm
- Holter monitoring if ECG unremarkable
- Event recorder to record infrequent events
- Implantable loop recorder if symptoms are rare but disabling

IMAGING STUDIES

- Echocardiogram in those with features of heart failure, aortic valve disease, and suspected infiltrative diseases

DIAGNOSTIC PROCEDURES

- Electrophysiologic study only if diagnostic uncertainty exists and symptoms are severe

TREATMENT

CARDIOLOGY REFERRAL

- Symptoms related to bradycardia
- Unexplained syncope and recurrent lightheadedness

HOSPITALIZATION CRITERIA

- Symptomatic bradycardia
- Complete heart block
- Mobitz type II heart block

MEDICATIONS

- Withdrawal of offending medications
- No treatment for most patients with Mobitz I block unless the condition progresses or patients develop symptoms

THERAPEUTIC PROCEDURES

- Pacemaker for symptoms of cerebral hypoperfusion
- Pacemaker for symptomatic patients with Mobitz II and complete heart block

SURGERY

- Epicardial pacemaker for patients with no access to transvenous insertion

MONITORING

- ECG monitoring in hospital

DIET AND ACTIVITY

- No restrictions other than general healthy life style

ONGOING MANAGEMENT

HOSPITAL DISCHARGE CRITERIA

- 24 hours after pacemaker insertion
- If an offending agent is withdrawn, patient should be observed until the heart rate is reasonable (resting heart rate > 50 bpm)

FOLLOW-UP

- After pacemaker insertion; monitor every 3 months for adequacy of pacemaker function

COMPLICATIONS

- If untreated, injuries secondary to syncope
- Rarely cardiac arrest
- Pacemaker complications such as infection rare

PROGNOSIS

- Once treated with pacemaker, prognosis is commensurate with age group and comorbidity

PREVENTION

- No known preventive strategy

RESOURCES

PRACTICE GUIDELINES

- Indications for pacemaker insertion: third-degree and advanced second-degree AV block with symptomatic bradycardia
- Aystole > 3 seconds or escape rate < 40 bpm in awake symptom-free patients
- Contraindication for pacemaker insertion: asymptomatic first-degree AV block and AV block expected to resolve

REFERENCES

- Barold SS, Hayes DL: Second-degree atrioventricular block: a reappraisal. Mayo Clin Proc 2001;76:44.
- Hayes DL: Evolving indications for permanent pacing. Am J Cardiol 1999;83:161D.

INFORMATION FOR PATIENTS

- www.drpen.com/426.0, 426.12, 426.11

WEB SITES

- www.americanheart.org
- www.hrsonline.org

Atrioventricular Nodal Reentrant Tachycardia

 ## KEY FEATURES

ESSENTIALS OF DIAGNOSIS

- Heart rate typically 160–190 bpm, but may be over 200 bpm or occasionally as slow as 120 bpm
- Most commonly a narrow QRS tachycardia (50–60%)
- P waves not visible in 90% of cases
- Occasionally, retrograde P waves seen after the QRS complex or buried within the end of the QRS complex
- Short RP tachycardia (RP interval shorter than PR interval)
- In atypical atrioventricular (AV) nodal reentrant tachycardia (< 10% of cases), long RP tachycardia (RP interval > PR interval) may be seen

GENERAL CONSIDERATIONS

- More common in females
- Polyuria not uncommon secondary to elevated atrial natriuretic peptide
- Age distribution is bimodal; initial episode during second decade of life, only to disappear and then reappear during the fourth and fifth decades
- Antegrade (slow pathway) and retrograde (fast pathway) limbs are within the AV node
- In atypical cases, fast pathway is antegrade limb
- Sudden death is reported in rare instances

CLINICAL PRESENTATION

SYMPTOMS AND SIGNS

- Rapid, regular pounding in the neck
- Palpitation
- Dizziness
- Occasionally syncope
- Polyuria

PHYSICAL EXAM FINDINGS

- Tachycardia: 120–200 bpm but usually > 160
- Occasionally hypotension
- Neck pulsations corresponding to the heart rate
- Tachycardia may occasionally terminate with vagal maneuver and carotid sinus pressure

DIFFERENTIAL DIAGNOSIS

- AV reentrant tachycardia
- Atrial tachycardia

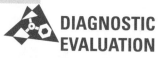 ## DIAGNOSTIC EVALUATION

LABORATORY TESTS

- CBC, basic metabolic panel

ELECTROCARDIOGRAPHY

- ECG and rhythm strip usually show a narrow QRS complex tachycardia without p waves. When p waves are visible, they are seen near the end of the QRS complex and usually a short RP (RP < PR) interval is noted.
- Holter monitoring to detect tachycardia
- Event recorder to detect tachycardia

IMAGING STUDIES

- In otherwise healthy patient no imaging required, although echocardiography is commonly performed to exclude structural heart disease

DIAGNOSTIC PROCEDURES

- Invasive electrophysiology (EP) study to confirm mechanism of tachycardia and its suitability for ablation

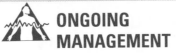

TREATMENT

CARDIOLOGY REFERRAL

- EP referral is recommended for all patients, although some physicians may try medications initially

HOSPITALIZATION CRITERIA

- If the diagnosis is certain and post-termination ECG is normal, hospitalization is not required

MEDICATIONS

- Acute termination occurs with adenosine 6-mg or 12-mg bolus injection
- Maintenance therapy includes beta blockers or calcium channel blockers to inhibit the slow pathway
- Class I drugs may be used to inhibit the fast pathway

THERAPEUTIC PROCEDURES

- EP study followed by slow pathway ablation

SURGERY

- None required in the modern era

MONITORING

- Once ablated, no long-term follow-up required unless there is recurrence
- Recurrence is rare (< 2%)

DIET AND ACTIVITY

- No restrictions other than general healthy life style

ONGOING MANAGEMENT

HOSPITAL DISCHARGE CRITERIA

- Discharge 24 hours after ablation; some physicians discharge patients same day after ablation

FOLLOW-UP

- Two to 4 weeks after ablation for a one-time visit
- No long-term follow-up required after ablation
- If medications are used without pursuing ablation, follow-up is required after symptomatic recurrence or semi-annually
- If pacemaker is implanted as a complication of ablation therapy (<1%), follow-up of pacemaker is required every 3 months

COMPLICATIONS

- Pacemaker requirement as a complication of ablative therapy

PROGNOSIS

- Generally excellent

PREVENTION

- None known

RESOURCES

PRACTICE GUIDELINES

- Guidelines on therapy: ablation or medication depends on patient's choice according to frequency and severity of symptoms and side effects/tolerance of medications
- Hemodynamic instability or recurrent symptomatic episodes are indications for ablation

REFERENCES

- Blomstrom-Lundqvist C, Scheinman MM, Aliot EM et al: ACC/AHA/ESC guidelines for the management of patients with supraventricular arrhythmias—executive summary. A report of the American College of Cardiology/American Heart Association Task Force on Practice Guidelines and the European Society of Cardiology Committee for Practice Guidelines (writing committee to develop guidelines for the management of patients with supraventricular arrhythmias) developed in collaboration with NASPE-Heart Rhythm Society. J Am Coll Cardiol 2003;42:1493.
- Tebbenjohannas J et al: Noninvasive diagnosis in patients with undocumented tachycardias: value of the adenosine test to predict AV nodal reentrant tachycardia. J Cardiovasc Electrophysiol 1999;10:916.

INFORMATION FOR PATIENTS

- www.drpen.com/427

WEB SITE

- www.hrsonline.org

KEY FEATURES

ESSENTIALS OF DIAGNOSIS

- Wolff-Parkinson-White syndrome
  - Short P-R interval (<120 ms)
  - Wide QRS complex caused by a delta wave due to pre-excitation over an AV bypass tract
  - Supraventricular tachycardia with heart rates of 140–250 bpm
- Atrioventricular reciprocating tachycardia (AVRT) with a narrow QRS is the most common arrhythmia

GENERAL CONSIDERATIONS

- AV bypass tracts or accessory pathways have a 2:1 male/female predominance, and may be familial
- Left ventricular free wall is the most common location for accessory pathways
- Right sided bypass tracts are commonly associated with structural heart disease
- 5–10% have structural heart disease (Ebstein anomaly is the most common)
- Fewer than half of those with documented bypass tracts sustain a clinical arrhythmia
- When the bypass tract conducts retrograde (antegrade conduction over the AV node), AVRT results
- Orthodromic AVRT (antegrade over AV node) accounts for 70-80% and antidromic (retrograde over AV node) accounts for 5–10%
- Orthodromic tachycardia has a narrow QRS complex, and antidromic tachycardia has a wide QRS complex
- Atrial fibrillation with antegrade conduction over the bypass tract can lead to ventricular fibrillation and sudden death
- Concealed bypass tracts conduct retrograde only and cause orthodromic AVRT, but cannot be detected during sinus rhythm

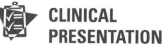 **CLINICAL PRESENTATION**

SYMPTOMS AND SIGNS

- Palpitations, chest pain, and dyspnea
- Dizziness
- Syncope
- Sudden death
- Asymptomatic

PHYSICAL EXAM FINDINGS

- Normal clinical exam in most patients
- If associated with Ebstein's anomaly, physical exam may be positive for tricuspid regurgitation and associated anomalies
- Mid systolic click and murmur are present if there is associated mitral valve prolapse (MVP)

DIFFERENTIAL DIAGNOSIS

- AV nodal reentrant tachycardia
- Supraventricular tachycardia with aberrancy
- Ventricular tachycardia (for antidromic tachycardia)

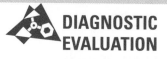 **DIAGNOSTIC EVALUATION**

LABORATORY TESTS

- Serum thyroid-stimulating hormone in atrial fibrillation patients

ELECTROCARDIOGRAPHY

- ECG during sinus rhythm (SR) or narrow QRS tachycardia
  - If there is preexcitation during SR, then antegrade conduction is present; otherwise concealed bypass tract)
  - Antidromic tachycardia usually has a wider QRS complex
- Holter monitoring or event recorder to document arrhythmia

IMAGING STUDIES

- Echocardiogram
  - If Ebstein's or MVP suspected
  - Recommended in patients with a presenting arrhythmia of atrial fibrillation

DIAGNOSTIC PROCEDURES

- Electrophysiologic study to define mechanism of the tachycardia

TREATMENT

CARDIOLOGY REFERRAL

- All patients should be evaluated by a cardiologist
- Referral to electrophysiology decided by a cardiologist

HOSPITALIZATION CRITERIA

- Patients presenting with syncope
- Sudden death survivors
- Atrial fibrillation in a patient with known antegrade conduction

MEDICATIONS

- For regular narrow QRS tachycardia, adenosine 6–12 mg is useful to terminate the arrhythmia
- Drugs that block the AV node, when used independently, may facilitate the conduction of atrial fibrillation through the accessory pathway, resulting in ventricular fibrillation
- Recurrent regular narrow QRS tachycardia may be treated with beta blockers or calcium channel blockers
- Class IA, class IC, or amiodarone may be tried to control arrhythmia with antidromic mechanism
- Digoxin must be avoided because it may improve conduction over the accessory pathway

THERAPEUTIC PROCEDURES

- For recurrent arrhythmia, radiofrequency ablation has a high success rate (95%)

SURGERY

- Seldom required today because of substantial advances in catheter-based techniques

MONITORING

- Those on medication may need periodic monitoring of drug side effects

DIET AND ACTIVITY

- No specific recommendations

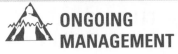

ONGOING MANAGEMENT

HOSPITAL DISCHARGE CRITERIA

- Symptomatically stable on medications or 24 hours after radiofrequency ablation

FOLLOW-UP

- If patient is on antiarrhythmic medication, follow-up every 6 months to evaluate symptoms and side effects
- After radiofrequency ablation, one-time visit 2 weeks after ablation; thereafter, generally no further follow-up required

COMPLICATIONS

- Complications from antiarrhythmic medications
- Sudden death (rare)

PROGNOSIS

- Generally very good except for the rare possibility of sudden cardiac death in Wolff-Parkinson-White syndrome

RESOURCES

PRACTICE GUIDELINES

- Indications for ablation: atrial fibrillation with rapid ventricular rate or poorly tolerated orthodromic reentrant tachycardia (ORT) or recurrent symptomatic arrhythmia
- Asymptomatic patients with preexcitation in general have a good prognosis and do not require prophylactic ablation

REFERENCES

- Al-Khatib SM, Pritchett EL: Clinical features of Wolff-Parkinson-White syndrome. Am Heart J 1999;138:403.
- Maury P, Zimmermann M, Metzger J: Distinction between atrioventricular reciprocating tachycardia and atrioventricular node re-entrant tachycardia in the adult population based on P wave location. Should we reconsider the value of some ECG criteria according to gender and age? Europace 2003;5:57.

INFORMATION FOR PATIENTS

- www.drpen.com/427

WEB SITES

- www.hrsonline.org
- www.theheart.org

Bicuspid Aortic Valve

 KEY FEATURES

ESSENTIALS OF DIAGNOSIS

- History of murmur since infancy, coarctation repair, or endocarditis
- Early systolic ejection click, harsh crescendo-decrescendo systolic murmur, or early decrescendo diastolic murmur
- Left ventricular hypertrophy
- Abnormal bicuspid or dysplastic aortic valve with stenosis or regurgitation on Doppler echocardiography

GENERAL CONSIDERATIONS

- Most common congenital heart disease with a prevalence of about 2% of the population
- Represents about 50% of all congenital outflow tract obstructive lesions
- Occurs more commonly in men than women by 3–5:1.0
- Associated lesions include
  - Patent ductus arteriosus
  - Coarctation of the aorta
  - Ventricular septal defects
- Hemodynamic distortions:
  - Leads to progressive valvular degeneration
  - Results in aortic stenosis in about 50% of patients by age 50
- Aortic regurgitation may also occur and, less commonly, is the dominant lesion

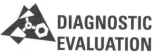 **CLINICAL PRESENTATION**

SYMPTOMS AND SIGNS

- Dyspnea
- Angina
- Effort syncope
- Sudden cardiac death

PHYSICAL EXAM FINDINGS

- Pulsus parvus et tardus
- Increased size, amplitude, and duration of the apical impulse
- Systolic ejection sound, diminished A_2 and S_4
- Harsh systolic ejection murmur radiating to the neck
- Often a high-pitched decrescendo murmur of aortic regurgitation
- Systolic murmur augmented in intensity in the beat after a premature beat
- Physical findings of associated lesions may be present

DIFFERENTIAL DIAGNOSIS

- Discrete subaortic stenosis
- Hypertrophic obstructive cardiomyopathy
- Marfan syndrome with aortic regurgitation
- Pulmonic stenosis
- Ventricular septal defect
- Mitral valve prolapse with mitral regurgitation

DIAGNOSTIC EVALUATION

LABORATORY TESTS

- No specific tests

ELECTROCARDIOGRAPHY

- Left ventricular hypertrophy if significant aortic stenosis is present

IMAGING STUDIES

- Chest x-ray often shows left ventricular enlargement
- Echocardiography demonstrates the bicuspid aortic valve
  - In most, the leaflet orientation is anterior and posterior
  - In some, it is right to left
  - Occasionally, a raphe on a leaflet may mimic a tricuspid leaflet arrangement and transesophageal echo is needed to diagnose bicuspid valve
- Doppler echocardiography can be used:
  - To measure the pressure gradient across the valve
  - To estimate orifice area size
- Color flow Doppler is useful for assessing associated lesions such as aortic regurgitation

DIAGNOSTIC PROCEDURES

- Cardiac catheterization
  - In pediatric patients, the peak-to-peak gradient on pullback of an end-hole catheter is used to assess the severity of aortic stenosis
  - < 50 mm Hg is mild, 50–80 is moderate, and > 80 is severe
- Catheterization and angiography are also useful for assessing the hemodynamic contribution of associated lesions

TREATMENT

CARDIOLOGY REFERRAL

- All patients suspected of having a bicuspid aortic valve should be assessed once by a cardiologist

HOSPITALIZATION CRITERIA

- Symptoms: dyspnea, angina, syncope
- Severe stenosis found by Doppler echocardiography with planned catheterization
- Heart failure

MEDICATIONS

- Diuretics to treat heart failure

THERAPEUTIC PROCEDURES

- In children, percutaneous aortic balloon valvuloplasty is often successful in relieving stenosis with a low mortality rate
- Long-term results in children are better than those observed in adults, but recurrent stenosis is common (at least 25%)

SURGERY

- Aortic valve replacement with a homograft (Ross procedure), bioprosthetic valve, or mechanical valve provides definitive therapy
- Surgery is the procedure of choice in adults

MONITORING

- ECG monitoring in the hospital

DIET AND ACTIVITY

- Low-sodium, cardiac diet
- Avoidance of strenuous or competitive exercise activities

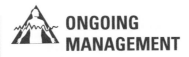 ## ONGOING MANAGEMENT

HOSPITAL DISCHARGE CRITERIA

- Resolution of symptoms
- After successful procedure or surgery

FOLLOW-UP

- Before surgery: periodically (every 3 years to 3 months), depending on the severity of stenosis
- After surgery: 2 weeks, 3 months, then every 6 months

COMPLICATIONS

- Sudden cardiac death
- Syncope
- Heart failure
- Infective endocarditis
- Aortic regurgitation after valvuloplasty

PROGNOSIS

- Most patients eventually develop significant hemodynamic abnormalities, usually stenosis
- Annual mortality rate for those with stenosis is up to 2% per year
- The risk of infective endocarditis is 27 per 10,000 person-years

PREVENTION

- Antibiotic prophylaxis for dental and other procedures to prevent endocarditis
- Bicuspid aortic valve is congenital

RESOURCES

PRACTICE GUIDELINES

- Valvuloplasty or replacement is indicated for:
  - Moderate to severe stenosis or regurgitation with symptoms
  - Left ventricular dysfunction
- Children with peak-to-peak gradient of > 75 mm Hg at catheterization should have the stenosis corrected

REFERENCES

- Ward C: Clinical significance of the bicuspid aortic valve. Heart 2000;83:81.

INFORMATION FOR PATIENTS

- www.drpen.com/hd424.1

WEB SITE

- www.emedicine.com/PED/topic2486.htm

Brugada Syndrome

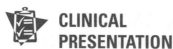 **KEY FEATURES**

ESSENTIALS OF DIAGNOSIS

- Life-threatening cardiac arrhythmia (ventricular fibrillation and ventricular tachycardia) with no demonstrable structural cardiac disease
- Apparent right bundle branch block with ST elevation in V1–V3 (V2 always present)
- The disease is secondary to a mutation in the sodium channel (*SCN5A*)
- Flecainide or procainamide may be used to unmask the ECG changes (ST elevation in V2)

GENERAL CONSIDERATIONS

- Spontaneous or inducible polymorphic VT
- Some patients remain asymptomatic despite Brugada type ECG
- QT interval is normal
- Young males and adolescents are most often affected
- Suggested to be a cause of "sleep death" among young Asian males
- The syndrome is familial and a mutation in chromosome 3 has been identified

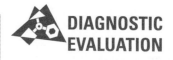 **CLINICAL PRESENTATION**

SYMPTOMS AND SIGNS

- Cardiac arrest
- Asymptomatic

PHYSICAL EXAM FINDINGS

- Normal physical exam

DIFFERENTIAL DIAGNOSIS

- Long QT syndrome
- Idiopathic ventricular arrhythmia
- ECG changes may mimic acute myocardial infarction (cardiac enzymes and regional wall motion are usually normal, but may be transiently abnormal after a cardiac arrest)

DIAGNOSTIC EVALUATION

LABORATORY TESTS

- Genetic testing in specialized labs

ELECTROCARDIOGRAPHY

- ECG with apparent right bundle branch block with ST elevation in V1–V3 (V2 always present)
- If the syndrome is suspected but the baseline ECG is normal, challenge with the administration of flecainide or procainamide is recommended

IMAGING STUDIES

- Echocardiogram to exclude structural heart disease

DIAGNOSTIC PROCEDURES

- Symptomatic or asymptomatic patients with abnormal ECG at baseline require electrophysiologic studies to determine whether sustained ventricular arrhythmia can be induced

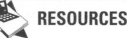

 TREATMENT

CARDIOLOGY REFERRAL

• All patients should be evaluated by a cardiac electrophysiologist

HOSPITALIZATION CRITERIA

• After a cardiac arrest, all patients are hospitalized to the cardiac intensive care unit
• Asymptomatic patients with abnormal ECG do not require hospitalization

THERAPEUTIC PROCEDURES

• Implantable cardioverter-defibrillator (ICD) is needed for patients with life-threatening arrhythmia or inducible sustained ventricular arrhythmias on electrophysiologic testing

SURGERY

• If there is no venous access, then epicardial placement of an ICD may be required

MONITORING

• ECG monitoring in hospital

DIET AND ACTIVITY

• General healthy life style

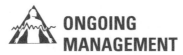 **ONGOING MANAGEMENT**

HOSPITAL DISCHARGE CRITERIA

• Discharge 24 hours after ICD implantation if clinically stable

FOLLOW-UP

• Every 3 months for patients implanted with an ICD
• Otherwise, role of regular follow-up is not clearly established

COMPLICATIONS

• Sudden cardiac death
• Complications of ICD implantation

PROGNOSIS

• Survivors of sudden cardiac death (SCD) and those with family history of SCD predict high-risk patients for sudden death
• Asymptomatic patients with abnormal ECG at baseline require electrophysiologic studies; inducibility is reported to predict high-risk patients for SCD
• Asymptomatic patients with normal baseline ECG have the best overall prognosis

PREVENTION

• None known

RESOURCES

PRACTICE GUIDELINES

• Survivors of SCD and high-risk patients should be referred to an electrophysiologist
• Asymptomatic patients with normal baseline ECG should be reassured until more data are available

REFERENCES

• Belhassen B, Viskin S, Antzelevitch C: The Brugada syndrome: is an implantable cardioverter defibrillator the only therapeutic option? Pacing Clin Electrophysiol 2002;25:1634.
• Wilde AA et al: Proposed diagnostic criteria for the Brugada syndrome. Eur Heart J 2002;23:1648.

INFORMATION FOR PATIENTS

• www.drpen.com/427.5
• www.nlm.nih.gov/medlineplus/arrhythmia.html

WEB SITES

• www.hrsonline.org
• www.theheart.org

Buerger's Disease (Thromboangiitis Obliterans)

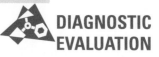 KEY FEATURES

ESSENTIALS OF DIAGNOSIS

- An inflammatory vasculopathy (arteries and veins) that predominantly involves the hands and is invariably associated with smoking
- Digital ulcers may be present
- Men younger than 50 years
- Thrombophlebitis may be the first sign of the disease
- Angiography shows disease of the small and median arteries with corkscrew collaterals; large arteries are unaffected
- Laboratory evidence of HLA antibodies, increased complement activity, and anticollagen antibodies

GENERAL CONSIDERATIONS

- The cause of Buerger's disease is unknown, but cigarette smoking plays a critical role in its genesis
- It occurs primarily in young men (< 40 years) and almost exclusively in smokers, ex-smokers, and passive smokers
- The inflammatory activity is seen in both arteries and veins with migratory thrombophlebitis
- Ischemia most often involves the digits
- Buerger's disease is more common in the eastern Mediterranean and Asia

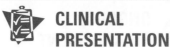 CLINICAL PRESENTATION

SYMPTOMS AND SIGNS

- The first sign is often thrombophlebitis in an extremity
- Inflammation of the digits with pain and swelling

PHYSICAL EXAM FINDINGS

- Pulse deficits in distal extremities
- Signs of ischemia, such as ulcers

DIFFERENTIAL DIAGNOSIS

- Atherosclerosis obliterans

DIAGNOSTIC EVALUATION

LABORATORY TESTS

- Positive HLA antigens DR4, A9, B5, and B8
- Increased complement
- Sensitivity to human collagen types 1 and 3
- Anticollagen antibodies

DIAGNOSTIC PROCEDURES

- Angiography is usually diagnostic:
  - Segmental lesions in otherwise normal arteries
  - Small- to medium-sized arteries involved with more disease distally
  - Corkscrew collaterals

TREATMENT

CARDIOLOGY REFERRAL
- Suspected thromboembolic disease

HOSPITALIZATION CRITERIA
- Complications, such as infection
- Gangrene

MEDICATIONS
- Stop smoking
- Prostaglandins may help ulcer healing

THERAPEUTIC PROCEDURES
- Hyperbaric oxygen may help ulcer healing

SURGERY
- Amputation may be necessary
- Thoracoscopic sympathectomy may benefit some cases
- Arterial bypass surgery may help some

ONGOING MANAGEMENT

HOSPITAL DISCHARGE CRITERIA
- Resolution of problem
- Successful surgery

FOLLOW-UP
- Depends on severity of disease and response to therapy

COMPLICATIONS
- Infection
- Limb loss

PROGNOSIS
- Good prognosis if the patient stops smoking and avoids smoke exposure

PREVENTION
- No smoking

RESOURCES

REFERENCES
- Bozkurt AK et al: Surgical treatment of Buerger's disease. Vasc Med 2004;12:192.
- De Giancomo T et al: Thoracoscopic sympathectomy for symptomatic arterial obstruction of the upper extremities. Ann Thorac Surg 2002;74:885.
- Ohta T et al: Clinical and social consequences of Buerger's disease. J Vasc Surg 2004;39:176.
- Olin JW: Thromboangiitis obliterans (Buerger's disease). N Engl J Med 2002;343:864.

INFORMATION FOR PATIENTS
- www.nlm.nih.gov/medlineplus/encyl/article/000172.htm

WEB SITE
- www.emedicine.com/med/topic253.htm

Bundle Branch Reentrant Ventricular Tachycardia

KEY FEATURES

ESSENTIALS OF DIAGNOSIS

- Rapid ventricular tachycardia (VT), usually with left bundle branch block morphology
- Generally occurs with advanced nonischemic dilated cardiomyopathy
- HV interval during the tachycardia is usually the same as in sinus rhythm

GENERAL CONSIDERATIONS

- The impulse reenters within the conduction system
- Right bundle antegrade of 90% and left bundle retrograde conduction
- Left bundle antegrade of 10% and right bundle retrograde conduction
- Intraventricular conduction system disease is common
- This type of VT is also occasionally seen in valvular cardiomyopathy
- Delay within the conduction system is critical for reentry to sustain this arrhythmia

CLINICAL PRESENTATION

SYMPTOMS AND SIGNS

- Syncope
- Cardiac arrest

PHYSICAL EXAM FINDINGS

- Features of cardiomyopathy
- During tachycardia, patients typically experience hypotension and tissue hypoperfusion
- S_3 may be present secondary to cardiomyopathy

DIFFERENTIAL DIAGNOSIS

- Intramyocardial reentrant VT
- Supraventricular tachycardia with aberrancy
- Mahaim tachycardia

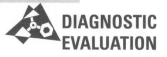 DIAGNOSTIC EVALUATION

LABORATORY TESTS

- Basal metabolic panel
- Thyroid-stimulating hormone
- Serum magnesium level

ELECTROCARDIOGRAPHY

- ECG during tachycardia typically shows left bundle branch block morphology tachycardia
- ECG in sinus rhythm usually shows intraventricular conduction delay

IMAGING STUDIES

- Echocardiography to evaluate left ventricular function and valvular abnormalities

DIAGNOSTIC PROCEDURES

- Invasive electrophysiologic study to establish mechanism of arrhythmia and determine feasibility of ablation

TREATMENT

CARDIOLOGY REFERRAL

- All patients with suspected bundle branch reentry VT should be referred to a cardiac electrophysiologist

HOSPITALIZATION CRITERIA

- All patients with this condition require hospitalization for management

MEDICATIONS

- No effective medication therapy exists

THERAPEUTIC PROCEDURES

- Invasive electrophysiologic study followed by ablation of the right bundle branch

SURGERY

- Implantable cardioverter-defibrillator (ICD) is recommended concurrent with ablation because of the risk of sudden death associated with poor left ventricular function

MONITORING

- Ablation is curative
- Patients with an ICD require follow-up of the device every 3 months

DIET AND ACTIVITY

- Once treated, no special restrictions required other than for the underlying heart disease

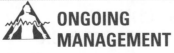

ONGOING MANAGEMENT

HOSPITAL DISCHARGE CRITERIA

- Twenty-four hours after successful ablation

FOLLOW-UP

- Follow-up for cardiomyopathy and ICD

COMPLICATIONS

- Once treated, no complications occur
- Patients remain at risk for sudden cardiac death secondary to the substrate of cardiomyopathy

PROGNOSIS

- Once the condition is identified and treated, prognosis reflects the underlying heart disease

PREVENTION

- None known

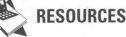

RESOURCES

PRACTICE GUIDELINES

- Bundle branch reentry should be considered in the differential diagnosis of VT associated with dilated cardiomyopathy
- Radiofrequency ablation is curative
- Because of poor left ventricular function even after RF ablation most patients are implanted with an ICD

REFERENCES

- Fisher JD: Bundle branch reentry tachycardia: why is the HV interval often longer than in sinus rhythm? The critical role of anisotropic conduction. J Interv Card Electrophysiol 2001;5:173.

INFORMATION FOR PATIENTS

- www.nlm.nih.gov/medlineplus/arrhythmia.html

WEB SITE

- www.hrsonline.org

Carcinoid and the Heart

 KEY FEATURES

ESSENTIALS OF DIAGNOSIS

- CT or other imaging of neuroendocrine tumor(s) in the gut, with possible liver or pulmonary metastases
- Elevated 5-hydroxyindoleacetic acid (HIAA) in the urine
- Cardiac auscultatory evidence of tricuspid regurgitation or pulmonic stenosis
- Echocardiographic evidence of thickened tricuspid or pulmonary valves

GENERAL CONSIDERATIONS

- Carcinoid tumors are neuroendocrine in origin and often secrete serotonin or its metabolites
- About 25% of carcinoid patients develop symptoms of flushing and diarrhea due to hepatic metastases (carcinoid syndrome)
- About 50% of carcinoid syndrome patients develop valvular heart disease, mainly of the right heart valves
- The endothelial lesion consists of distinctive fibrotic plaques that adhere to the valves and chamber walls
- Valvular plaques usually result in tricuspid regurgitation and pulmonic stenosis
- Bronchial tumors can result in left heart valve disease

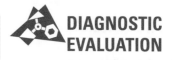 **CLINICAL PRESENTATION**

SYMPTOMS AND SIGNS

- Symptoms range from flushing to diarrhea to profound hypotension

PHYSICAL EXAM FINDINGS

- The murmur of tricuspid regurgitation or pulmonic stenosis may be present
- Signs of right heart failure may be present

DIFFERENTIAL DIAGNOSIS

- Other causes of pulmonic stenosis, tricuspid regurgitation, and right-heart failure
- Consumption of serotonin-rich foods can give false-positive urine screening test results

DIAGNOSTIC EVALUATION

LABORATORY TESTS

- Twenty-four–hour urine for 5-HIAA:
  - > 30 mg is diagnostic
  - < 10 mg is normal on a diet devoid of serotonin-rich foods

ELECTROCARDIOGRAPHY

- Some patients demonstrate right ventricular hypertrophy or right atrial enlargement

IMAGING STUDIES

- Abdominal CT is indicated to locate the primary tumor and hepatic or other metastases
- Echocardiography shows the characteristic diffuse thickening of the right heart valves with an echogenic material
  - Doppler echo shows tricuspid regurgitation and pulmonic stenosis

DIAGNOSTIC PROCEDURES

- Cardiac catheterization may be required in selected patients

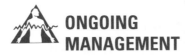

TREATMENT

CARDIOLOGY REFERRAL

- Evidence of significant valvular disease
- Right heart failure
- Endocarditis

HOSPITALIZATION CRITERIA

- Right heart failure
- Endocarditis
- Profound hypotension

MEDICATIONS

- Somatostatin therapy to shrink metastases:
  - Octreotide 50–150 µg 2–4 times a day SC or IV; maximum dose 1500 µg/day
  - Octreotide 50–500 µg IV prn carcinoid crisis or 250–500 µg IV preoperatively to prevent crisis

THERAPEUTIC PROCEDURES

- Valvuloplasty has met with mixed success

SURGERY

- Surgical removal of tumor if it has not metastasized
- Valve replacement in selected patients with slowly progressive disease

MONITORING

- ECG and blood pressure monitoring in hospital as appropriate

DIET AND ACTIVITY

- Low-sodium diet if right heart failure
- Restrict activity if heart failure

ONGOING MANAGEMENT

HOSPITAL DISCHARGE CRITERIA

- Resolution of symptoms
- Successful surgery

FOLLOW-UP

- Cardiology every 3–6 months

COMPLICATIONS

- Right heart failure
- Endocarditis
- Syncope

PROGNOSIS

- Progression can be slow, so patients may live many years, making valve surgery to relieve symptoms a viable option
- Heart disease does not regress with reducing serotonin levels

PREVENTION

- Octreotide is most effective for preventing symptoms
- The serotonin receptor antagonists, such as cyproheptadine, have *not* been very effective

RESOURCES

PRACTICE GUIDELINES

- Mortality rate with valve replacement surgery is higher than that observed in noncarcinoid patients, so the decision to operate on the heart must be carefully thought out

REFERENCE

- Ganim RB, Norton JA: Recent advances in carcinoid pathogenesis, diagnosis and management. Surg Oncol 2000;9:173.

INFORMATION FOR PATIENTS

- www.nlm.nih.gov/medlineplus/ency/article/000347.htm

WEB SITE

- www.emedicine.com/med/topic271.htm

Cardiac Allograft Vasculopathy

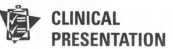 KEY FEATURES

ESSENTIALS OF DIAGNOSIS

- Major long-term problem after cardiac transplantation
- Possible causes: myocardial infarction (MI), impaired left ventricular function with heart failure, arrhythmias, and sudden death
- Angina pectoris is rare because of allograft denervation
- Diffuse, concentric coronary artery narrowing on angiography

GENERAL CONSIDERATIONS

- Incidence is 20–50% at 5 years
- It is the main cause of late post-transplantation deaths and is the main factor limiting long-term survival
- Noninvasive tests (except possibly dobutamine stress echocardiography) are not useful in assessing this disease
- Recipient characteristics (eg, hypertension, hyperlipidemia, insulin resistance, and cytomegalovirus infection) and donor characteristics (eg, preexisting coronary disease, donor ischemic time) may play a role
- Cyclosporine-based immunosuppression has not reduced the frequency of this entity

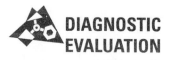 CLINICAL PRESENTATION

SYMPTOMS AND SIGNS

- Dyspnea
- Sudden death
- Ventricular arrhythmia
- Angina is rare despite advanced graft vasculopathy

PHYSICAL EXAM FINDINGS

- Features of heart failure may be present

DIFFERENTIAL DIAGNOSIS

- Acute rejection
- Cytomegalovirus infection

DIAGNOSTIC EVALUATION

LABORATORY TESTS

- No specific lab tests
- Cardiac biomarker elevation if there is acute MI

ELECTROCARDIOGRAPHY

- ECG may indicate acute MI
- Ventricular arrhythmias may signify allograft vasculopathy

IMAGING STUDIES

- Dobutamine echocardiography (DSE) may offer reasonable sensitivity and specificity
- DSE may also provide prognostic value

DIAGNOSTIC PROCEDURES

- Coronary angiography:
  - The disease is diffuse and concentric and easy to miss on angiogram
  - Diameter comparison with prior angiogram is critical in recognizing the condition
  - Collateral vessel formation is uncommon
- Intravascular ultrasound is a promising tool for early recognition of allograft vasculopathy

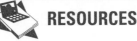
 TREATMENT

CARDIOLOGY REFERRAL

- All patients are usually followed by a transplantation cardiologist

HOSPITALIZATION CRITERIA

- Heart failure
- Acute MI
- Symptomatic arrhythmia

MEDICATIONS

- Diltiazem and lipid-lowering agents (statins), regardless of lipid levels, are useful for prevention
- Risk factor modification and aspirin may help in prevention
- Retransplantation is a choice for diffuse vasculopathy, but is associated with a low survival rate

THERAPEUTIC PROCEDURES

- Percutaneous coronary intervention may be useful in some cases if discrete proximal lesions are noted

SURGERY

- Retransplantation: rarely bypass grafting may be attempted

MONITORING

- ECG monitoring in hospital

DIET AND ACTIVITY

- Cardiac, low-fat diet
- Regular exercise
- Cessation of smoking

ONGOING MANAGEMENT

HOSPITAL DISCHARGE CRITERIA

- Symptomatically stable
- Hemodynamic stability

FOLLOW-UP

- Depending on clinical status
- Follow-up every week to once in 3 months

COMPLICATIONS

- Heart failure
- Arrhythmias, sudden death
- MI

PROGNOSIS

- Poor
- One-year survival rate is 67%; 2-year rate is 44%

PREVENTION

- Statins
- Diltiazem
- Aspirin
- Regular exercise
- Cessation of smoking
- Maintenance of ideal body weight
- Low-fat diet

RESOURCES

PRACTICE GUIDELINES

- Prevention of allograft vasculopathy is the best strategy

REFERENCES

- Valantine HA: Cardiac allograft vasculopathy: central role of endothelial injury leading to transplant "atheroma" transplantation. 2003;76:891.
- Weis M: Cardiac allograft vasculopathy: prevention and treatment options. Transplant Proc 2002;34:1847.

INFORMATION FOR PATIENTS

- www.nlm.nih.gov/medlineplus/cardiomyopathy.html

WEB SITES

- www.americanheart.org
- www.unos.org

Cardiac Cachexia

KEY FEATURES

ESSENTIALS OF DIAGNOSIS

- Chronic severe heart failure
- Unintentional loss of more than 6% of previous nonedematous weight with body mass index < 24 kg/m^2
- Muscle wasting, weakness
- Decreased serum transferrin and elevated triglycerides

GENERAL CONSIDERATIONS

- Affects up to 15% of patients with congestive heart failure (CHF)
- Associated with very poor survival
- Inflammatory cytokine activation and neuroendocrine abnormalities play a role in the pathogenesis of wasting
- No established, proven therapy

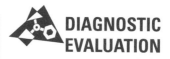 CLINICAL PRESENTATION

SYMPTOMS AND SIGNS

- Elderly (most common) patient with a history of chronic CHF
- Fatigue
- Muscle weakness
- Unintentional non-edematous weight loss of > 6% over at least 6 months
- Preserved or deteriorating appetite

PHYSICAL EXAM FINDINGS

- Body mass index < 24 kg/m^2
- Muscle-wasting/atrophy
- Loss of adipose tissue

DIFFERENTIAL DIAGNOSIS

- Cancer
- Hyperthyroidism
- Acquired immunodeficiency syndrome
- Intentional weight loss
- Diuresis
- Starvation

DIAGNOSTIC EVALUATION

LABORATORY TESTS

- Serum electrolytes (hyponatremia)
- Serum uric acid elevation
- C-reactive protein and erythrocyte sedimentation rate elevations
- Serum creatinine
- Triglycerides (elevated)
- Serum transferrin level (decreased)
- Digoxin level (exclude digoxin toxicity)

ELECTROCARDIOGRAPHY

- Sinus rhythm/sinus tachycardia
- Atrial fibrillation
- Low-voltage QRS or evidence of ventricular hypertrophy

IMAGING STUDIES

- Chest x-ray: normal or enlarged cardiac silhouette, pulmonary vascular congestion and/or curly B lines may be present; osteopenia with or without vertebral body compression fractures may be present
- Echocardiography: biventricular and/or right ventricular enlargement and reduced contractility; atrial enlargement; color Doppler evidence of valvular regurgitation due to annular dilatation; mitral, pulmonary venous, and tissue Doppler evidence of left ventricular diastolic dysfunction with elevated filling pressures; elevated Doppler tricuspid regurgitant peak velocity indicating pulmonary hypertension; the IVC may be dilated
- Other diagnostic tests directed at excluding malignancy and other noncardiac causes of cachexia

DIAGNOSTIC PROCEDURES

- No specific diagnostic procedures

TREATMENT

CARDIOLOGY REFERRAL

- Most patients with chronic CHF should be followed up by a cardiologist

HOSPITALIZATION CRITERIA

- Syncope
- Decompensated CHF
- Severe or symptomatic hypotension

MEDICATIONS

- Traditional heart failure medications
- Fish oil
- Antioxidants (vitamins C and E)
- Anabolic steroids
- Recombinant human growth hormone
- Avoid drugs that worsen anorexia

MONITORING

- Weight
- Fluid and nutritional intake

DIET AND ACTIVITY

Nutritional support (40–50 kcal/m^2 of body surface/hour including 1.5–2 g/kg/hour protein)
- Two-gram dietary sodium restriction
- Exercise training for CHF patients in New York Heart Association (NYHA) functional classes I–III

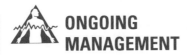 **ONGOING MANAGEMENT**

HOSPITAL DISCHARGE CRITERIA

- Adequate nutritional intake

FOLLOW-UP

- Nutritionist within 1–2 weeks
- Cardiologist within 2–4 weeks
- Primary care physician within 2 weeks

COMPLICATIONS

- Progressive weight loss and debilitation
- Death

PROGNOSIS

- High natural and perioperative morbidity and mortality
- Approximately 50% 18-month mortality rate

PREVENTION

- ACE inhibitor and beta-blocker therapy for CHF appear to help prevent cardiac cachexia

RESOURCES

PRACTICE GUIDELINES

- Cachexia is a common complication of chronic CHF, which is associated with very poor survival
- It can be diagnosed by demonstration of > 6% of previous nonedematous weight over at least 6 months
- No definitive treatment exists, but nutritional supplementation along with moderate exercise for CHF patients with NYHA functional class I–III symptoms are recommended

REFERENCES

- Anker SD et al: Prognostic importance of weight loss in chronic heart failure and the effect of angiotensin-converting enzyme inhibitors: an observational study. Lancet 2003;361:1077.
- Anker SD et al: Cardiac cachexia. Ann Med. 2004;36:518–529.

INFORMATION FOR PATIENTS

- http://www.clevelandclinic.org/health/health-info/docs/1800/1834.asp
- http://www.americanheart.org/presenter.jhtml?identifier=1444

WEB SITES

- http://www.medscape.com/viewarticle/429276?src=search
- http://www.emedicine.com/med/topic3552.htm

Cardiac Contusion/Blunt Trauma

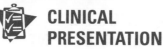 **KEY FEATURES**

ESSENTIALS OF DIAGNOSIS

- Injuries may range from minor myocardial bruise to cardiac rupture
- Chest pain not responding to nitrates may suggest contusion
- There may be evidence of other injuries, such as rib fracture or impression of the steering wheel on the anterior chest wall
- Hemodynamic response to appropriate resuscitative measures is inadequate
- Clinically significant myocardial injury with intact pericardium presents as cardiac tamponade
- When the pericardium is not intact, extrapericardial bleeding causes hypovolemic shock
- Valvular dysfunction secondary to tear or rupture may not cause acute symptoms, but later may present as heart failure
- ECG abnormalities, most commonly nonspecific repolarization changes, consistently accompany contusion
- Cardiac enzymes may be elevated but do not have prognostic value

GENERAL CONSIDERATIONS

- Blunt cardiac trauma most frequently results from motor vehicle accidents
- Significant blunt chest trauma results in cardiac injury in 15% of cases
- Almost any structure in the heart may be injured, but myocardial contusion, valve disruption, and aortic disruption are the most common injuries
- Abnormal ECG is the best predictor of complications
- Hemodynamically stable patients with normal ECG require no additional testing

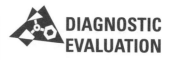 **CLINICAL PRESENTATION**

SYMPTOMS AND SIGNS

- Angina-like pain not responding to nitrates
- Dyspnea

PHYSICAL EXAM FINDINGS

- Evidence of chest wall trauma
- Hypotension, especially if unresponsive to resuscitative measures
- Elevated jugular veins with tamponade
- Pulsus paradoxus with tamponade
- Signs of heart failure
- Hypovolemic shock
- Murmurs of valvular dysfunction, usually regurgitation

DIFFERENTIAL DIAGNOSIS

- ECG changes secondary to coronary artery disease
- Noncardiac intrathoracic trauma
- Cardiac enzyme elevation secondary to noncardiac trauma

DIAGNOSTIC EVALUATION

LABORATORY TESTS

- CBC
- Cardiac biomarkers, such as troponins, creatine kinase MB

ELECTROCARDIOGRAPHY

- Nonspecific repolarization abnormalities
- Sinus tachycardia, atrial tachyarrhythmias, and ventricular premature beats are common

IMAGING STUDIES

- Echocardiography is useful for identifying left ventricular, valvular, or pericardial abnormalities
- Gated equilibrium scintigraphy can identify ventricular wall motion abnormalities and reduced function
  - Especially useful for the right ventricle

DIAGNOSTIC PROCEDURES

- Transesophageal echocardiography is especially useful if great vessel involvement is suspected

TREATMENT

CARDIOLOGY REFERRAL

- Suspected cardiac trauma, such as abnormal ECG
- Unresolved hypotension or shock

HOSPITALIZATION CRITERIA

- Suspected cardiac trauma
- Hypotension/shock
- Heart failure

MEDICATIONS

- Drugs to control heart rate in atrial tachyarrhythmias, such as diltiazem 20 mg IV over 2 minutes, then 5–15 mg/hour IV for 24 hours
- Pharmacologic agents to suppress ventricular arrhythmia
- Appropriate treatment for heart failure
- Fluid resuscitation
- Pressor support if necessary

THERAPEUTIC PROCEDURES

- Pericardiocentesis for patients with cardiac tamponade
- Intra-aortic balloon pump in selected cases, such as acute mitral regurgitation

SURGERY

- Definitive treatment in critical patients: thoracotomy (or sternotomy) and appropriate surgical repair

MONITORING

- Invasive hemodynamic monitoring in hemodynamically unstable patients
- ECG monitoring for patients with minor trauma but abnormal ECG

DIET AND ACTIVITY

- Low-sodium diet for heart failure
- Restricted activities as appropriate for injuries

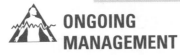

ONGOING MANAGEMENT

HOSPITAL DISCHARGE CRITERIA

- Hemodynamic stability
- Definitive treatment accomplished

FOLLOW-UP

- As appropriate for the injury

COMPLICATIONS

- Sudden death
- Heart failure
- Shock
- Cardiac tamponade
- Arrhythmias

PROGNOSIS

- Myocardial contusion rarely results in significant permanent sequelae
- Other injuries have a prognosis similar to that of naturally occurring disease of the same variety

PREVENTION

- Avoidance of blunt trauma
- Use of protective devices, such as chest protectors, seatbelts, airbags

RESOURCES

PRACTICE GUIDELINES

- Recommended screening of blunt chest trauma patients:
  1. ECG: if abnormal, admit patient for 24–48 hours of observation; if normal, significant cardiac trauma is unlikely and no further evaluation is necessary if hemodynamically stable
  2. Echocardiogram for hemodynamically unstable patient: if abnormal, admit; if normal, consider further diagnostic testing, such as transesophageal echo, CT scan
  3. Cardiac biomarkers confirm myocardial injury, but do not predict outcomes and are not useful for triage
  4. Sternal fracture does not predict cardiac trauma
  5. Delaying necessary emergency surgery for a cardiac evaluation (catheterization, stress testing) is not advisable because most patients do well if properly monitored, which may include a right heart catheter

REFERENCES

- Salim A et al: Clinically significant blunt cardiac trauma: role of serum troponin levels combined with electrocardiographic findings. J Trauma 2001;50:237.
- Sybrandy KC et al: Diagnosing cardiac contusion: old wisdom and new insights. Heart 2003;89:485.

INFORMATION FOR PATIENTS

- www.nlm.nih.gov/medlineplus/ency/article/000202.htm

WEB SITE

- www.emedicine.com/emerg/topic932.htm

Cardiac Syndrome X (Microvascular Angina Pectoris)

KEY FEATURES

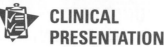

ESSENTIALS OF DIAGNOSIS

- Angina pectoris
- Positive stress test for myocardial ischemia, especially exercise ECG or stress myocardial perfusion abnormalities
- Normal or near-normal epicardial coronary arteries
- Usually occurs in women (75%); many also have neuropsychological symptoms
- No evidence of coronary spasm on ambulatory ECG monitoring or coronary angiography

GENERAL CONSIDERATIONS

- This syndrome is different from metabolic syndrome X
- True ischemia as evidenced by increased myocardial lactate production occurs in some patients
- Many patients have no metabolic evidence of ischemia
- Microvascular dysfunction, altered pain perception, and autonomic imbalance may play a variable role either alone or in combination as the causative mechanism for angina
- This syndrome is more common in women

CLINICAL PRESENTATION

SYMPTOMS AND SIGNS

- Atypical chest pain in most patients
- Classic angina in a minority
- Chest pain possibly severe and disabling
- Angina may occur with exertion or at rest but seldom at night
- Attacks persist for a long time after cessation of exertion
- Poor or worsening response to nitrates

PHYSICAL EXAM FINDINGS

- Positive findings uncommon
- Third heart sound heard in an occasional patient

DIFFERENTIAL DIAGNOSIS

- Variant angina pectoris
- Missed coronary artery lesions because of inadequate angiography
- Other causes of chest pain with a false-positive stress test, such as esophageal dysmotility
- Neuropsychiatric disorder

DIAGNOSTIC EVALUATION

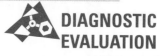

LABORATORY TESTS

- CBC to exclude anemia as an etiology for chest pain
- Metabolic panel
- Lipid panel
- Fasting glucose

ELECTROCARDIOGRAPHY

- ECG may be abnormal
- Holter monitoring may show ST depression even if stress test was negative

IMAGING STUDIES

- Stress echocardiogram and nuclear stress tests may be abnormal

DIAGNOSTIC PROCEDURES

- Coronary angiogram to exclude epicardial lesions or vasospasm

Cardiac Syndrome X (Microvascular Angina Pectoris)

 TREATMENT

CARDIOLOGY REFERRAL

- Patients with angina are referred to cardiologists on most occasions

HOSPITALIZATION CRITERIA

- Persistent severe pain
- Prior to coronary arteriogram

MEDICATIONS

- Reassurance; prognosis is good
- Calcium channel blockers
- Nitrates and beta blockers for selected patients
- Aminophylline for selected patients
- Imipramine for refractory cases
- Spinal cord stimulation in selected cases
- Estrogen in some cases

MONITORING

- Reevaluation during exacerbation

DIET AND ACTIVITY

- Cardiac low-fat diet
- Physical exercise as tolerated

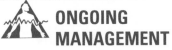 ONGOING MANAGEMENT

HOSPITAL DISCHARGE CRITERIA

- Post-coronary angiogram
- After angiogram findings are known, patients may be managed as outpatients

FOLLOW-UP

- Periodic follow-up during exacerbations or every 6 months

COMPLICATIONS

- None

PROGNOSIS

- Very good
- Survival no different from age-matched general population

PREVENTION

- Avoid smoking
- Risk factor modification

RESOURCES

PRACTICE GUIDELINES

- Prognosis is very good
- Reassurance

REFERENCES

- Crea F, Lanza GA: Angina pectoris and normal coronary arteries: cardiac syndrome X. Heart 2004;90(4):457.

INFORMATION FOR PATIENTS

- www.nhlbi.nih.gov/health/dci/ Diseases/Angina/Angina_WhatIs.html

WEB SITE

- www.americanheart.org

Cardiac Tamponade

KEY FEATURES

ESSENTIALS OF DIAGNOSIS

- Increased jugular venous pressure with an obliterated y descent
- Pulsus paradoxus
- Echocardiographic evidence of right atrial and ventricular collapse
- Equal diastolic pressures in all four cardiac chambers

GENERAL CONSIDERATIONS

- Cardiac tamponade occurs when the intrapericardial pressure exceeds the intracardiac pressures and causes the following:
  - Collapse of the cardiac chamber(s)
  - Impedance of filling of the heart
  - Reduced cardiac output
- The volume of pericardial fluid required to cause tamponade depends on the speed of fluid accumulation
- Severe tamponade may ensue with a modest effusion (as in the setting of trauma) in a brief time
- Low-pressure cardiac tamponade occurs when an effusion that is ordinarily insufficient to cause hemodynamic compromise becomes significant when intravascular volume is depleted
  - This typically occurs in a patient with chronic renal failure during dialysis

CLINICAL PRESENTATION

SYMPTOMS AND SIGNS

- Dyspnea
- Chest discomfort
- Impaired consciousness
- Signs of reduced cardiac output
- Shock may be present

PHYSICAL EXAM FINDINGS

- Hypotension
- Diminished pulse pressure
- Tachycardia until the terminal stages, when bradycardia ensues
- Pulsus paradoxus
- Elevated jugular venous pressure with blunted or obliterated y descent
- Diminished heart sounds
- Rarely, a pericardial rub

DIFFERENTIAL DIAGNOSIS

- Cardiogenic shock
- Severe obstructive airway disease
- Congestive heart failure
- Pulmonary embolus
- Constrictive pericarditis
- Tension pneumothorax

DIAGNOSTIC EVALUATION

LABORATORY TESTS

- Fluid obtained at pericardial drainage should be examined using the following texts:
  - Gram's stain
  - Bacterial cultures
  - Acid-fast bacilli stain and culture
  - Polymerase chain reaction
  - Cytology and carcinoembryonic antigen (CEA)

ELECTROCARDIOGRAPHY

- Low-voltage QRS complex
- Electrical alternans with large effusions

IMAGING STUDIES

- Chest x-ray findings:
  - Enlarged cardiac silhouette
  - Lung fields frequently oligemic
- Echocardiography, an invaluable adjunctive tool:
  - Confirms the presence of pericardial fluid
  - Provides evidence of increased intrapericardial pressure such as diastolic collapse of the right atrium and right ventricle
- Two-dimensional echo is helpful in guiding pericardiocentesis

DIAGNOSTIC PROCEDURES

- Cardiac catheterization findings:
  - Elevated and equal or near-equal diastolic pressures in all four cardiac chambers
  - Loss of the normal y descent in atrial pressure tracings
  - Reduced cardiac output

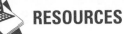

TREATMENT

CARDIOLOGY REFERRAL

- In-hospital emergent referral is indicated in patients with suspected cardiac tamponade for urgent pericardiocentesis

HOSPITALIZATION CRITERIA

- Suspected cardiac tamponade

MEDICATIONS

- Intravenous fluids until drainage can be accomplished

THERAPEUTIC PROCEDURES

- Percutaneous pericardiocentesis of even modest amounts (100–200 mL) of fluid may result in striking improvement
- Drainage is most common in the subxiphoid position, with the patient in the semi-upright position to allow inferior pooling of the effusion
- Leaving a pericardial catheter in place for continuous drainage may be helpful until the rate of drainage decreases or a pericardial window is created
- Echocardiography to guide pericardiocentesis can decrease the incidence of cardiac puncture
- A percutaneous balloon technique for creating a pleuropericardial opening is primarily used in patients with malignant effusions in whom quality of the remaining life is of paramount importance

SURGERY

- In selected cases, surgical drainage is required with creation of a pericardial-to-pleural opening
  - This also permits pericardial biopsy in cases of suspected malignant effusion
- Some conditions may require surgical removal of the pericardium

MONITORING

- Close hemodynamic monitoring is required
- ECG monitoring

DIET AND ACTIVITY

- No dietary restrictions
- Bed rest for patients with tamponade

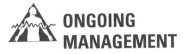

ONGOING MANAGEMENT

HOSPITAL DISCHARGE CRITERIA

- After successful pericardial fluid removal and no significant pericardial fluid re-accumulation as shown by echocardiography
- Stable hemodynamics

FOLLOW-UP

- Repeat echocardiography within 1–2 weeks with periodic echo thereafter as clinically indicated
- Follow-up with cardiologist within 1–2 weeks

COMPLICATIONS

- Right ventricular puncture or laceration with pericardiocentsis
- Pneumothorax
- Intrahepatic hemorrhage
- Re-accumulation of pericardial fluid and tamponade
- Effusive-constrictive pericarditis
- Constrictive pericarditis, sometimes requiring pericardiectomy

PROGNOSIS

- Most patients experience immediate relief or improvements in symptoms after percutaneous or surgical drainage of the pericardial fluid
- Overall prognosis depends on the underlying condition associated with the pericardial disease, if any
- Some patients eventually develop constrictive pericarditis that may require surgical pericardiectomy

RESOURCES

PRACTICE GUIDELINES

- The presence of at least 1 cm of echo-free space anterior to the heart has been recommended as the minimum volume of fluid that should be present before pericardiocentesis is undertaken
- Pericardiocentesis is ideally carried out in the cardiac catheterization lab with fluoroscopic guidance and concomitant right heart catheterization in most circumstances
- Subsequent monitoring with two-dimensional and Doppler echo is warranted to ensure adequate fluid removal, to ascertain re-accumulation of fluid, or to diagnose early constriction

REFERENCES

- Lindenberger M et al: Pericardiocentesis guided by 2-D echocardiography: the method of choice for treatment of pericardial effusion. J Intern Med 2003;253:411.
- Maisch B et al: Guidelines on the diagnosis and management of pericardial diseases, executive summary: the Task Force on the Diagnosis and Management of Pericardial Diseases of the European Society of Cardiology. Eur Heart J 2004;25:587.

INFORMATION FOR PATIENTS

- http://www.nlm.nih.gov/medlineplus/ency/article/000194.htm
- http://www.mayoclinic.com/invoke.cfm?id=AN00438

WEB SITE

- http://www.emedicine.com/med/topic283.htm

Cardiogenic Shock

 KEY FEATURES

ESSENTIALS OF DIAGNOSIS

- Tissue hypoperfusion: depressed mental status, cool extremities, urine output < 30 mL/hour
- Hypotension: systolic blood pressure < 80 mm Hg
- Cardiac index < 2.2 L/min/m^2
- Pulmonary artery wedge pressure > 18 mm Hg

GENERAL CONSIDERATIONS

- Causes and contributors: right or left ventricular failure, mechanical complications of acute myocardial infarction (MI; ventricular septal rupture, papillary muscle rupture or dysfunction, and myocardial rupture), hypovolemia, valve disease, arrhythmias, and abnormalities of diastolic filling
- Shock resulting from an acute MI typically involves ≥40% of the myocardium
- More than two-thirds of patients dying of cardiogenic shock have severe three-vessel coronary artery disease

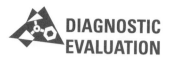 **CLINICAL PRESENTATION**

SYMPTOMS AND SIGNS

- History of chest pain associated with myocardial infarction within hours or up to a week
- Cardiac arrest associated with an acute MI
- Shortness of breath or acute respiratory distress
- Syncope
- Palpitations
- Nausea, vomiting
- Diaphoresis
- Obtundation and lethargy

PHYSICAL EXAM FINDINGS

- Systolic blood pressure < 80 mm Hg or < 90 mm Hg on pressors
- Tachycardia
- Tachypnea
- Pulmonary rales
- Jugular venous distention
- Displaced and diffuse apical impulse
- Muffled heart sounds in the presence of a pericardial effusion or cardiac tamponade
- S$_3$ and S$_4$
- Short, slight systolic murmur in patients with acute, severe mitral regurgitation
  - Systolic murmur and associated parasternal thrill may indicate a ventricular septal rupture
- Hepatomegaly; pulsatile liver with severe tricuspid regurgitation
- Ascites in cases of longstanding right heart failure
- Peripheral edema
- Peripheral pulses are rapid and faint
- Mottled extremities
- Cool, ashen, or cyanotic skin

DIFFERENTIAL DIAGNOSIS

- Septic shock
- Hypovolemia

DIAGNOSTIC EVALUATION

LABORATORY TESTS

- Troponin, creatine kinase
- Electrolytes, blood urea nitrogen, creatinine, and serum lactate
- CBC
- Bilirubin, alanine transaminase, aspartate transaminase, lactate dehydrogenase, partial thromboplastin time, prothrombin time
- Arterial blood gases

ELECTROCARDIOGRAPHY

- Sinus tachycardia or atrial tachyarrhythmias
- Q waves may indicate prior myocardial infarction
- ST and T waves suggestive of an acute MI

IMAGING STUDIES

- Chest x-ray:
  - Cardiomegaly and pulmonary vascular congestion or edema
  - Heart size may be normal in patients with a first infarction
  - Pulmonary congestion may be less prominent or absent in patients with predominant right ventricular failure or hypovolemia
- Echocardiography:
  - Provides assessment of left and right ventricular size and function, global and segmental wall motion, valvular function (stenosis or regurgitation), right ventricular systolic pressures, detection of ventricular septal shunts and pericardial fluid

DIAGNOSTIC PROCEDURES

- Right heart catheterization: (generally useful to exclude other causes of shock and monitor therapy); hemodynamic indicators of cardiogenic shock are: pulmonary capillary wedge pressure > 15 mm Hg and a cardiac index < 2.2 L/min/m^2
- Coronary angiography: to assess the anatomy of the coronary arteries and need for urgent revascularization

TREATMENT

CARDIOLOGY REFERRAL

- Urgent cardiology referral for patients with suspected or confirmed cardiogenic shock, especially with evidence of myocardial ischemia or MI

HOSPITALIZATION CRITERIA

- All patients should be hospitalized in the critical care unit

MEDICATIONS

Intubation, ventilation, and oxygen supplementation

Swan-Ganz catheter:

- Pulmonary wedge pressure < 18 mm Hg: administer fluids
- Pulmonary wedge pressure > 18 mm Hg: administer inotropic agents

Inotropic and vasoactive agents:

- Dopamine 5–10 μg/kg/min IV
- Dobutamine: 2–20 μg/kg/min IV if systolic blood pressure > 80 mm Hg *or*
- Milrinone: load with 50 μg/kg IV over 10 minutes, then 0.375–0.75 μ/kg/min if SPB is >80 mm Hg
- Norepinephrine (if needed for pressor support): 0.2–1.5 μ/kg/min
- Nitroprusside (if needed for afterload reduction): 0.25–10 μg/kg/min

THERAPEUTIC PROCEDURES

- Intra-aortic balloon pump to stabilize for coronary intervention
- A percutaneous left ventricular assist device
- Percutaneous coronary revascularization in patients with MI

SURGERY

- Emergent coronary artery bypass graft surgery for patients with multivessel or left main disease to improve survival
- Valve repair for patients with severe ischemic mitral regurgitation

MONITORING

- Intensive monitoring in the critical care unit for all patients
- Fluid and nutritional support as appropriate

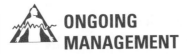

ONGOING MANAGEMENT

HOSPITAL DISCHARGE CRITERIA

- After successful medical therapy and revascularization
- Stable vital signs and evidence of adequate organ perfusion

FOLLOW-UP

- Cardiology follow-up within 2 weeks of discharge
- Follow-up cardiac imaging studies to be determined by the cardiologist on an individual basis

COMPLICATIONS

- Mortality rate is high
- Vascular complications from percutaneous catheters
- Infections
- Sternal wound complications in patients who undergo cardiac surgery
- Stroke

PROGNOSIS

- Over 70% mortality rate in patients with acute MI and cardiogenic shock who are medically treated
- Forty-to-sixty percent mortality rate with aggressive, prompt supportive therapy, including intra-aortic balloon pump insertion and coronary artery revascularization in patients with MI
- Patients > 75 years with myocardial ischemia or MI and cardiogenic shock do not appear to benefit from coronary revascularization

PREVENTION

- Primary and secondary prevention against MI and aggressive treatment of any cardiomyopathic process may help reduce the incidence of cardiogenic shock

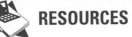

RESOURCES

PRACTICE GUIDELINES

- Patients who develop cardiogenic shock should be transferred immediately to an institution with capabilities of invasive monitoring, coronary revascularization, and skilled personnel who can provide expert care
- Intra-aortic balloon pump insertion may be a useful adjunct to thrombolysis for initial stabilization and transfer of patients to a tertiary care facility
- Revascularization is the only definite therapy shown to decrease mortality in patients who develop cardiogenic shock after an MI, except in the elderly

REFERENCES

- Hasdai D et al: Cardiogenic shock complicating acute coronary syndromes. Lancet 2000;356:749.
- Webb JG: Percutaneous coronary intervention for cardiogenic shock in the SHOCK trial. J Am Coll Cardiol 2003;42:1380.

INFORMATION FOR PATIENTS

- http://www.nlm.nih.gov/medlineplus/ency/article/000185.htm

WEB SITE

- http://www.emedicine.com/med/topic285.htm

Cardiomyopathy, Alcoholic

KEY FEATURES

ESSENTIALS OF DIAGNOSIS

- Heavy, chronic alcohol consumption: 80 g/day for 10 years or more
- Symptoms and signs of biventricular congestive heart failure
- Proximal myopathy common
- Regression of cardiomegaly with alcohol cessation

GENERAL CONSIDERATIONS

- Mechanism of alcohol-induced cardiac damage remains unclear but is likely a direct toxic result of ethanol and/or its metabolites (eg, acetaldehyde and fatty acid ethyl esters)
- Higher prevalence among males than females (due to a higher rate of alcohol abuse in men), but females appear more sensitive to alcohol's cardiotoxic affects
- May be the cause of up to one-third of cases of dilated cardiomyopathy
- Light to moderate alcohol consumption (ie, 1–2 drinks per day or 3–9 drinks per week) decreases the risk of myocardial infarction

CLINICAL PRESENTATION

SYMPTOMS AND SIGNS

- A person of at least middle age (less common in people < 40 years)
- Dyspnea, orthopnea, and paroxysmal nocturnal dyspnea
- Fatigue
- Palpitations
- Chest discomfort
- Dizziness, syncope
- Anorexia

PHYSICAL EXAM FINDINGS

- Generalized cachexia
- Reduced pulse pressure
- Pulmonary rales
- Tachycardia
- Laterally displaced, diffuse point of maximal impulse
- Holosystolic murmurs of mitral and tricuspid regurgitation
- S_3 and S_4
- Elevated jugular venous pressure
- Hepatomegaly
- Peripheral edema
- Cool extremities
- Muscle atrophy and weakness

DIFFERENTIAL DIAGNOSIS

- Certain heavy metals (cobalt, lead, iron) found in illegally produced alcoholic beverages
- Metabolic disturbances in alcoholics: hypermagnesemia, hypokalemia, selenium deficiency, thiamine deficiency
- Hypertensive heart disease common in alcoholics
- Other causes of cardiomyopathy

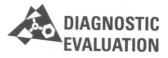 DIAGNOSTIC EVALUATION

ELECTROCARDIOGRAPHY

- Premature atrial or ventricular contractions
- Supraventricular tachycardia
- First- or second-degree atrioventricular block
- Left or right bundle branch block
- Voltage criteria for left ventricular hypertrophy
- Prolonged QT interval
- Nonspecific ST- and T-wave changes
- Abnormal Q waves also possible

IMAGING STUDIES

- Chest x-ray:
  - Enlarged cardiac silhouette
  - Pulmonary vascular congestion
  - Pleural effusions
- Echocardiogram:
  - Four-chamber cardiac enlargement with reduced left and right ventricular systolic function in a global pattern
  - Doppler evidence of left ventricular diastolic dysfunction, left ventricular hypertrophy, and intracardiac thrombi in the atria or ventricles
- Stress nuclear imaging of echo imaging can screen for coronary artery disease

DIAGNOSTIC PROCEDURES

- Cardic catheterization: not always necessary, but may be useful to exclude other causes of heart failure

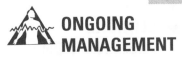

 TREATMENT

CARDIOLOGY REFERRAL

- Suspected alcoholic cardiomyopathy
- Congestive heart failure

HOSPITALIZATION CRITERIA

- Decompensated congestive heart failure
- Tachyarrhythmias
- Syncope

MEDICATIONS

- Cessation of alcohol consumption
- Correction of metabolic and nutritional deficiencies (thiamine, vitamin B_{12}, folate)
- Treatment of hypertension if present
- Vasodilators (angiotensin-converting enzyme-inhibitor, angiotensin receptor blocker, nitrates, hydralazine)
- Loop diuretics
- IV inotropic agents if necessary acutely
- Beta blockers once heart failure is compensated
- Spironolactone or eplerenone for patients with severe heart failure
- Anticoagulation for atrial fibrillation or flutter

THERAPEUTIC PROCEDURES

- No specific therapeutic procedures

SURGERY

- Cardiac transplantation may be an option for some patients with end-stage cardiomyopathy who can demonstrate abstinence from alcohol

MONITORING

- ECG monitoring during hospitalization
- Fluid balance

DIET AND ACTIVITY

- Abstinence from alcohol
- Fluid- and sodium-restricted diet
- No activity restrictions

ONGOING MANAGEMENT

HOSPITAL DISCHARGE CRITERIA

- Stable cardiac rhythm
- Compensated heart failure

FOLLOW-UP

- Cardiologist within 2–4 weeks of hospital discharge
- Serial echocardiography may demonstrate progressive improvement and even normalization of cardiac function in patients who remain abstinent from alcohol

COMPLICATIONS

- Progressive heart failure
- Arrhythmias
- Stroke, presumably embolic in origin

PROGNOSIS

- Approximately 50% of patients continue to deteriorate, 25% improve, and 25% remain stable
- Survival rates are the same or better than patients with idiopathic dilated cardiomyopathy

PREVENTION

- Abstinence from alcohol

RESOURCES

PRACTICE GUIDELINES

- Complete alcohol intake history should be obtained from every patient with heart failure
- Other than abstinence from alcohol, treatment is the same as for other forms of dilated cardiomyopathy
- Cardiac transplantation remains an option for patients who continue to deteriorate despite medical therapy and who demonstrate continued abstinence from alcohol

REFERENCES

- Lee WK: Alcoholic cardiomyopathy: is it dose-dependent?. Congest Heart Fail. 2002;8:303.
- Nicolas JM et al: The effect of controlled drinking in alcoholic cardiomyopathy. Ann Intern Med 2002;16:192.
- Piano MR: Alcoholic cardiomyopathy: incidence, clinical characteristics, and pathophysiology. Chest. 2002;121:1638.

INFORMATION FOR PATIENTS

- http://www.nlm.nih.gov/medlineplus/ency/article/000174.htm
- http://www.heartcenteronline.com/myheartdr/common/articles.cfm?ARTID=428

WEB SITE

- http://www.emedicine.com/med/topic286.htm

Cardiomyopathy, Hypertrophic

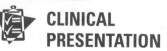

KEY FEATURES

ESSENTIALS OF DIAGNOSIS

- Dyspnea
- Systolic ejection murmur with characteristic changes during bedside maneuvers
- Markedly asymmetric left ventricular hypertrophy on echocardiogram
- Normal or hyperkinetic left ventricular systolic function

GENERAL CONSIDERATIONS

- Hypertrophic cardiomyopathy is an autosomnal genetic disorder caused by abnormalities in the genes that encode myocardial sarcomeric proteins
- The clinical manifestations of the disease vary from asymptomatic carriers to severely disabled patients
- The corresponding genetic abnormalities are also heterogeneous
- Two thirds of affected individuals have asymmetric hypertrophy often involving the intraventricular system but occasionally limited to the apex of the left ventricle
- One third of those affected have diffuse concentric hypertrophy
- Microscopically, the affected myocardium shows myofiber disarray with undersized intramural arteries for the mass of myocardium
- The left ventricle cavity is usually small and shows hyperdynamic function
- Patients with symmetric hypertrophy may demonstrate intracavitary gradients that worsen with increased contractile stimuli and improve with increased afterload
- Asymmetric septal hypertrophy often results in systolic anterior motion of the anterior mitral valve leaflet, which narrows the left ventricular outflow tract, producing a gradient and a characteristic systolic murmur that varies in intensity with loading conditions
- Systolic anterior movement of the mitral valve often leads to mitral regurgitation

CLINICAL PRESENTATION

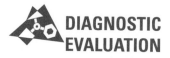

SYMPTOMS AND SIGNS

- May be asymptomatic
- Dyspnea, fatigue
- Chest pain
- Syncope
- Palpitation

PHYSICAL EXAM FINDINGS

- May be unremarkable
- Left ventricle lift; may be bifid
- S_4
- Systolic ejection murmur that increases in intensity with maneuvers that decrease left ventricular filling, such as standing; and softens with increased filling, such as squatting

DIFFERENTIAL DIAGNOSIS

- Left ventricular hypertrophy secondary to other conditions (eg, hypertension)
- Aortic stenosis with marked left ventricular hypertrophy
- Restrictive cardiomyopathy with hypertrophy, such as amyloidosis
- Ischemic heart disease with compensatory septal hypertrophy
- Athlete's heart

DIAGNOSTIC EVALUATION

LABORATORY TESTS

- Elevated brain natriuretic peptide
- Appropriate genetic abnormality

ELECTROCARDIOGRAPHY

- Almost all patients have an abnormal ECG, but the patterns are nonspecific
- Voltage criteria for left ventricular hypertrophy with repolarization abnormalities are common
- Some patients have giant negative T waves in the precordium, especially the apical variant

IMAGING STUDIES

- Echocardiography:
  - Shows the hypertrophy
  - Demonstrates any mitral valve motion abnormalities
  - Doppler detects any intracavitary gradients, mitral regurgitation, and diastolic dysfunction
- Radionuclide perfusion imaging: may show areas of fixed and reversible tracer uptake deficits in the absence of epicardial coronary artery disease

DIAGNOSTIC PROCEDURES

- Cardiac catheterization for diagnosing hypertrophic cardiomyopathy has been supplanted by echocardiography
- Coronary angiography may be necessary to exclude epicardial coronary artery disease
- Exercise testing may demonstrate exercise induced hypotension

TREATMENT

CARDIOLOGY REFERRAL

- Suspected hypertrophic cardiomyopathy
- Exercise hypotension
- Syncope

HOSPITALIZATION CRITERIA

- Significant arrhythmias
- Syncope
- Heart failure

MEDICATIONS

- Beta blockers, calcium channel blockers, and antiarrhythmic agents as appropriate

THERAPEUTIC PROCEDURES

- Intracoronary ethanol septal ablation
- Pacemaker to set atrioventricular delay to minimize left ventricular outflow tract gradient
- Automatic implantable cardioverter-defibrillator

SURGERY

- Septal myectomy to relieve left ventricular outflow tract obstruction
- Mitral valve replacement in selected cases

MONITORING

- ECG as appropriate in hospital
- Ambulatory ECG in outpatients with suspected arrhythmias

DIET AND ACTIVITY

- Avoid dehydration

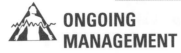

ONGOING MANAGEMENT

HOSPITAL DISCHARGE CRITERIA

- Resolution of problem
- Successful procedure or surgery

FOLLOW-UP

- Three months, then every 6 months

COMPLICATIONS

- Sudden cardiac death
- Atrial fibrillation
- Heart failure
- Infective endocarditis

PROGNOSIS

- The risk of sudden death is 1–4% annually
- Risk predictors:
  - The younger the disease presents
  - Ventricular arrhythmias or syncope
  - Family history of sudden death
  - Marked left ventricular hypertrophy
  - Hypotension with exercise

PREVENTION

- Genetic counseling
- Endocarditis prophylaxis

RESOURCES

PRACTICE GUIDELINES

- The major indication for treatment is the presence of symptoms
- The only potential prophylactic therapy to prolong life is an implantable cardioverter-defibrillator. Patients with several high-risk features (?) should be considered for this therapy

REFERENCE

- Elliott PM et al: Relation between severity of left-ventricular hypertrophy and prognosis in patients with hypertrophic cardiomyopathy. Lancet 2001;357:420.

INFORMATION FOR PATIENTS

- www.drpen.com/425.1

WEB SITE

- www.emedicine.com/med/topic290.htm

Cardiomyopathy, Idiopathic Dilated

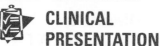 KEY FEATURES

ESSENTIALS OF DIAGNOSIS

- Dilatation of both ventricles with diffusely reduced contractile function
- No identifiable cause of the cardiomyopathy

GENERAL CONSIDERATIONS

- Estimated prevalence rate is 0.04%
- Disease is three times more common in blacks and males as in whites and females
- Familial linkage is common and may be close to 20%
- Affects patients of any age
- Some patients may have had an undetected viral myocarditis

CLINICAL PRESENTATION

SYMPTOMS AND SIGNS

- Decreased exercise tolerance
- Dyspnea
- Orthopnea
- Paroxysmal nocturnal dyspnea
- Fatigue
- Palpitations
- Presyncope or syncope

PHYSICAL EXAM FINDINGS

- Tachycardia
- Tachypnea
- Jugular venous distention may be present
- Pulmonary rales
- Laterally displaced and diffuse point of maximal impulse; left and right ventricular lifts
- Soft S_1, paradoxically split S_2 with a left bundle branch block
- S_3 and S_4 gallops
- Hepatomegaly due to elevated venous pressures; the liver may be pulsatile with severe tricuspid regurgitation
- Ascites, peripheral edema
- Muscle wasting or other signs of cardiac cachexia

DIFFERENTIAL DIAGNOSIS

- Ischemic cardiomyopathy
- Valvular heart disease
- Hypertensive heart disease
- Alcoholic cardiomyopathy
- Cardiomyopathy related to thyroid dysfunction
- HIV cardiomyopathy

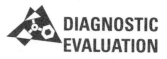 DIAGNOSTIC EVALUATION

LABORATORY TESTS

- Electrolytes, blood urea nitrogen, and creatinine
- CBC
- Liver function tests: elevations may be due to hepatic congestion
- Cardiac enzymes: to exclude acute or recent myocardial injury (elevated CKMB levels may be seen in persons with muscular dystrophy)
- Thyroid function tests
- Urine pregnancy test: in women of childbearing age
- Urine toxicology screen

ELECTROCARDIOGRAPHY

- Supraventricular tachycardia
- Premature ventricular complexes
- Nonspecific ST- and T-wave changes
- Left ventricular hypertrophy or biventricular hypertrophy
- Left bundle branch block common
- Varying degrees of atrioventricular block may be present

IMAGING STUDIES

- Chest x-ray:
  - Enlarged cardiac silhouette
  - Pulmonary vascular congestion
  - Pleural effusions
- Echocardiography:
  - All four cardiac chambers are typically enlarged, and ventricular contractile function is reduced
  - Varying degrees of mitral and tricuspid regurgitation due to annular dilatation

DIAGNOSTIC PROCEDURES

- Noninvasive stress testing with nuclear imaging: can screen for coronary artery disease
- Left heart catheterization with coronary angiography: typically performed to exclude coronary artery disease
- Endomyocardial biopsy: not routinely indicated except for suspected cardiac amyloidosis in patients considered for heart transplantation

TREATMENT

CARDIOLOGY REFERRAL

- Any patient with symptomatic or asymptomatic ventricular dysfunction

HOSPITALIZATION CRITERIA

- Decompensated heart failure
- Atrial fibrillation with rapid ventricular response
- Syncope
- Cardiac arrest

MEDICATIONS

- Angiotensin-converting enzyme (ACE) inhibitors or angiotensin receptor blockers
- Beta blockers
- Diuretics and digoxin for symptomatic relief
- Spironolactone 25 mg/day PO for advanced heart failure

THERAPEUTIC PROCEDURES

- Implantable cardioverter-defibrillator and/or cardiac resynchronization therapy (biventricular pacemaker) in patients meeting criteria

SURGERY

- Left and right ventricular assist devices may be used as a bridge to cardiac transplantation or as destination therapy in some who are not candidates for heart transplantation
- Cardiac transplantation in patients with severe progressive disease despite optimal therapy

MONITORING

- ECG monitoring in the hospital
- Fluid balance

DIET AND ACTIVITY

- Low-sodium, fluid-restricted diet
- Mild to moderate regular exercise is encouraged; cardiac rehabilitation has been shown to improve patient outcomes
- Low-potassium diet for patients with hyperkalemia due to ACE inhibitor therapy

ONGOING MANAGEMENT

HOSPITAL DISCHARGE CRITERIA

- After medical stabilization and optimization of heart failure medications
- After successful implantation of a cardiac defibrillator and/or biventricular pacemaker device

FOLLOW-UP

- Every 3 months or more, depending on severity of disease
- Appropriate follow-up with an electrophysiologist as needed
- Serial echocardiography not indicated unless there has been a change in the patient's clinical status

COMPLICATIONS

- Progressive heart failure
- Arrhythmias
- Sudden death
- Complications of device implantation: perforation with myocardial rupture and cardiac tamponade, infection, and bleeding

PROGNOSIS

- Depends on severity of symptoms
  - Generally, approximately 50–80% 5-year survival rate
  - Patients with advanced disease have ≤50% 1-year survival rate
- Approximately 10% of patients have spontaneous improvement and normalization of cardiac function
- Cardiopulmonary exercise testing to determine when to list a patient for cardiac transplantation
  - Peak oxygen consumption of < 14 mL/kg/min signifies a poor prognosis and is generally used as the cut-off for listing a patient

PREVENTION

- Avoidance of all known cardiotoxic agents and treatment of any underlying condition that has been associated with dilated cardiomyopathy

RESOURCES

PRACTICE GUIDELINES

- Patients with NYHA class III–IV symptoms and intraventricular conduction delay should be considered for cardiac resynchronization therapy
- Patients with left ventricular ejection fraction ≤ 35% should be considered for an implantable cardioverter-defibrillator device
- Patients with NYHA class III or IV symptoms despite optimal medical management should be referred for possible cardiac transplantation

REFERENCE

- Cooper LT Jr, Gersh BJ: Viral infection, inflammation, and the risk of idiopathic dilated cardiomyopathy: can the fire be extinguished? Am J Cardiol 2002;90:751.

INFORMATION FOR PATIENTS

- http://www.nlm.nih.gov/medlineplus/ency/article/000190.htm

WEB SITE

- http://www.emedicine.com/med/topic289.htm

Cardiomyopathy, Peripartum

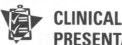 KEY FEATURES

ESSENTIALS OF DIAGNOSIS

- Development of heart failure during the last month of pregnancy or within 5 months of delivery
- Absence of other causes of cardiomyopathy
- No history of heart disease
- Reduced left ventricular systolic function on cardiac imaging

GENERAL CONSIDERATIONS

- No identifiable cause, but risk factors may include preeclampsia and selenium deficiency
- More common in multiparous women
- Affects women of any age
- More common in African-American women

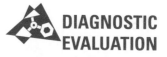 CLINICAL PRESENTATION

SYMPTOMS AND SIGNS

- Symptoms may be difficult to differentiate from those of normal pregnancy
- Dyspnea
- Dizziness
- Fatigue
- Orthopnea
- Reduced exercise capacity
- Cough
- Palpitations
- Hemoptysis
- Chest pain
- Abdominal pain

PHYSICAL EXAM FINDINGS

- Tachypnea
- Tachycardia
- Elevated jugular venous pressure
- Pulmonary rales
- Diffuse, sustained apical impulse
- Murmurs of tricuspid and mitral regurgitation
- S_3 gallop
- Accentuated P_2
- Hepatomegaly
- Abdominal ascites
- Peripheral edema

DIFFERENTIAL DIAGNOSIS

- Heart failure due to other causes
- Pulmonary embolus
- Aortic dissection with coronary artery compromise or cardiac tamponade

DIAGNOSTIC EVALUATION

LABORATORY TESTS

- Tests to exclude preeclampsia (CBC, liver enzymes, urinalysis for proteinuria)
- Electrolytes, blood urea nitrogen, creatinine
- Thyroid function tests
- Serologic tests to exclude myocarditis (viral, HIV, rickettsial infection, syphilis, Chagas' disease, diphtheria toxin) in suspected cases
- Serologic tests to exclude collagen vascular disease when indicated
- Urine toxicology to exclude cocaine and ethanol
- Urine metanephrines to exclude pheochromocytoma in suspected cases

ELECTROCARDIOGRAPHY

- Sinus tachycardia
- Atrial fibrillation (rare)
- Low-voltage QRS
- Left ventricular hypertrophy
- Nonspecific ST- and T-wave abnormalities

IMAGING STUDIES

- Chest x-ray:
  - Findings include cardiomegaly, pulmonary vascular congestion, pleural effusions
- Echocardiography findings include:
  - Abnormal enlargement of the left and sometimes the right ventricle
  - Reduced systolic ventricular function of varying degrees in a global pattern
  - Valvular regurgitation common
  - Elevated continuous-wave Doppler tricuspid regurgitant velocity indicating elevated pulmonary artery systolic pressure

DIAGNOSTIC PROCEDURES

- Stress echocardiography: test of choice during pregnancy for patients with suspected coronary artery disease

TREATMENT

CARDIOLOGY REFERRAL

- Reduced left ventricular function
- Congestive heart failure
- Tachyarrhythmias

HOSPITALIZATION CRITERIA

- Congestive heart failure
- Syncope
- Arrhythmia
- Labor and delivery

MEDICATIONS

- Angiotensin-converting enzyme (ACE) inhibitors and angiotensin receptor blockers (ARBs) are contraindicated prepartum, but should be used postpartum
- Hydralazine and nitrates during
- Digoxin
- Loop diuretics
- Anticoagulants are indicated because of the high risk of thromboemboli and should be continued until left ventricular function improves
- Beta blockers (carvedilol) or metoprolol) should be used postpartum
- Intravenous inotropes when clinically indicated

THERAPEUTIC PROCEDURES

- Intra-aortic balloon pump when indicated
- Left ventricular assist devices should be considered for progressive or severe cases despite medical therapy

SURGERY

- Cardiac transplantation may be needed

MONITORING

- Telemetry during hospitalization
- Vital signs
- Fluid balance
- Pulse oximetry

DIET AND ACTIVITY

- Activity as tolerated (strict bedrest may increase risk of thrombosis)

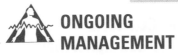

ONGOING MANAGEMENT

HOSPITAL DISCHARGE CRITERIA

- Compensated heart failure
- Stable vital signs
- Stable cardiac rhythm

FOLLOW-UP

- Cardiologist within 2 weeks
- ACE inhibitors should replace nitrate and hydralazine postpartum
- Echocardiography in 2 months and again within the year for persistent left ventricular dysfunction; thereafter depends on the clinical situation

COMPLICATIONS

- Progressive heart failure
- Arrhythmias
- Thromboembolic events
- Fetal distress due to maternal hypoxia or placental perfusion

PROGNOSIS

- Best prognosis among all causes of dilated cardiomyopathy
- Variable prognosis that depends on recovery of ventricular function
- Fifty percent of deaths occur in the first 3 postpartum months
- Thirty percent have normalization of ventricular function within 6 months
- Fifty percent have improvement in symptoms and ventricular function
- Dobutamine-induced contractile reserve during stress echocardiography at presentation may predict patients with subsequent recovery of ventricular function on follow-up

PREVENTION

- Avoidance of pregnancy reduces the risk of recurrent of left ventricular dysfunction

RESOURCES

PRACTICE GUIDELINES

- Patients with persistent ventricular dysfunction should be treated with standard heart failure therapy
- Morbidity and mortality rates with subsequent pregnancies are high for patients with persistent ventricular dysfunction; pregnancies should be avoided
- Patients with normalization of ventricular function have an excellent prognosis
- Dobutamine stress echocardiography should be considered before subsequent pregnancies in patients with normalized ventricular function; those with reduced contractile reserve may not tolerate the hemodynamic stressors of pregnancy

REFERENCES

- Dorbala S et al: Risk stratification of women with peripartum cardiomyopathy at initial presentation: a dobutamine stress echocardiography study. J Am Soc Echocardiogr 2005;18:45.
- Elkayam U et al: Maternal and Fetal Outcomes of subsequent pregnancies in women with peripartum cardiomyopathy. N Engl J Med 2001;344:1567.
- Elkayam U et al: Pregnancy-associated cardiomyopathy: clinical characteristics and a comparison between early and late presentation. Circulation 2005;111:2050.

INFORMATION FOR PATIENTS

- http://www.americanheart.org/presenter.jhtml?identifier=4468
- http://www.heartcenteronline.com/myheartdr/common/artprn_rev.cfm?filename=&ARTID=428

WEB SITE

- http://www.emedicine.com/med/topic292.htm

Cardiomyopathy, Restrictive

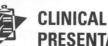 **KEY FEATURES**

ESSENTIALS OF DIAGNOSIS

- Symptoms and signs of heart failure with predominantly right-sided findings
- Normal left and right ventricular size and systolic function with dilated atria
- Abnormalities of diastolic ventricular function suggestive of reduced ventricular compliance
- Increased ventricular filling pressure (left > right) and reduced cardiac output

GENERAL CONSIDERATIONS

- Rare disease of the myocardium accounting for approximately 5% of all cases of primary cardiomyopathies
- Causes include: idiopathic, endomyocardial fibrosis, eosinophilic endomyocarditis, infiltrative processes (eg, amyloidosis, hemochromatosis, sarcoidosis, glycogen storage disease), metastatic malignancy, carcinoid heart disease, mediastinal radiation, and following heart transplantation
- Disease course varies depending on the pathology
- Important to distinguish from constrictive pericarditis, which may have similar clinical and hemodynamic findings
- Pathophysiology involves abnormal myocardial stiffness leading to a precipitous rise in ventricular diastolic filling pressures with a reduction in left ventricular filling volume and cardiac output

CLINICAL PRESENTATION

SYMPTOMS AND SIGNS

- Gradually progressive dyspnea and exercise intolerance
- Fatigue and weakness
- Chest pain
- Palpitations
- Dizziness and syncope
- Increasing abdominal girth (ascites)
- One third of patients may present with thromboembolic events

PHYSICAL EXAM FINDINGS

- Reduced pulse pressure
- Tachycardia
- Increased jugular venous pressure with rapid X and Y descents
- Kussmaul sign in the jugular venous pulse (increase with inspiration)
- Loud S_3
- Murmurs of mitral and tricuspid regurgitation may be present
- Evidence of abdominal ascites
- Liver may be palpable and pulsatile
- Peripheral edema
- Decreased breath sounds due to pleural effusions
- Pulmonary rales may be heard

DIFFERENTIAL DIAGNOSIS

- Dilated cardiomyopathy with restrictive physiology
- Hypertrophic cardiomyopathy
- Constrictive pericarditis

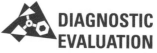 **DIAGNOSTIC EVALUATION**

LABORATORY TESTS

- Complete blood count with peripheral smear: to rule out eosinophilia
- Serum iron concentrations, percent saturation of total iron binding capacity, and serum ferritin levels to exclude hemochromatosis
- Serum protein electrophoresis and serum and urine immunofixation to exclude light-chain deposition disease

ELECTROCARDIOGRAPHY

- Sinus rhythm, sinus tachycardia, or atrial arrhythmias may be present
- Varying degrees of atrioventricular block may be present
- Low QRS voltage
- Nonspecific ST-segment and T-wave abnormalities

IMAGING STUDIES

- Chest x-ray:
  - Increased cardiothoracic ratio due to dilated atria with normal ventricular size
  - Increased pulmonary vasculature and interstitial edema with Kerley B lines
  - Pleural effusions may be present
- Two-dimensional echocardiography findings:
  - Normally contracting right and left ventricles with normal or increased (infiltrative diseases) wall thickness with normal or reduced ventricular cavity size
  - Markedly dilated left and right atria
  - A ventricular mural thrombus may be present
  - Color Doppler evidence of mitral, tricuspid, or pulmonic valve regurgitation may be present
  - Mitral inflow, pulmonary venous, and tissue Doppler evidence of restrictive diastolic filling pattern

DIAGNOSTIC PROCEDURES

- Right and left heart catheterization:
  - Elevated right atrial, left and right ventricular diastolic, and pulmonary artery pressures

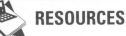

Cardiomyopathy, Restrictive

– Rapid X and Y descents in the right atrial pressure tracing ("dip-plateau" or "square-root" contour of the ventricular diastolic pressures with the left ventricular diastolic pressure being ≥ 5 mm Hg more than the right ventricular filling pressures)

– Right ventricular end diastolic pressure less than one third the right ventricular systolic pressure, right ventricular systolic pressure > 50 mm Hg

• Contrast left ventriculography: may show a small, thick-walled cavity in eosinophilic endomyocardial disease that may be distorted by a mural thrombus

• Endomyocardial biopsy: may be useful to establish the diagnosis in cases of endomyocardial or infiltrative disease where noninvasive studies have failed to establish a clear-cut diagnosis

• Cardiac MRI may demonstrate significant cardiac iron infiltration in patients with hemochromatosis

TREATMENT

CARDIOLOGY REFERRAL

• Congestive heart failure
• Arrhythmias
• High-risk patients suspected of having an infiltrative myocardial process

HOSPITALIZATION CRITERIA

• Decompensated congestive heart failure
• Tachy- or bradyarrhythmias
• Syncope

MEDICATIONS

• Low-dose loop diuretics and nitrates to lower the ventricular preload
• Maintenance of sinus rhythm to preserve atrial contribution to left ventricular filling
• Rate control, if atrial fibrillation persists, to provide adequate time for left ventricular filling
• Management of ventricular tachyarrhythmias
• Anticoagulation for those with atrial fibrillation and endocardial fibrosis
• Treatment of the underlying systemic disease

THERAPEUTIC PROCEDURES

• Pacing for extreme bradycardia or conduction block

SURGERY

• Cardiac transplantation may be considered for some patients with severe, refractory heart failure, depending on the underlying systemic disease
• Surgical resection of endocardial fibrosis in selected cases

MONITORING

• ECG monitoring during hospitalization
• Fluid balance

DIET AND ACTIVITY

• Two-gram dietary sodium restriction
• Activity as tolerated

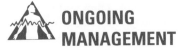

ONGOING MANAGEMENT

HOSPITAL DISCHARGE CRITERIA

• Compensated heart failure
• Stable cardiac rhythm and vital signs

FOLLOW-UP

• Cardiologist within 2 weeks of hospital discharge
• Follow-up cardiac imaging studies, depending on the clinical course

COMPLICATIONS

• Progressive heart failure
• Atrial and ventricular tachyarrhythmias
• Heart block
• Sudden death
• Thromboembolic events
• Syncope

PROGNOSIS

• Largely depends on the underlying pathology
• Survival is limited for most patients

PREVENTION

• Treatment of systemic diseases may help prevent myocardial deposition and the development of infiltrative restrictive cardiomyopathy

RESOURCES

PRACTICE GUIDELINES

• Restrictive cardiomyopathy should be considered in patients with signs and symptoms of progressive congestive heart failure and preserved ventricular systolic function
• The clinical and hemodynamic findings of restrictive cardiomyopathy and pericardial constriction are often similar
• Hemodynamic findings useful to distinguish restriction from constriction include: right ventricular systolic pressure > 50 mm Hg, right ventricular end diastolic pressure to systolic pressure ratio ≤ 0.33, ≥ 5 mm Hg difference between right and left ventricular end-diastolic pressures, absence of respirophasic variation in left-sided filling pressures, marked atrial dilatation, and absence of pericardial thickening and calcification

REFERENCES

• Ammash NM et al: Clinical profile and outcome of idiopathic restrictive cardiomyopathy. Circulation 2000;101:2490.
• Ha JW et al: Differentiation of constrictive pericarditis from restrictive cardiomyopathy using mitral annular velocity by tissue Doppler echocardiography. Am J Cardiol 2004;94:316.
• Morshedi-Meibodi A: Is it constrictive pericarditis or restrictive cardiomyopathy? A systematic approach. Congest Heart Fail 2004;10:309.

INFORMATION FOR PATIENTS

• http://www.heartcenteronline.com/myheartdr/common/articles.cfm?ARTID=433

WEB SITE

• http://www.emedicine.com/MED/topic291.htm

Cardiomyopathy, Tachycardia Induced

 KEY FEATURES

ESSENTIALS OF DIAGNOSIS

- Typical dilated cardiomyopathy with reduced systolic function
- Supraventricular tachycardia (not sinus tachycardia) for more than 15% of the day

GENERAL CONSIDERATIONS

- Atrial tachyarrhythmias with persistently elevated ventricular rates (120–180 beats per minute) can lead to progressive left ventricle dilatation and systolic dysfunction
- The cardiomyopathy develops slowly (over months or longer)
- The mechanism of tachycardia cardiomyopathy is poorly understood, but it can be created in animals by rapid atrial pacing

CLINICAL PRESENTATION

SYMPTOMS AND SIGNS

- Typical symptoms of congestive heart failure, such as dyspnea

PHYSICAL EXAM FINDINGS

- Typical findings of congestive heart failure, such as, pulmonary rales
- Tachycardia > 120 beats per minute at rest

DIFFERENTIAL DIAGNOSIS

- Idiopathic dilated cardiomyopathy should be suspected if left ventricular function does not improve with control or termination of the tachyarrhythmia
- Other forms of heart failure with sinus tachycardia

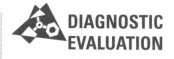 **DIAGNOSTIC EVALUATION**

LABORATORY TESTS

- Electrolytes, creatinine, brain natriuretic peptide

IMAGING STUDIES

- Chest x-ray
  - Pulmonary edema with cardiomegaly
- Echocardiography
  - Dilated, hypokinetic left ventricle
  - Functional mitral regurgitation, tricuspid regurgitation, and mildly elevated pulmonary pressures on Doppler

DIAGNOSTIC PROCEDURES

- Coronary angiography may be necessary in some cases to exclude other causes of heart failure and coronary artery disease

TREATMENT

CARDIOLOGY REFERRAL

- Suspected tachycardia cardiomyopathy

HOSPITALIZATION CRITERIA

- Moderate or worse heart failure

MEDICATIONS

- Pharmacologic therapy to control the rate, such as a beta blocker
- Pharmacologic therapy to eliminate the tachyarrhythmia, such as sotalol

THERAPEUTIC PROCEDURES

- Cardioversion of ventricular tachycardia, atrial fibrillation, or atrial flutter
- Atrioventricular node ablation plus a pacemaker

MONITORING

- ECG in hospital as appropriate

DIET AND ACTIVITY

- Low-sodium diet
- Restricted activity until problem corrected

ONGOING MANAGEMENT

HOSPITAL DISCHARGE CRITERIA

- Resolution of heart failure
- Successful ablation

FOLLOW-UP

- Depends on therapy

COMPLICATIONS

- Death, cardiac arrest
- Pulmonary edema
- Antiarrhythmic drug toxicity
- Chamber perforation during ablation

PROGNOSIS

- Excellent with prompt, effective treatment

PREVENTION

- Refer patients with persistent tachycardia to a cardiologist

RESOURCES

PRACTICE GUIDELINES

- The approach to treatment will be predicated by the underlying tachyarrhythmia.
- Atrioventricular node ablation with subsequent permanent pacing is reserved for those refractory to pharmacologic therapy

INFORMATION FOR PATIENTS

- www.drpen.com/425

WEB SITE

- www.emedicine.com/med/topic289.htm

Cardiomyopathy, Tako-Tsubo

KEY FEATURES

ESSENTIALS OF DIAGNOSIS

- Women older than age 60 years
- Chest discomfort, dyspnea, or both during or within hours of emotional or physical stress
- ECG evidence of myocardial infarction
- Left ventricular apical "balloon" dilation and dysfunction with preserved basal wall motion on cardiac imaging
- No significant stenosis or slow flow in epicardial coronary arteries on angiography
- Mild elevation of cardiac enzymes
- Complete normalization of left ventricular function within weeks

GENERAL CONSIDERATIONS

- Transient left ventricular apical ballooning named for shape of Japanese octopus fishing pot
- Mechanism unknown but probably related to sympathetic activation and catecholamine release
- Probably shares a similar mechanism to "neurogenic stunned myocardium" described after subarachnoid hemorrhage and stroke

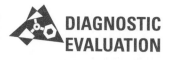

CLINICAL PRESENTATION

SYMPTOMS AND SIGNS

- Typically a woman over age 60 years
- Chest discomfort, dyspnea, or both occurring during or within hours of emotional or physical stress
- Syncope
- Ventricular fibrillation cardiac arrest

PHYSICAL EXAM FINDINGS

- Tachypnea
- Tachycardia
- Hypertension or hypotension
- Cardiogenic shock
- Elevated jugular venous pressure
- Pulmonary rales
- Prominent, diffuse, and sustained apical impulse
- Gallop rhythms may be present
- Edema

DIFFERENTIAL DIAGNOSIS

- Acute myocardial infarction
- Myocarditis
- Cardiomyopathy following subarachnoid hemorrhage

DIAGNOSTIC EVALUATION

LABORATORY TESTS

- Cardiac enzymes may be normal or mildly elevated
- Serum brain type natriuretic peptide levels are elevated

ELECTROCARDIOGRAPHY

- Sinus tachycardia
- Prolonged PR interval in one-quarter
- Prolonged QT interval in one-quarter
- ST-segment elevations in the anterior precordial leads in 15–20%
- Q waves in the anterior precordial leads in > one third
- Diffuse, deep T-wave inversions develop within 48 hours

IMAGING STUDIES

- Chest x-ray:
  - Cardiac silhouette may be normal or enlarged
  - Pulmonary vascular congestion or edema may be present
- Echocardiography: apical "balloon" dilation with akinesis or dyskinesis and moderate-to-severe dysfunction of the midventricle and normal or hyperkinetic contractility of the basilar segments

DIAGNOSTIC PROCEDURES

- Cardiac catheterization:
  - No angiographically significant epicardial coronary artery disease or spasm
  - Left ventriculography reveals apical and midventricular akinesis to dyskinesis
  - Elevated left ventricular end-diastolic pressure
  - Right heart catheterization demonstrates variable elevations in pulmonary capillary wedge pressure, pulmonary artery pressure, right atrial pressure, and reduced cardiac output

TREATMENT

CARDIOLOGY REFERRAL

- All patients

HOSPITALIZATION CRITERIA

- Suspected acute coronary syndrome
- Congestive heart failure
- Syncope
- Arrhythmias

MEDICATIONS

- Supportive therapy including diuretics and vasodilators until spontaneous recovery occurs
- Pressors and beta agonists are typically avoided in favor of mechanical support when needed

THERAPEUTIC PROCEDURES

- Intra-aortic balloon pump (IABP): may be needed in severe cases

SURGERY

- Left ventricular assist device may be considered in severe cases in patients who do not stabilize with an IABP

DIET AND ACTIVITY

- Fluid and sodium restriction
- Activity restricted to walking or lifting < 5–10 lb until after recovery of ventricular function

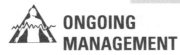 ## ONGOING MANAGEMENT

HOSPITAL DISCHARGE CRITERIA

- Stable cardiac rhythm
- Compensated heart failure and/or improvement of ventricular function

FOLLOW-UP

- Cardiologist within 2 weeks
- Serial echocardiography to demonstrate recovery (usually within 2 weeks) of ventricular function

COMPLICATIONS

- Cardiogenic shock
- Rarely death
- Ventricular tachycardia requiring defibrillator implantation has been described

PROGNOSIS

- Prognosis is excellent
- Recurrence has not been reported

PREVENTION

- No preventive measures identified

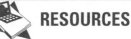 ## RESOURCES

PRACTICE GUIDELINES

- Standard supportive therapy for congestive heart failure with diuretics and vasodilators is recommended
- In cases of severe hemodynamic compromise, mechanical support is favored over pressors and beta agonists because of the association of massive catecholamine release with the disease

REFERENCES

- Akashi Y et al: The clinical features of *takotsubo* cardiomyopathy. Q J Med 2003;96:563.
- Kurisu S et al: Tako-tsubo-like left ventricular dysfunction with ST-segment elevation: a novel cardiac syndrome mimicking acute myocardial infarction. Am Heart J 2002;143:448
- Wittstein I et al: Neurohumoral features of myocardial stunning due to sudden emotional stress. N Engl J Med 2005;352:539.

INFORMATION FOR PATIENTS

- http://www.heartcenteronline.com/ myheartdr/common/articles.cfm? ARTID=442

WEB SITES

- http://www.gpnotebook.co.uk/ simplepage.cfm?ID=x20050315100032 411760
- http://www.emedicine.com/radio/ topic128.htm

Carotid Sinus Hypersensitivity (CSH)

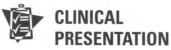 ## KEY FEATURES

ESSENTIALS OF DIAGNOSIS

- Syncope or near syncope occurring during carotid sinus stimulation
- Precipitating events such as shaving or looking up may be reported
- Syncope tends to be abrupt, and the patient may not recall a specific maneuver
- Occurs in older patients
- Bradycardia and vasodepressor element may both play a role

GENERAL CONSIDERATIONS

- Pure cardioinhibitory response is most common (60–80%)
- Pure vasodepressor response is rare (5–10%)
- The remainder is of a mixed variety
- Syncope or near syncope may occur during carotid sinus stimulation or fortuitous Holter monitoring showing asystole during maneuvers of carotid sinus stimulation
- Increased vagal activity and inhibition of peripheral sympathetic activity occur as part of carotid sinus reflex
- Heightened response to carotid sinus pressure
- Frequently associated with coronary artery disease
- Tendency to occur in older patients
- Maneuvers that precipitate syncope may include:
  - Tight collars
  - Heavy lifting
  - Trumpet playing
  - Sometimes the pressure of a seatbelt
- May be a cause of symptoms such as shortness of breath, angina, and syncope in patients with atrial fibrillation
- Carotid aneurysm and head-neck tumors can predispose to CSH

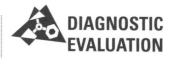 ## CLINICAL PRESENTATION

SYMPTOMS AND SIGNS

- Dizziness
- Presyncope
- Syncope
- May present as unexplained falls

PHYSICAL EXAM FINDINGS

- No specific features other than reproduction of symptoms on carotid sinus pressure
- May have features of coexistent coronary heart disease or carotid bruit

DIFFERENTIAL DIAGNOSIS

- Neurocardiogenic syncope
- Ventricular tachycardia may coexist with carotid sinus hypersensitivity, particularly in patients with previous myocardial infarction or systolic dysfunction

DIAGNOSTIC EVALUATION

LABORATORY TESTS

- CBC, basic metabolic panel

ELECTROCARDIOGRAPHY

- ECG to identify previous myocardial infarction and arrhythmic disorders
- Holter monitoring to document episodes and detect rhythm disturbances

IMAGING STUDIES

- Generally not required unless there is evidence of underlying structural heart disease

DIAGNOSTIC PROCEDURES

- Carotid sinus massage (contraindicated if there is a bruit, history of stroke, or carotid surgery)
- The carotid sinus massage should be done with ECG and hemodynamic monitoring
- The duration of the massage should not exceed 5–10 seconds
- Comprehensive evaluation includes both supine and upright carotid sinus massage
- Cardioinhibitory response is defined as ≥ 3 seconds ventricular standstill (terminate carotid pressure at the onset of asystole)
- Vasodepressor response is defined as a drop in systolic blood pressure of ≥ 50 mm Hg

TREATMENT

CARDIOLOGY REFERRAL

- All patients with a clinical suspicion of carotid sinus hypersensitivity should be evaluated by an cardiac electrophysiologist

HOSPITALIZATION CRITERIA

- If marked asystole is documented (>3 seconds), then hospitalization is warranted until definitive treatment
- A patient with concomitant structural heart disease may undergo electrophysiologic study for risk stratification

MEDICATIONS

- Elimination of triggers such as tight collars
- Avoidance of diuretics and negative chronotropic drugs when feasible
- Adjuvant treatment with serotonin reuptake inhibitors in patients with a substantial vasodepressor element

THERAPEUTIC PROCEDURES

- Atrioventricular (AV) sequential pacemaker (reduces morbidity but may not influence mortality)

SURGERY

- Generally, none required

MONITORING

- ECG monitoring in hospital

DIET AND ACTIVITY

- No specific restrictions

ONGOING MANAGEMENT

HOSPITAL DISCHARGE CRITERIA

- After definitive treatment

FOLLOW-UP

- Pacemaker follow-up

COMPLICATIONS

- Injuries secondary to fall

PROGNOSIS

- After pacemaker implantation, patients have a substantial reduction in syncope

PREVENTION

- Not applicable

RESOURCES

PRACTICE GUIDELINES

- Indication for pacemaker insertion:
  - Recurrent syncope or minimal carotid sinus pressure leads to ventricular asystole of more than 3 seconds' duration in the absence of medications that depress the sinus node or AV conduction

REFERENCES

- Kenny RA, Richardson DA: Carotid sinus syndrome and falls in older adults. Am J Geriatr Cardiol 2001;10:97.

INFORMATION FOR PATIENTS

- www.nlm.nihgov/medlineplus/arrhythmia.html
- www.drpen.com/780.2

WEB SITES

- www.acc.org
- www.hrsonline.org

Cerebral Vascular Disease

 KEY FEATURES

ESSENTIALS OF DIAGNOSIS

- Rapid development of focal or global disturbance of cerebral function:
  - Duration < 24 hours is a transient ischemic attack
  - Duration > 24 hours is a stroke
- Early CT scan is negative, which excludes intracerebral or subarachnoid hemorrhage
- Duplex ultrasound or angiography shows large-vessel disease

GENERAL CONSIDERATIONS

- Acute cerebrovascular disorders cause more morbidity and mortality than any other disease in those over age 45 years
- In North America, about 80% of strokes are ischemic and are caused by thrombosis in cerebral arteries, emboli to the brain arteries, or hypertension
- Hemorrhagic strokes are more common in East Asia and are due to rupture of an intracerebral artery
- About 20% of ischemic strokes are from cardiac emboli
- Ten to 20% are lacunar (deep brain and small)
- Watershed infarcts from hypotension account for < 5%
- The remaining two thirds are due to large-vessel disease
- Risk factors for stroke include:
  - Hypertension (most important)
  - Smoking
  - Atrial fibrillation

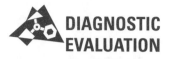 CLINICAL PRESENTATION

SYMPTOMS AND SIGNS

- *Transient ischemic attack* (TIA):
  - Focal neurologic defects last < 24 hours and are presumed to be ischemic
- *Minor stroke:*
  - Focal defects last > 24 hours but without significant functional impairment at 1 week
- *Progressing stroke:*
  - Worsening neurologic defects over 2–3 days
- *Brain infarction:*
  - Stable or gradually improving neurologic defects with functionality significant impairment at 1 week

PHYSICAL EXAM FINDINGS

- Unilateral or bilateral motor defects
- Unilateral or bilateral sensory defects
- Aphasia or dysphagia
- Monocular vision problems
- Hemianopia
- Atypical— confusion, vertigo

DIFFERENTIAL DIAGNOSIS

- Subdural hematoma
- Epilepsy
- Migraine
- Hypoglycemia
- Hypertension
- Hypertensive encephalopathy
- Cerebral infection
- Brain tumor
- Multiple sclerosis
- Hysterical conversion

DIAGNOSTIC EVALUATION

LABORATORY TESTS

- CBC, electrolytes, glucose
- Lipid panel, homocysteine
- Cardiac biomarkers (troponins, creatine kinesis

ELECTROCARDIOGRAPHY

- ECG abnormalities are common but specific findings may suggest the cause of the stroke, such as myocardial infarction or atrial fibrillation
- Prolonged QT and torsades de pointes can occur as a result of a stroke

IMAGING STUDIES

- CT scan to distinguish ischemia from hemorrhage
- MR angiography in selected patients to detect vascular occlusion
- Duplex ultrasonography to assess extra cranial blood vessels

DIAGNOSTIC PROCEDURES

- Digital subtraction angiography is the gold standard for evaluating extra and intracranial arteries, but it carries some risk
- Transesophageal echocardiography is useful to detect intracardiac sources of emboli

Cerebral Vascular Disease

TREATMENT

CARDIOLOGY REFERRAL

- Suspected cardiac emboli

HOSPITALIZATION CRITERIA

- Progressive stroke
- Brain infarction
- Acute myocardial infarction
- Rapid atrial fibrillation

MEDICATIONS

- Transient ischemic attack:
  - Antiplatelet agents (aspirin 160 mg/day, clopridogrel 75 mg/day, dipyridamole 150–400 mg/day, usually with aspirin)
- Stroke:
  - Thrombolysis in appropriate candidates (alteplase 0.9 mg/kg IV over 60 minutes, 10% as bolus over 1 minute; maximum dose 90 mg IV)
- Secondary prevention measures for atherosclerosis
- Antihypertensive therapy if blood pressure > 175/115 mm Hg
- Anticoagulants for atrial fibrillation

THERAPEUTIC PROCEDURES

- Carotid surgery or stenting for symptomatic patients with > 70% diameter narrowing
- Intracranial percutaneous arterial embolectomy

SURGERY

- Carotid endarterectomy

MONITORING

- Stoke unit to monitor neurologic status

DIET AND ACTIVITY

- Adequate fluids, low-fat diet
- Bed rest acutely

ONGOING MANAGEMENT

HOSPITAL DISCHARGE CRITERIA

- Adequate recovery to move to a rehab unit
- Successful therapy, procedure, or surgery

FOLLOW-UP

- Close follow-up of secondary prevention interventions is necessary to prevent recurrences

COMPLICATIONS

- Death
- Seizures
- Delirium
- Neuropsychiatric problems such as depression

PROGNOSIS

- The risk of recurrent stroke is 10–15% the first year, then declines to half that value thereafter
- Long-term mortality rate is more closely related to coronary artery disease

PREVENTION

- Reduce risk factors for atherosclerosis
- Control blood pressure
- Control diabetes
- Anticoagulants for atrial fibrillation
- Antiplatelet agents

RESOURCES

PRACTICE GUIDELINES

- The approach to stroke involves three phases:
  - Restoration of blood flow
  - Protection of the brain from ischemia
  - Prevention of further thromboembolism

REFERENCES

- Derex L et al: Clinical and imaging predictors of intracerebral hemorrhage in stroke patients treated with intravenous tissue plasminogen activator. J Neurol Neourosurg Psychiatry 2005;76:70.
- Jin PH et al: Carotid artery stenting with routine cerebral protection in high-risk patients. Am J Surg 2004;188:644.
- Kastrup A et al: Comparison of angioplasty and stenting with cerebral protection versus endarterectomy for treatment of internal carotid artery stenosis in elderly patients. J Vasc Surg 2004;40:945.

INFORMATION FOR PATIENTS

- www.strokeassociation.org/ presenter.jhtml?identifier=11402

WEB SITES

- www.emedicine.com/neuro/topic9.htm
- www.emedicine.com/neuro/topic702.htm
- www.emedicine.com/neuro/topic370.htm

Chagas' Heart Disease

 KEY FEATURES

ESSENTIALS OF DIAGNOSIS

- Remote history of residence in rural Central or South America
- ECG evidence of conduction system disease, especially right bundle branch block and left anterior fascicular block, and ST-segment elevation, suggesting ventricular aneurysm
- Premature ventricular contractions and nonsustained ventricular tachycardia (VT)
- Echocardiographic evidence of an apical left ventricular aneurysm
- Positive serology for Chagas' disease

GENERAL CONSIDERATIONS

- Caused by the protozoan *Trypanosoma cruzi*
- Most common cause of cardiomyopathy in South and Central America
- Three phases of Chagas' disease: acute, indeterminate, and chronic
- Pericarditis-myocarditis may develop in the acute phase with variable signs of cardiac failure that often resolve
- Patients are asymptomatic during the indeterminate phase, which lasts 10–30 years
- Thirty percent of patients in the indeterminate phase eventually develop chronic heart failure
- Cardiomyopathy occurs in the chronic phase of *Trypanosoma cruzi* infection

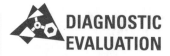 **CLINICAL PRESENTATION**

SYMPTOMS AND SIGNS

- Remote history of residence in South or Central America
- Fatigue
- Palpitations
- Dizziness and syncope
- Stokes-Adams attacks due to arrhythmias
- Chest pain
- Dyspnea
- Dysphasia in patients with mega-esophagus
- Severe constipation and abdominal discomfort in patients with megacolon

PHYSICAL EXAM FINDINGS

- Tachypnea
- Tachycardia
- Hypotension
- Elevated jugular venous pressure
- Pulmonary rales
- Diffuse, sustained apical impulse
- Wide splitting of S_2 due to right bundle branch block
- Systolic murmurs of mitral and tricuspid insufficiency
- S_3 and S_4
- Hepatomegaly and pulsatile liver
- Abdominal ascites
- Peripheral edema
- Signs of thromboemboli phenomenon

DIFFERENTIAL DIAGNOSIS

- Coronary artery disease
- Dilated cardiomyopathy
- Isolated conduction system disease
- Other causes of ventricular arrhythmias

DIAGNOSTIC EVALUATION

LABORATORY TESTS

- Laboratory findings are nonspecific
- CBC demonstrates leukocytosis with an absolute increase in lymphocyte count
- Serologic tests for *T. cruzi*

ELECTROCARDIOGRAPHY

- Sinus rhythm or sinus bradycardia
- Atrial fibrillation
- VT
- First- to third-degree atrioventricular (AV) block
- Right bundle branch block
- Left anterior fascicular block

IMAGING STUDIES

- Chest x-ray: variable degrees of cardiomegaly, pulmonary vascular redistribution and pulmonary edema
- Echocardiography: variable ventricular dilatation and reduced systolic function; a ventricular apical aneurysm may be present; mural thrombi may be present; mitral and tricuspid regurgitation are often present

DIAGNOSTIC PROCEDURES

- Cardiac catheterization and angiography: can exclude coronary artery disease
- Electrophysiologic study: indicated in selected cases to assess sinus node function and AV conduction in symptomatic patients; may be useful in patients with sustained VT to determine prognosis and select the appropriate anti-arrhythmic therapy

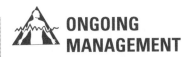

TREATMENT

CARDIOLOGY REFERRAL

- Heart failure
- Arrhythmias

HOSPITALIZATION CRITERIA

- Decompensated congestive heart failure
- Syncope
- Thromboembolic events and stroke
- Arrhythmias
- Symptomatic bradycardia

MEDICATIONS

- Standard medical therapy for heart failure (angiotensin-converting enzyme inhibitors/angiotensin receptor blockers, beta blockers, digoxin, diuretics)
- Amiodarone is effective for ventricular arrhythmias
- Role of antiparasite therapy in patients with chronic Chagas cardiomyopathy has not been demonstrated

THERAPEUTIC PROCEDURES

- Dual-chamber or biventricular pacemaker with or without defibrillator device implantation in appropriate candidates
- Pacemaker often required
- Implanted cardioverter-defibrillator in patients who meet criteria
- VT catheter ablation may be considered

SURGERY

- Aneurysmectomy in selected cases
- Heart transplantation is an option for patients with persistent, severe disease and poor quality of life

MONITORING

- Telemetry during hospitalization
- Fluid balance

DIET AND ACTIVITY

- Sodium and fluid restriction for patients with congestive heart failure
- Activity as tolerated

ONGOING MANAGEMENT

HOSPITAL DISCHARGE CRITERIA

- Compensated heart failure
- Stable cardiac rhythm

FOLLOW-UP

- Cardiologist within 2 weeks
- Serial echocardiography depending on the patient's clinical course
- Electrophysiology clinic for patients with devices

COMPLICATIONS

- Arrhythmias
- Progressive heart failure
- Sudden death
- Thromboembolic events including stroke

PROGNOSIS

- Dependent on the degree of myocardial dysfunction
- Fifty percent 4-year mortality rate for patients presenting with chronic heart failure
- Fifty-five to 65% mortality rate from sudden cardiac death in patients with chronic heart failure
- Approximately one fourth to one third die from progressive heart failure
- Ten to 15% mortality rate from stroke

PREVENTION

- Avoidance of endemic areas in South and Central America

RESOURCES

PRACTICE GUIDELINES

- Treatment of arrhythmias is largely empiric but generally similar to that of other forms of cardiomyopathy
- Some patients benefit from surgical excision of fibrotic tissue, aneurysmectomy, or VT ablation
- Medical treatment for Chagas cardiomyopathy is similar to other causes of cardiomyopathy
- Outcomes after cardiac transplantation are at least as good as for other causes of heart failure

REFERENCES

- Bocchi EA et al: The paradox of survival results after heart transplantation for cardiomyopathy caused by *Trypanosoma cruzi*. First Guidelines Group for Heart Transplantation of the Brazilian Society of Cardiology. Ann Thorac Surg 2001;71:1833.
- Davila DF et al: Effects of metoprolol in chagasic patients with severe congestive heart failure. Int J Cardiol 2002;85:255.
- Elizari MV: Arrhythmias associated with Chagas' heart disease. Card Electrophysiol Rev 2002;6:115.
- Higuchi ML et al: Pathophysiology of the heart in Chagas' disease: current status and new developments. Cardiovasc Res 2003;60:96.

Chemotherapy-Induced Cardiac Disease

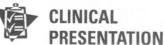 KEY FEATURES

ESSENTIALS OF DIAGNOSIS

- Past or present treatment with chemotherapeutic agents associated with cardiotoxicity
- Patients with arrhythmias, chest pain, or symptoms and signs of congestive heart failure

GENERAL CONSIDERATIONS

- Anthracycline antibiotics (doxorubicin, daunorubicin) are the most common agents, and cardiotoxicity risk increases with increasing cumulative dosage
- 5-Fluorouracil may cause vasospastic or thrombotic occlusion and acute myocardial infarction
- Cisplatin, bleomycin, and vinca alkaloids may cause myocardial infarction secondary to vasospastic effects
- Cyclophosphamide (> 2000 mg/m^2) may cause severe cardiomyopathy; interferon-alpha and trastuzumab rarely cause cardiomyopathy
- Interleukin-2 may cause capillary leak syndrome, noncardiogenic pulmonary edema, and occasionally myocardial infarction

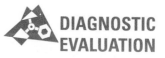 CLINICAL PRESENTATION

SYMPTOMS AND SIGNS

- Palpitations
- Chest pain
- Fatigue
- Dyspnea
- Reduced exercise tolerance
- Orthopnea and paroxysmal nocturnal dyspnea
- Syncope
- Weight gain

PHYSICAL EXAM FINDINGS

- Tachypnea
- Tachycardia
- Elevated jugular venous pressure
- Pulmonary rales
- Diffuse, sustained apical impulse
- Murmurs of tricuspid and mitral insufficiency
- S_3 and S_4
- Pericardial rub
- Hepatomegaly; pulsatile liver from tricuspid regurgitation
- Abdominal ascites
- Peripheral edema
- Reduced pulse pressure

DIFFERENTIAL DIAGNOSIS

- Coexistent cardiomyopathy such as ischemic and dilated cardiomyopathies should be in the differential diagnosis

DIAGNOSTIC EVALUATION

LABORATORY TESTS

- Electrolytes (hyponatremia portends a poor prognosis)
- Blood urea nitrogen and creatinine
- CBC (anemia should be worked up)
- Liver function tests (elevations may be due to hepatic congestion)
- Cardiac enzymes to exclude acute or recent myocardial injury (elevated CKMB levels may be seen with muscular dystrophy)
- Thyroid function tests

ELECTROCARDIOGRAPHY

- Sinus tachycardia or atrial fibrillation
- Varying degrees of atrioventricular block may be present
- Premature ventricular complexes
- ST elevations indicative of acute myocardial infarction
- Nonspecific ST- and T-wave changes
- Q waves

IMAGING STUDIES

- Chest x-ray: enlarged cardiac silhouette; pulmonary vascular congestion; curly B lines; pleural effusions
- Echocardiography typical findings:
  - Four-chamber cardiac enlargement
  - Mild to severe left and often right ventricular systolic dysfunction with global hypokinesis (sometimes with segmental variation)
  - Thrombi may be noted in the atria or ventricles
  - Spontaneous echo contrast within the cardiac chambers (indicates a high thrombotic potential)
  - Varying degrees of mitral and tricuspid regurgitation due to annular dilatation
- Elevated tricuspid regurgitant peak velocity indicates pulmonary hypertension
- Noninvasive stress testing with nuclear imaging: can screen for coronary artery disease

DIAGNOSTIC PROCEDURES

- Cardiopulmonary exercise testing with oxygen consumption: used to determine when to list a patient for cardiac transplantation; peak oxygen consumption of < 14 mL/kg/min signifies a poor prognosis and is generally used as the cut-off for listing a patient

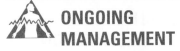

- Left heart catheterization with coronary angiography: indicated for patients with acute myocardial infarction or to exclude coronary artery disease; the left ventricular end-diastolic pressure is typically elevated

TREATMENT

CARDIOLOGY REFERRAL

- Reduced ventricular function
- Arrythmias
- Myocardial infarction

HOSPITALIZATION CRITERIA

- Congestive heart failure
- Tachy- or bradyarrhythmias
- Acute myocardial infarction

MEDICATIONS

- Limit the dose of anthracycline and use new formulations (liposome-encapsulated)
- Calcium channel blockers, beta blockers, and iron-chelating agents are cardioprotective
- Modified dosing schedules may also be protective
- Other agents may be cardioprotective, such as probucol, mesna, and vitamin E
- Once cardiomyopathy develops, prognosis is poor, and treatment is similar to that for heart failure from other causes

THERAPEUTIC PROCEDURES

- Pacemaker for bradycardia
- Implantable cardioverter-defibrillator and/or cardiac resynchronization therapy (biventricular pacemaker) in patients meeting criteria

SURGERY

- Prior malignancy is a relative contraindication to cardiac transplantation but may be considered in patients with severe, progressive heart failure and poor quality of life who have a relatively good oncologic prognosis

MONITORING

- ECG monitoring in the hospital
- Fluid balance

DIET AND ACTIVITY

- Sodium and water restriction
- Activity as tolerated

ONGOING MANAGEMENT

HOSPITAL DISCHARGE CRITERIA

- After medical stabilization and optimization of heart failure medications

FOLLOW-UP

- Cardiologist every 3 months or more, depending on severity of disease
- Appropriate follow-up with an electrophysiologist as needed
- Serial echocardiography during chemotherapy recommended

COMPLICATIONS

- Progressive heart failure
- Arrhythmias
- Sudden death
- Myocardial infarction
- Thromboembolic events including stroke

PROGNOSIS

- Generally poor

PREVENTION

- Use of novel infusion protocols, new anthracycline compounds, liposome encapsulation, adjunctive agents, and noninvasive serial monitoring of cardiac function may reduce the risk of anthracycline cardiotoxicity
- Use of other cardioprotective agents during chemotherapy

RESOURCES

PRACTICE GUIDELINES

- Every effort should be made to prevent and screen for chemotherapy-induced cardiotoxicity
- Once chemotherapy-induced ventricular dysfunction develops, the prognosis is generally poor, and standard heart failure therapy is indicated

REFERENCES

- Gharib MI, Burnett AK: Chemotherapy-induced cardiotoxicity: current practice and prospects of prophylaxis. Eur J Heart Fail 2002;4:235.
- Grande AM et al: Heart transplantation in chemotherapeutic dilated cardiomyopathy. Transplant Proc 2003;35:1516.

INFORMATION FOR PATIENTS

- http://www.americanheart.org/presenter.jhtml?identifier=4468

WEB SITE

- http://www.emedicine.com/med/topic289.htm

Coarctation of the Aorta

KEY FEATURES

ESSENTIALS OF DIAGNOSIS

- Elevated systolic blood pressure in the upper extremities (always in right arm)
- Normal systolic blood pressure in lower extremities (often in left arm)
- Radial–femoral pulse delay
- Left ventricular prominence, "3" sign, rib-notching on chest radiograph
- Coarctation visible by imaging
- Distal aortic pressure drop by Doppler echocardiography or catheterization

GENERAL CONSIDERATIONS

- Male predominance
- Most commonly located distal to the left subclavian artery
- May coexist with bicuspid aortic valve
- Usually diagnosed in childhood by routine physical examination
- Symptoms may arise during the second and third decade of life
  - Coarctation should be suspected in the patient in his 20s or 30s presenting with hypertension
- Seen in more than 10% of patients with Turner's syndrome
- Early detection and repair are important to forestall the accelerated development of coronary artery disease and congestive heart failure

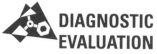 CLINICAL PRESENTATION

SYMPTOMS AND SIGNS

- Usually asymptomatic
- Nonspecific symptoms:
  - Exertional dyspnea
  - Headache
  - Hepistaxis
  - Leg fatigue
- Hemorrhagic cerebrovascular accidents
- Endarteritis
- Possible congestive heart failure in the adult with longstanding hypertension related to coarctation
- Aortic rupture or dissection
- Aortic aneurysm distal to the coarctation
- Infective endocarditis of an associated bicuspid aortic valve

PHYSICAL EXAM FINDINGS

- Elevated systolic blood pressure in the right arm
- Reduced systolic blood pressure in the legs
- Radial–femoral pulse delay
- Palpable intercostal arteries (collaterals)
- Brisk carotid upstroke
- Hyperdynamic left ventricular impulse
- Late systolic murmur between the scapulae to the left of the spine
- Ejection click and systolic ejection murmur (with or without diastolic murmur of aortic insufficiency) with associated bicuspid aortic valve

DIFFERENTIAL DIAGNOSIS

- Other causes of systemic hypertension
- Aortoiliac disease

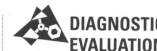 DIAGNOSTIC EVALUATION

LABORATORY TESTS

- No specific studies

ELECTROCARDIOGRAPHY

- ECG findings:
  - Left ventricular hypertrophy
  - Left atrial enlargement
  - Atrial fibrillation

IMAGING STUDIES

- Chest x-ray:
  - Rib notching
  - "3" sign (dilated left subclavian artery and dilated distal aorta forming the upper and lower curvatures, respectively)
  - Left ventricular and left atrial enlargement
- Echocardiography:
  - Precordial two-dimensional echocardiogram from the suprasternal notch may reveal the coarctation
  - Color-flow Doppler acceleration in the descending aorta with persistent diastolic forward flow
- Magnetic resonance angiography:
  - Can localize and define the extent of narrowing with a high degree of accuracy
  - Also used for postoperative evaluation

DIAGNOSTIC PROCEDURES

- Cardiac catheterization(rarely necessary):
  - When noninvasive imaging cannot fully define the anatomy
  - When concomitant coronary artery disease is suspected

TREATMENT

CARDIOLOGY REFERRAL

- When aortic coarctation is diagnosed or suspected
- After repair of aortic coarctation for routine follow-up evaluation

HOSPITALIZATION CRITERIA

- Congestive heart failure
- Suspected aortic dissection or rupture
- Suspected endarteritis or endocarditis
- Stroke
- Unstable angina

MEDICATIONS

- Antibiotic prophylaxis
- One third of patients operated on after age 14 years require therapy for persistent hypertension

THERAPEUTIC PROCEDURES

- Angioplasty is generally not indicated for uncomplicated native coarctation
- Recurrent coarctation after surgical correction can usually be treated with balloon angioplasty with or without a stent

SURGERY

- Surgical correction is indicated at the time of diagnosis
- End-to-end anastomosis is preferred
- Interposition graft and/or subclavian flap may be required

MONITORING

- Blood pressure monitoring

DIET AND ACTIVITY

- Low-sodium diet
- Avoidance of heavy lifting and strenuous exercise in patients with uncorrected coarctation, significant recoarctation, or an aneurysm
- Patients with surgically corrected coarctation without significant recoarctation have no activity restrictions

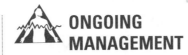

ONGOING MANAGEMENT

HOSPITAL DISCHARGE CRITERIA

- After successful aortic coarctation repair

FOLLOW-UP

- Regular annual or biannual follow-up visits
- With no clinical evidence of recoarctation, MRI/MR angiography every 1–2 years

COMPLICATIONS

- Aortic aneurysm, rupture, or dissection
- Endarteritis
- Recoarctation in 5–10% of cases
- Systemic hypertension

PROGNOSIS

- Mortality rate in patients with *uncorrected* coarctation is approximately 50% by age 30 and 90% by age 60
- Major determinants of survival following repair of coarctation:
  - Age at operation
  - Presence of associated lesions
- Survival is nearly normal if surgery is performed before age 20 years
- Twenty-five–year survival rate is 75% if surgery is performed between the ages of 20 and 40 years
- Fifteen-year survival rate is 50% if surgery is performed after age 40 years
- Postsurgical mortality rate in patients > 20 years old with isolated coarctation repair is 5%
- Ten percent of patients require additional cardiovascular surgery (usually aortic valve replacement)
- Rate of recoarctation is 5 – 14%

PREVENTION

- Antibiotic prophylaxis before dental and other nonsterile procedures is recommended

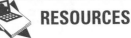

RESOURCES

PRACTICE GUIDELINES

- Management of coarctation depends on patient's age, presentation, and morphology
- Surgery (preferred) or balloon angioplasty should be performed early in childhood to prevent hypertension
- Close follow-up of patients with a history of aortic coarctation for complications, including recoarctation, is mandatory

REFERENCES

- Brickner ME et al: Congenital heart disease in adults. First of two parts. N Engl J Med 2000;342:256.
- Toro-Salazar OH et al: Long-term follow-up of patients after coarctation of the aorta repair. Am J Cardiol 2002;89:541.

INFORMATION FOR PATIENTS

- http://www.americanheart.org/presenter.jhtml?identifier=11069
- http://www.heartcenteronline.com/myheartdr/common/articles.cfm?ARTID=202

WEB SITES

- http://www.emedicine.com/med/topic154.htm
- http://www.emedicine.com/ped/topic2504.htm
- http://www.emedicine.com/ped/topic2824.htm

Cocaine-Induced Cardiovascular Disease

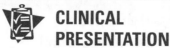 KEY FEATURES

ESSENTIALS OF DIAGNOSIS

- Chest pain and myocardial infarction
- Features of congestive heart failure secondary to cocaine cardiomyopathy
- Hypertension
- Positive history or urine drug screen for cocaine (history of cocaine use may be denied and urine drug screen may be negative)
- ECG is often nonspecific (non–Q-wave infarction is more common than Q-wave infarction in cocaine users)

GENERAL CONSIDERATIONS

- Cocaine is the most common illicit drug with major actions on the cardiovascular system
- Cocaine increases vasoactive and cardiac-stimulating substances, causing peripheral and coronary artery constriction, tachycardia, and increased cardiac contractility
- Myocardial ischemia and life-threatening ventricular arrhythmias may ensue

CLINICAL PRESENTATION

SYMPTOMS AND SIGNS

- Chest pain
- Dyspnea
- Syncope

PHYSICAL EXAM FINDINGS

- Hypertension
- Tachycardia
- Increased respiratory rate

DIFFERENTIAL DIAGNOSIS

- Atherosclerotic coronary artery disease
- Spontaneous coronary artery spasm

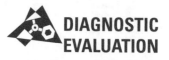 DIAGNOSTIC EVALUATION

LABORATORY TESTS

- Cocaine blood or urine screen
- Elevated cardiac biomarkers, such as troponin

ELECTROCARDIOGRAPHY

- Nonspecific ST-T–wave changes
- Ischemic ST-T–wave changes
- Q-wave myocardial infarction less common

IMAGING STUDIES

- Echocardiography: may show segmental wall motion abnormalities and reduced left ventricular function
- Nuclear perfusion studies: may show patchy defects

DIAGNOSTIC PROCEDURES

- Coronary angiography may be needed to exclude coronary artery disease

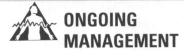

TREATMENT

CARDIOLOGY REFERRAL

- Suspected myocardial ischemia/infarction
- Serious ventricular arrhythmias
- Cardiomyopathy present

HOSPITALIZATION CRITERIA

- Acute coronary syndromes
- Syncope or collapse
- Significant arrhythmias
- Severe hypertension

MEDICATIONS

- Nitrates, alpha-adrenoreceptor blockers, and verapamil for acute ischemia
- Aspirin
- Thrombolytic therapy in acute ST-elevation myocardial infarction
- Beta blockers should be avoided
- Lidocaine should be used cautiously because it lowers the seizure threshold

THERAPEUTIC PROCEDURES

- Emergent coronary angiography and primary angioplasty may be used as alternative means of establishing perfusion, particularly when diagnosis is uncertain because of early repolarization

MONITORING

- ECG monitoring in hospital as appropriate

DIET AND ACTIVITY

- Low-sodium, low-fat diet
- Restricted activities initially, then cardiac rehabilitation

ONGOING MANAGEMENT

HOSPITAL DISCHARGE CRITERIA

- Resolution of problems

FOLLOW-UP

- Depends on residual disease severity

COMPLICATIONS

- Sudden death
- Myocardial infarction
- Aortic dissection
- Stroke

PROGNOSIS

- Good, with abstinence from cocaine

RESOURCES

PRACTICE GUIDELINES

- Cocaine abuse should be suspected in young individuals with acute coronary syndromes and no apparent risk factors for coronary atherosclerosis
  - Mortality rate is very low if the correct diagnosis is made
  - Beta-blockers are contraindicated

REFERENCE

- Kloner RA, Rezkalla SH: Cocaine and the heart. N Engl J Med 2003;348:487.

INFORMATION FOR PATIENTS

- www.drpen.com/305.60

WEB SITE

- www.emedicine.com/med/topic400.htm

Congestive Heart Failure: Diastolic Dysfunction

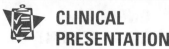 KEY FEATURES

ESSENTIALS OF DIAGNOSIS

- Clinical presentation of congestive heart failure
- Normal left ventricular systolic function
- Abnormal left ventricular diastolic function

GENERAL CONSIDERATIONS

- About one third of patients presenting with congestive heart failure have normal systolic function, but up to 50% in the elderly
- The basic pathophysiologic problem is the inability of the left ventricle to fill at normal filling pressures
- This reduction in ventricular compliance can be due to hypertrophy, infiltrative diseases such as amyloid, restriction from fibrosis such as radiation damage, or segmental fibrosis and hypertrophy from chronic ischemic heart disease
- Many patients with predominant diastolic left ventricular dysfunction have systolic dysfunction as well, but it is mild
- Because diastolic left ventricular dysfunction has no specific treatment, it is important to detect reversible causes of heart failure with normal systolic function such as transient myocardial ischemia

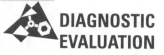 CLINICAL PRESENTATION

SYMPTOMS AND SIGNS

- Dyspnea and fatigue with exertion
- Orthopnea

PHYSICAL EXAM FINDINGS

- Elevated jugular venous pressure, edema
- Pulmonary rales
- S_4

DIFFERENTIAL DIAGNOSIS

- Pulmonary hypertension
- Mitral valve disease
- Transient myocardial ischemia
- Volume overload

DIAGNOSTIC EVALUATION

ELECTROCARDIOGRAPHY

- Left ventricular and atrial hypertrophy is common

IMAGING STUDIES

- Echocardiography:
  - Normal or near-normal left ventricular systolic function
  - Abnormal left ventricular diastolic function with elevated filling pressures on Doppler
  - The cause of the diastolic dysfunction may be identified, such as left ventricular hypertrophy, amyloid, or myocardial scarring

DIAGNOSTIC PROCEDURES

- Stress testing with echo or radionuclide perfusion imaging may be necessary to exclude myocardial ischemia
- Coronary angiography may be necessary to exclude coronary artery disease
- Myocardial biopsy may be necessary to diagnose infiltrative diseases, eg, amyloid

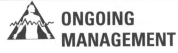 TREATMENT

CARDIOLOGY REFERRAL

- Heart failure
- Abnormal left ventricular diastolic function

HOSPITALIZATION CRITERIA

- Pulmonary edema
- Suspected acute myocardial ischemia
- Rapid atrial fibrillation

MEDICATIONS

- Diuretics
- Beta blockers
- Heart rate–lowering calcium channel blockers
- Treatment of underlying cause (eg, hypertension, myocardial ischemia)
- Antiarrhythmic drugs to preserve sinus rhythm

MONITORING

- ECG monitoring in hospital as appropriate

DIET AND ACTIVITY

- Low-sodium diet
- Restricted activity until heart failure treated

ONGOING MANAGEMENT

HOSPITAL DISCHARGE CRITERIA

- Resolution of problem

FOLLOW-UP

- Three months, then every 6 months if stable

COMPLICATIONS

- Atrial fibrillation
- Acute pulmonary edema

PROGNOSIS

- In general, the mortality rate is lower in patients with heart failure and diastolic dysfunction compared with systolic dysfunction, but this varies widely with the underlying cause

PREVENTION

- Control hypertension
- Prevent myocardial ischemia

RESOURCES

PRACTICE GUIDELINES

- The treatment of diastolic heart failure has three goals:
  - Eliminate congestion (eg, diuretics)
  - Eliminate or reverse the causes of diastolic dysfunction (treat hypertension)
  - Maintain optimal left ventricular filling at as low a filling pressure as possible (control heart rate)

REFERENCE

- Argeja B, Grossman W: Evaluation and management of diastolic heart failure. Circulation 2003;107:659.

INFORMATION FOR PATIENTS

- www.drpen.com/428.3

WEB SITE

- www.emedicine.com/med/topic3552.htm

Congestive Heart Failure: Systolic Dysfunction

KEY FEATURES

ESSENTIALS OF DIAGNOSIS

- Dyspnea on exertion, paroxysmal nocturnal dyspnea, orthopnea, and dyspnea at rest (late stage)
- Jugular venous distention, peripheral edema, sinus tachycardia, pulmonary rales, cardiomegaly, S_3, and liver enlargement
- Left ventricular (LV) systolic dysfunction

GENERAL CONSIDERATIONS

- Affects more than 2 million patients in the United States
- Approximately 400,000 new patients each year
- Complex clinical syndrome characterized by dysfunction of the left, right, or both ventricles and changes in neurohumoral regulation
- Effort intolerance, fluid retention, and shortened survival
- Principal clinical manifestations result from inadequate forward cardiac output
- Neurohumoral activation responsible for fluid retention, peripheral edema, and an increase in peripheral resistance
- Manifestations depend on the rate of heart failure development with adaptive mechanisms minimizing symptoms and chronic heart failure
- Causes:
  - Coronary artery disease
  - Idiopathic dilated cardiomyopathy
  - Metabolic causes (alcohol, nutritional and thyroid disorders, pheochromocytoma)
  - Drugs and toxins
  - Infectious organisms
  - Connective tissue diseases
  - Neurologic diseases
  - Inherited storage diseases
  - Infiltrative diseases

CLINICAL PRESENTATION

SYMPTOMS AND SIGNS

- Dyspnea
- Paroxysmal nocturnal dyspnea
- Orthopnea
- Cough
- Fatigue and weakness
- Nocturia and oliguria
- Abdominal bloating and discomfort

PHYSICAL EXAM FINDINGS

- Tachycardia
- Hypotension
- Tachypnea
- Diaphoresis
- Elevated jugular venous pressure
- Pulmonary rales
- Reduced breath sounds and dullness to percussion consistent with pleural effusions
- Laterally displaced, enlarged, and sustained ventricular impulse
- Murmurs of tricuspid and mitral regurgitation
- S_3 and sometimes S_4
- Hepatomegaly, pulsatile liver with tricuspid regurgitation
- Abdominal fluid wave due to ascites
- Peripheral edema
- Pulses alternans
- Reduced pulse pressure
- Cool, clammy skin

DIFFERENTIAL DIAGNOSIS

- Chronic lung disease
- Pneumonia
- Pulmonary emboli
- Pericardial disease—tamponade or constriction
- Nephrosis
- Hepatic cirrhosis
- Hypothyroidism

DIAGNOSTIC EVALUATION

LABORATORY TESTS

- CBC: to exclude anemia or infection
- Electrolyte, blood urea nitrogen, creatinine (may have hyponatremia and/or renal failure)
- Liver function tests: may be elevated from passive liver congestion
- Calcium, magnesium, phosphate levels
- Thyroid function tests

ELECTROCARDIOGRAPHY

- Sinus tachycardia
- Atrial fibrillation
- Ventricular premature beats
- Intraventricular conduction delay
- Nonspecific ST- and T-wave segment changes

IMAGING STUDIES

- Chest x-ray findings:
  - Ccardiomegaly
  - Cephalization
  - Interstitial and perivascular edema
  - Kerley B lines
  - P\leural effusions
- Typical transthoracic echocardiography findings:\
  - Biatrial enlargement
  - Left and/or right ventricular enlargement and reduced contractility
  - Eccentric hypertrophy
  - Functional mitral and tricuspid regurgitation
- Doppler: oulmonary artery systolic pressure can be estimated by the peak tricuspid regurgitant velocity

DIAGNOSTIC PROCEDURES

- Cardiac catheterization and angiography
  - Can determine the extent of coronary artery disease
  - Right heart catheterization may be useful to guide medical therapy in patients with refractory heart failure

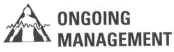

TREATMENT

CARDIOLOGY REFERRAL

- Reduced LV systolic function
- Decompensated congestive heart failure
- Arrhythmias

HOSPITALIZATION CRITERIA

- Decompensated congestive heart failure
- Hypotension
- Syncope
- Arrhythmias

MEDICATIONS

- Diuretics
- Digoxin
- Angiotensin-converting enzyme (ACE) inhibitors or angiotensin-receptor blockers (ARBs)
- Beta blockers
- Aldosterone antagonists
- Nitrates and hydralazine in patients who are not taking ACE inhibitors or ARBs
- Antiarrhythmic drugs
- Anticoagulation in patients with mural thrombi or severe LV dysfunction
- Intravenous vasodilators and/or inotropes may be needed in acutely decompensated or severe cases

THERAPEUTIC PROCEDURES

- Automatic implantable cardioverter-defibrillator
- Biventricular pacing for patients with intraventricular conduction delay
- Percutaneous coronary revascularization
- Extracorporeal ultrafiltration (hemofiltration) is effective for removing excess fluid in refractory heart failure
- Intra-aortic balloon pump for acutely decompensated, severe heart failure

SURGERY

- Coronary artery bypass surgery
- Ventricular aneurysmectomy
- Cardiac transplantation
- Ventricular assist devices as a bridge to recovery or cardiac transplantation

MONITORING

- Telemetry monitoring
- Fluid balance
- Pulse oximetry
- Blood pressure

DIET AND ACTIVITY

- Two-gram sodium and fluid restriction
- Modest exercise training may be beneficial in stable patients without unstable coronary syndromes

ONGOING MANAGEMENT

HOSPITAL DISCHARGE CRITERIA

- Compensated heart failure
- Stable vital signs

FOLLOW-UP

- Cardiologist within 2 weeks of hospital discharge
- Serial echocardiography for changes in clinical status

COMPLICATIONS

- Progressive heart failure
- Syncope
- Ventricular arrhythmias
- Sudden death

PROGNOSIS

- High morbidity and mortality (approximately 900,000 patients are hospitalized and up to 200,000 patients die annually)
- Approximately one-third to one-half of deaths in patients with congestive heart failure are due to progressive heart failure; the remainder die suddenly (presumably from ventricular arrhythmias)
- Annual mortality rate has improved to approximately 20–38% with current medical therapy

PREVENTION

- Primary prevention against myocardial infarction with control of risk factors
- Avoidance of cardiotoxic agents
- Treatment of disease associated with the development of heart failure

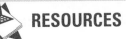

RESOURCES

PRACTICE GUIDELINES

- All patients with LV systolic dysfunction should be on therapeutic doses of ACE inhibitors or ARBs, beta blockers (Coreg or metoprolol), digoxin, and spironolactone in advanced cases except where contraindicated
- Diuretics should be given in doses to adequately control congestive symptoms without overdiuresis
- Electrophysiologic referral for possible implantable cardioverter defibrillator device implantation with or without biventricular pacing in patients with LV ejection fractions ≤ 30–35%
- Ventricular assist devices as a bridge to cardiac transplantation or for destination therapy in patients ineligible for cardiac transplantation

REFERENCES

- Drazner MH et al: Prognostic importance of elevated jugular venous pressure and a third heart sound in patients with heart failure. N Engl J Med 2001;345:574.
- Hunt S et al: ACC/AHA Guidelines for the Evaluation and Management of Chronic Heart Failure in the Adult: executive summary. J Am Coll Cardiol 2001;38:2007.

INFORMATION FOR PATIENTS

- http://www.americanheart.org/presenter.jhtml?identifier=1486
- http://www.emedicinehealth.com/Articles/10929-1.asp

WEB SITE

- http://www.emedicine.com/ped/topic2636.htm

Contrast Nephropathy

KEY FEATURES

ESSENTIALS OF DIAGNOSIS

- The peak rise in serum creatinine occurs within 2–5 days after the diagnostic procedure using IV contrast, and it returns to baseline in most cases
- Increase in serum creatinine of > 50% represents clinically important acute renal failure

GENERAL CONSIDERATIONS

- Most commonly seen after cardiac catheterization, especially if left ventricular angiography is carried out
- May be seen after CT scans or other diagnostic tests using contrast agents
- Hypoxic tubular injury due to vasoconstriction with release of free oxygen radicals is the likely mechanism
- Major risk factors:
  - Prior renal insufficiency
  - Diabetes mellitus
- Minor risk factors:
  - Congestive heart failure
  - Dehydration
  - Hypotension
  - Hypoxia
  - Large amount of contrast
  - Ionic and high osmolar contrast
  - Repeated examinations at short intervals
  - Abdominal examination
- Other possible risk factors:
  - Age
  - Smoking
  - Hypercholesterolemia
  - Use of nonsteroidal anti-inflammatory drugs

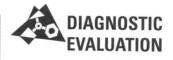

CLINICAL PRESENTATION

SYMPTOMS AND SIGNS

- No specific symptoms or signs

PHYSICAL EXAM FINDINGS

- No specific findings

DIFFERENTIAL DIAGNOSIS

- Atheroembolic renal failure
- Prerenal azotemia secondary to low cardiac output

DIAGNOSTIC EVALUATION

LABORATORY TESTS

- Increased serum creatinine over baseline before procedure using contrast
- Serum electrolytes: may be abnormal

ELECTROCARDIOGRAPHY

- Nonspecific ST-T–wave changes can occur
- Signs of hyperkalemia may occur

TREATMENT

HOSPITALIZATION CRITERIA

- Rising creatinine following procedure

MEDICATIONS

- When contrast nephropathy occurs, treatment is similar to that for any other cause of acute renal insufficiency
- Most patients improve spontaneously with conservative management

THERAPEUTIC PROCEDURES

- A few patients require temporary dialysis
- Need for long-term dialysis purely for contrast nephropathy is rare

SURGERY

- Shunt placement if long-term dialysis is needed

MONITORING

- ECG monitoring in hospital

DIET AND ACTIVITY

- As appropriate for renal and cardiac condition

ONGOING MANAGEMENT

HOSPITAL DISCHARGE CRITERIA

- Falling serum creatinine
- Resolution of the problem

FOLLOW-UP

- Visit in 4–8 weeks to confirm stable renal function

COMPLICATIONS

- Persistent renal dysfunction
- Chronic dialysis

PROGNOSIS

- Good if renal function returns to normal
- Persistent renal dysfunction decreases survival

PREVENTION

- Adequate hydration (0.45% normal saline at 1 mL/kg/hour for 12 hours before and 12 hours after the procedure): the most important therapy for preventing contrast nephropathy in high-risk patients
- *N*-acetylcysteine 600 mg orally twice daily before and after administration of the contrast agent is a useful adjunct for prevention in high-risk patients
- Fenoldopam (0.1 µg/kg/min), the dopamine-1 receptor agonist, is a useful adjunct in high-risk patients
- Iodixanol, an iso-osmolar contrast agent, is useful for prevention in high-risk patients

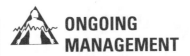 **RESOURCES**

PRACTICE GUIDELINES

- With creatinine levels > 2.0 mg/dL, the advisability of studies using contrast agents should be considered
- In those with creatinine levels above normal but below 2.0 mg/dL, precautions should be taken to prevent contrast nephropathy

REFERENCE

- Lindholt JS: Radiocontrast induced nephropathy. Eur J Vasc Endovasc Surg 2003;25:296.

Cor Pulmonale/Right-Heart Failure

 KEY FEATURES

ESSENTIALS OF DIAGNOSIS

- Respiratory or pulmonary vascular disease
- Elevated jugular venous pressure, hepatomegaly, peripheral edema
- Normal or near-normal LV function and filling pressures

GENERAL CONSIDERATIONS

- Alteration in the structure and function of the right ventricle (RV) caused by pulmonary hypertension (PH) due to a respiratory disorder or pulmonary vascular disease
- Pathophysiology: pulmonary vasoconstriction due to alveolar hypoxia or blood acidemia, reduced cross-sectional area of the pulmonary vascular bed
- Causes:
  - Lung disorders (eg, emphysema
  - Pulmonary embolism
  - Interstitial lung disease)
  - Increased blood viscosity (eg, polycythemia vera, sickle cell disease, macroglobulinemia)
  - Pulmonary arterial hypertension
- Acute right-heart failure may accompany acute respiratory failure or pulmonary embolism
- RV hypertrophy predominates in chronic pulmonary hypertensive states
- RV dilatation and dysfunction predominantly occur with acute cor pulmonale
- > 50% of cases are due to chronic obstructive pulmonary disease (COPD)
- Acute cor pulmonale is usually due to acute pulmonary thromboembolism

 CLINICAL PRESENTATION

SYMPTOMS AND SIGNS

- Symptoms may be vague and subtle, especially in the early stages
- Fatigue
- Dyspnea
- Syncope
- Chest discomfort (usually exertional)
- Palpitations
- Dizziness
- Cough
- Hemoptysis

PHYSICAL EXAM FINDINGS

- Tachypnea
- Tachycardia
- Systemic hypotension
- Elevated jugular venous pressure
- Labored respiratory efforts with retractions of the chest wall
- Hyperresonance to lung percussion
- Diminished breath sounds
- Pulmonary wheezes
- Left parasternal lift
- Distant heart sounds
- Accentuated pulmonic component of the S_2
- Split second heart sound that increases with inspiration
- Holosystolic murmur at the lower sternal border (tricuspid regurgitation)
- Diastolic murmur along the left sternal border due to pulmonary regurgitation may be present
- Right-sided S_3 and S_4
- Hepatomegaly; pulsatile liver (with severe tricuspid regurgitation)
- Abdominal fluid wave from ascites
- Peripheral edema
- Cyanosis

DIFFERENTIAL DIAGNOSIS

- Right-heart failure due to left-heart failure
- RV myocardial infarction
- Constrictive pericarditis
- Other cardiac causes of right-heart failure, such as pulmonic stenosis or atrial septal defect

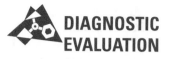 **DIAGNOSTIC EVALUATION**

LABORATORY TESTS

- CBC (polycythemia may be present)
- Electrolytes (hypokalemia from furosemide)
- Blood urea nitrogen and creatinine (prerenal azotemia due to decreased filling of the LV)
- Test for calcium, magnesium, and phosphate levels
- Serum uric acid level (may be elevated from diuretics)
- Liver function tests (elevated with hepatic congestion)
- Coagulation studies
- Antinuclear antibody and rheumatoid factor, hypercoagulability laboratories, HIV test, thyroid function test, serum alpha$_1$-antitrypsin (if deficiency is suspected) to exclude causes of PH

ELECTROCARDIOGRAPHY

- Sinus tachycardia
- Atrial fibrillation or flutter
- Premature atrial contractions
- Multifocal atrial tachycardia
- Junctional tachycardia
- Low-voltage QRS in patients with COPD
- Right atrial enlargement (P pulmonale)
- Right bundle branch block
- RV hypertrophy: R/S amplitude ratio > 1 mV in lead V1 and right-axis deviation (QRS axis of +110°)

IMAGING STUDIES

- Chest x-ray findings vary with underlying disorder
- Transthoracic echocardiography: RV hypertrophy may be present
  - RV dilatation with reduced systolic function
  - Septal deviation toward the LV during systole
  - Color-flow Doppler evidence of mild to severe functional tricuspid regurgitation
  - Pulmonary artery systolic pressure can be estimated by the tricuspid regurgitant jet
- Ventilation-perfusion lung scanning, contrast chest CT scan, or pulmonary angiography: exclude pulmonary emboli as an underlying cause of PH

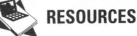

DIAGNOSTIC PROCEDURES

- Right-heart catheterization:
  - The gold standard method for diagnosis and quantification of PH
  - Required in patients in whom pulmonary vasodilator therapy is being considered

TREATMENT

CARDIOLOGY REFERRAL

- Acute or chronic right-heart failure
- Arrhythmias

HOSPITALIZATION CRITERIA

- Hypoxia
- Acute-onset or decompensated right-heart failure
- Syncope
- Tachy- or bradyarrhythmias
- Pulmonary embolism

MEDICATIONS

- Oxygen should be used liberally (including high-flow oxygen)
- CPAP for patients with sleep apnea
- Diuretics
- Correction of bronchospasm or other reversible pulmonary conditions
- Pulmonary vasodilators in selected patients with PH
- Theophylline may be considered for COPD
- Low-dose inotropes may be needed to facilitate diuresis
- Anticoagulation for pulmonary arterial hypertension and pulmonary emboli

THERAPEUTIC PROCEDURES

- Phlebotomy with saline replacement should be considered for an hematocrit > 65

SURGERY

- Lung or heart-lung transplantation for eligible patients
- Embolectomy for pulmonary thromboemboli
- Uvulopalatopharyngoplasty for selected patients with sleep apnea

MONITORING

- Pulse oximetry
- Telemetry
- Systemic blood pressure
- Fluid balance
- Pulmonary arterial catheter: may be helpful in critical patients

DIET AND ACTIVITY

- Fluid and sodium restriction
- Activity as tolerated

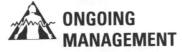
ONGOING MANAGEMENT

HOSPITAL DISCHARGE CRITERIA

- Adequate oxygenation
- Stable vital signs
- Compensated right-heart failure

FOLLOW-UP

- Close follow-up with pulmonologist and cardiologist
- Some patients may benefit from pulmonary rehabilitation program

COMPLICATIONS

- Progressive right-heart failure
- Arrrythmias
- Hypoxia
- Syncope
- Death

PROGNOSIS

- Related to underlying disease
- Five-year survival rate of 30% in patients with cor pulmonale due to COPD

PREVENTION

- Avoidance of tobacco smoke, air pollution, and other risk factors for respiratory disease
- Avoidance of risk factors for pulmonary arterial hypertension (anorexigens, amphetamines/cocaine)
- Oxygen therapy for hypoxic respiratory disease
- Appropriate treatment of sleep apnea

RESOURCES

PRACTICE GUIDELINES

- Appropriate treatment of the underlying pulmonary disease and adequate oxygenation can improve morbidity and mortality

REFERENCES

- Vieillard-Baron A, Sebastien P, Chergui K et al: Echo-Doppler demonstration of acute cor pulmonale at the bedside in the medical intensive care unit. Am J Respir Crit Care Med 2002;166:1310.
- Weitzenblum E. Chronic cor pulmonale. Heart 2003;89(2):225.

INFORMATION FOR PATIENTS

- http://www.nlm.nih.gov/medlineplus/ency/article/000129.htm

WEB SITE

- http://www.emedicine.com/med/topic449.htm

Coronary Artery Disease, Symptomatic Non-Revascularizable

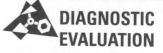 KEY FEATURES

ESSENTIALS OF DIAGNOSIS

- Persistent angina pectoris despite maximally tolerated doses of nitrates, beta blockers, and calcium channel blockers
- Diffuse coronary atherosclerosis not amenable to revascularization
- Relatively normal left ventricular function, which excludes heart transplantation

GENERAL CONSIDERATIONS

- This situation is uncommon
- Diffuse disease of the target vessels is the usual problem

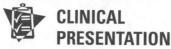 CLINICAL PRESENTATION

SYMPTOMS AND SIGNS

- Angina on exertion or at rest
- Shortness of breath

PHYSICAL EXAM FINDINGS

- S_4

DIFFERENTIAL DIAGNOSIS

- Precipitating or aggravating conditions such as hypertension, anemia, thyrotoxicosis
- Less than maximal medical therapy
- Second opinion on lack of feasibility of revascularization
- Patients with noncardiac advanced disease that prohibits revascularization

DIAGNOSTIC EVALUATION

LABORATORY TESTS

- CBC, metabolic panel
- Thyroid-stimulating hormone
- Lipid panel
- High sensitive C-reactive protein (hS-CRP)

ELECTROCARDIOGRAPHY

- 12-lead ECG (may show ST-segment depression)

IMAGING STUDIES

- Echocardiogram to evaluate left ventricular function (if left ventriculogram not done during angiogram)

DIAGNOSTIC PROCEDURES

- Coronary angiogram to define coronary anatomy

Coronary Artery Disease, Symptomatic Non-Revascularizable

 TREATMENT

CARDIOLOGY REFERRAL

- Refractory symptoms or need for hospitalization

HOSPITALIZATION CRITERIA

- Chest pain active and persistent
- Chest pain at rest or on minimal exertion

MEDICATIONS

- Antianginal medications titrated to maximal tolerated doses
- Statin group of medications to reduce low-density lipoproteins < 100 and hS-CRP below 1.0
- Narcotic analgesics if necessary

THERAPEUTIC PROCEDURES

- Enhanced external counterpulsation (EECP)
- Spinal cord stimulation
- Gene therapy locally, such as vascular endothelial growth factor, is under investigation

SURGERY

- Transmyocardial laser revascularization
- Transplantation is theoretically possible but seldom done if left ventricular function is normal

MONITORING

- ECG monitoring in hospital

DIET AND ACTIVITY

- Cardiac low-fat diet
- Exercise as tolerated

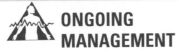 **ONGOING MANAGEMENT**

HOSPITAL DISCHARGE CRITERIA

- When symptoms are stable

FOLLOW-UP

- Depending on symptoms, every 4–12 weeks follow-up

COMPLICATIONS

- Myocardial infarction
- Frequent hospitalization secondary to unstable angina or non–ST-segment elevation myocardial infarction

PROGNOSIS

- Prognosis is generally guarded

PREVENTION

- Similar to atherosclerosis
- Low-fat diet
- Regular exercise
- Statins

RESOURCES

PRACTICE GUIDELINES

- EECP is the most available option with some benefit

REFERENCES

- Arora RR et al: The multicenter study of enhanced external counterpulsation (MUST-EECP): effect of EECP on exercise-induced myocardial ischemia and angina episodes. J Am Coll Cardiol 1999;33:1833.
- Roguin A, Beyar R: Interventional cardiology: promises and challenges. Isr Med Assoc J 1999;1:104.

INFORMATION FOR PATIENTS

- www.nhlbi.nih.gov/health/dci/Diseases/Cad/cad_WhatIs.html

WEB SITES

- www.americanheart.org

Cushing's Syndrome

 KEY FEATURES

ESSENTIALS OF DIAGNOSIS

- Excess cortisol in the circulation
- Central obesity
- Hypertension
- Hyperlipidemia
- Hyperglycemia

GENERAL CONSIDERATIONS

- Cushing's syndrome can be caused by an adrenocorticotropic hormone (ACTH)-producing pituitary tumor (Cushing's disease); ACTH production by other tumors, such as lung; glucocorticoid-secreting adrenal tumors; or exogenous steroid use
- Because of associated central obesity, hypertension, hyperglycemia, and hyperlipidemia, affected patients are at risk for coronary artery disease

 CLINICAL PRESENTATION

SYMPTOMS AND SIGNS

- Fatigue, dyspnea, and chest pain

PHYSICAL EXAM FINDINGS

- Central obesity, dorsal hump, plethoric facies, striae
- Signs of cardiac dysfunction

DIFFERENTIAL DIAGNOSIS

- Pseudo-Cushing's syndrome: patients appear cushingoid but have normal screening laboratory tests
- Other causes of obesity, hypertension, hyperlipidemia, and hyperglycemia

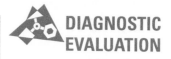 **DIAGNOSTIC EVALUATION**

LABORATORY TESTS

- Twenty-four-hour urine for free cortisol
- Overnight dexamethasone suppression test
- ACTH level if above tests are positive, to determine cause

ELECTROCARDIOGRAPHY

- Signs of myocardial ischemia/infarction may be present

IMAGING STUDIES

- CT scan usually identifies the tumor(s)

TREATMENT

CARDIOLOGY REFERRAL

• Suspected cardiac disease

HOSPITALIZATION CRITERIA

• Acute coronary syndrome
• Planned surgery

MEDICATIONS

• If surgery is not feasible, adrenolytic or adrenocortical-blocking pharmacologic agents can be used

SURGERY

• Surgical removal of the pituitary, adrenal, or ectopic tumor is usually definitive

MONITORING

• ECG monitoring in hospital as appropriate

DIET AND ACTIVITY

• Low-fat diet
• Restricted activity if heart disease is present

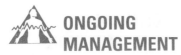

ONGOING MANAGEMENT

HOSPITAL DISCHARGE CRITERIA

• Resolution of problem
• Successful surgery

FOLLOW-UP

• Depends on condition

COMPLICATIONS

• Myocardial infarction
• Heart failure
• Cardiovascular death

PROGNOSIS

• Good with recognition and treatment. The longer the condition persists, the more likely coronary artery disease will occur

RESOURCES

PRACTICE GUIDELINES

• Diagnosis requires three steps:–Screening for excess cortisol–Confirmation to exclude exogenous steroid ingestion
  – Determination of the cause (ACTH levels)

REFERENCE

• Boscaro M et al: The diagnosis of Cushing's syndrome: atypical presentations and laboratory shortcomings. Arch Intern Med 2000;160:3045.

INFORMATION FOR PATIENTS

• www.nlm.nih.gov/medlineplus/ency/article/000410.htm

WEB SITE

• www.emedicine.com/med/topic485.htm

Deep Venous Thrombosis

 KEY FEATURES

ESSENTIALS OF DIAGNOSIS

- Lower leg pain, swelling, erythema
- Palpable chord, especially in the calf
- Duplex ultrasound evidence of thrombus
- Evidence of thrombus on CT or magnetic resonance angiography

GENERAL CONSIDERATIONS

- There are three basic mechanisms of venous thrombus formation (Virchow's triad):
  - Venous stasis
  - Vessel wall damage
  - Hypercoagulability
- Venous stasis is usually caused by:
  - Extrinsic compression from adenopathy or tumors
  - Fibrosis or tumors
  - Also can be caused by low flow states, such as heart failure
- Endothelial damage, such as during limb surgery, exposes blood to the arterial media that contains tissue factors that initiate the cascade leading to blood clotting
- Hypercoagulability can be genetic or acquired
  - Genetic examples are deficiencies in factors V Leiden and protein C or S
  - Acquired examples are estrogen therapy and antiphospholipid antibody syndrome

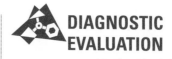 **CLINICAL PRESENTATION**

SYMPTOMS AND SIGNS

- Pain and swelling in an extremity, usually a lower leg
- Bilateral swelling less likely thrombotic in origin

PHYSICAL EXAM FINDINGS

- Pitting edema
- Tenderness to palpation along the deep vein distribution
- Homan's sign (pain on dorsiflexion of the foot) is uncommon
- A palpable venous chord is unusual unless there is also superficial venous involvement
- Phlegmasia cerulea dolens is rare (ie, severe pain and swelling accompanied by cyanosis [tissue ischemia])

DIFFERENTIAL DIAGNOSIS

- Ruptured Baker's cyst
- Abscesses
- Ruptured plantaris tendon
- Muscle strain
- Tumors

DIAGNOSTIC EVALUATION

LABORATORY TESTS

- D-dimer (thrombin breakdown products) positivity is nonspecific, but a negative test is very specific
- Factors II, VIII, and V Leiden; protein S and C; antithrombin III; anticardiolipin antibodies, and homocysteine levels

ELECTROCARDIOGRAPHY

IMAGING STUDIES

- Duplex ultrasonography can identify thrombus in veins
- MRI is useful for distinguishing new from old thrombi
- CT scan of the leg is becoming more widely used in conjunction with CT scans of the chest for pulmonary emboli

DIAGNOSTIC PROCEDURES

- Contrast venography

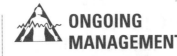

TREATMENT

CARDIOLOGY REFERRAL

- Suspected pulmonary embolus

HOSPITALIZATION CRITERIA

- Any suspected deep venous thrombosis

MEDICATIONS

- Systemic anticoagulation for 3–6 months
- Locally delivered thrombolysis in selected cases

THERAPEUTIC PROCEDURES

- Inferior vena cava filter placement early to prevent pulmonary emboli in selected patients with later removal in some

SURGERY

- Inferior vena cava ligation is rarely done today
- Thrombectomy in selected patients

MONITORING

- Anticoagulation with unfractionated heparin or warfarin

DIET AND ACTIVITY

- Bed rest until leg pain gone

ONGOING MANAGEMENT

HOSPITAL DISCHARGE CRITERIA

- Pain resolved
- Adequate anticoagulation achieved—INR 2.0–3.0—unless on unfractionated heparin

FOLLOW-UP

- Three months, 6 months, 12 months, then yearly

COMPLICATIONS

- Pulmonary embolus in up to 40%
- Chronic venous insufficiency in 20%
- Anticoagulation related bleeding in 1–3%

PROGNOSIS

- Depends on cause of venous disease

PREVENTION

- Low molecular weight heparin 1–1.5 mg/kg subcutaneously every 12 hours
- Early ambulation after surgery
- Intermittent pneumatic compression of the legs if at bed rest
- Elastic stockings

RESOURCES

PRACTICE GUIDELINES

- Venous thromboembolism is the most common disorder of veins
- The cornerstone of deep venous thrombosis prevention and treatment is anticoagulant therapy
- Although serious complications from deep venous thrombosis can occur, such as pulmonary embolus and chronic venous insufficiency, most patients do well

REFERENCES

- Bush RL et al: Pharmacomechanical thrombectomy for treatment of symptomatic lower extremity deep venous thrombosis: safety and feasibility study. J Vasc Surg 2004;40:965.
- Hoff WS et al: Early experience with retrievable inferior vena cava filters in high-risk trauma patients. J Am Coll Surg 2004;199:869.

INFORMATION FOR PATIENTS

- www.drpen.com/453.9

WEB SITE

- www.emedicine.com/med/topic2785.htm

Diabetic Cardiomyopathy

KEY FEATURES

ESSENTIALS OF DIAGNOSIS

- Diabetes mellitus type 2, especially in women
- Unexplained heart failure without hypertension or large epicardial coronary artery disease
- Left ventricular hypertrophy with systolic and diastolic dysfunction by echocardiography

GENERAL CONSIDERATIONS

- In addition to being a risk factor for macrovascular atherosclerosis, diabetes produces a microvascular disease that can involve the heart leading to left ventricular hypertrophy
- Microvascular disease is associated with endothelial dysfunction
- Insulin sensitivity, lipid-lowering agents, and angiotensin-modulating drugs improve endothelial function
- Because diabetics often have painless myocardial infarction, macrovascular coronary artery disease must be excluded in diabetics with heart failure
- Diabetes frequently coexists with hypertension, which can lead to left ventricular hypertrophy and heart failure

CLINICAL PRESENTATION

SYMPTOMS AND SIGNS

- Dyspnea, fatigue
- Chest pain

PHYSICAL EXAM FINDINGS

- Hypertension in some
- Left ventricular lift
- S_3 or S_4

DIFFERENTIAL DIAGNOSIS

- Atherosclerotic cardiovascular disease with silent infarction
- Hypertensive heart disease
- Other causes of heart failure

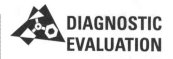 DIAGNOSTIC EVALUATION

LABORATORY TESTS

- Glucose, hemoglobin A_{1c}
- Lipid panel
- Liver function tests

ELECTROCARDIOGRAPHY

- ECG findings:
  - left ventricular hypertrophy
  - Left atrial abnormality

IMAGING STUDIES

- Echocardiogram:
  - Left ventricular, left atrial enlargement
  - Systolic and diastolic dysfunction may be seen

DIAGNOSTIC PROCEDURES

- Coronary angiography may be necessary to exclude macrovascular coronary artery disease

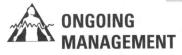

 TREATMENT

CARDIOLOGY REFERRAL

- Suspected cardiac disease

HOSPITALIZATION CRITERIA

- Heart failure
- Significant tachyarrhythmias

MEDICATIONS

- Tight control of blood glucose (hemoglobin A_{1c} < 7.0%)
- Angiotensin-converting enzyme inhibitors titrated to achieve blood pressure < 130/85 mm Hg
- Correction of dyslipidemia
- Other treatment for heart failure as needed
- Aspirin 81 mg/day PO

THERAPEUTIC PROCEDURES

- Percutaneous coronary revascularization may be indicated in some

SURGERY

- Coronary bypass surgery may be required

MONITORING

- ECG monitoring in hospital

DIET AND ACTIVITY

- Diabetic diet plus low-sodium diet
- Exercise as tolerated

ONGOING MANAGEMENT

HOSPITAL DISCHARGE CRITERIA

- Resolution of problem
- After successful procedure or surgery

FOLLOW-UP

- Careful management of diabetes is important

COMPLICATIONS

- Heart failure
- Serious arrhythmias
- Myocardial infarction

PROGNOSIS

- Diabetic cardiomyopathy reduces survival

PREVENTION

- Tight diabetes and blood pressure control reduces cardiac event rates

RESOURCES

PRACTICE GUIDELINES

- To prevent microvascular disease hemoglobin A_{1c} should be maintained at < 7.0%, blood pressure < 130/85 mm Hg, low-density lipoprotein cholesterol < 100 mg/dL, triglycerides < 150 mg/dL, high-density lipoprotein cholesterol > 45 mg/dL in women and > 55 mg/dL in men

REFERENCE

- Sowers JR et al: Diabetes, hypertension, and cardiovascular disease: an update. Hypertension 2001;37:1053.

INFORMATION FOR PATIENTS

- www.nlm.nih.gov/medlineplus/ency/article/000313.htm

WEB SITE

- www.emedicine.com/med/topic547.htm

Digitalis Toxicity

 KEY FEATURES

ESSENTIALS OF DIAGNOSIS

- Elevated serum level of a digitalis compound
- Gastrointestinal symptoms with altered color vision
- Cardiac arrhythmias, especially premature ventricular beats and heart block

GENERAL CONSIDERATIONS

- May occur in up to 30% of patients hospitalized for heart failure
- Common clinical features:
  - Nausea and vomiting
  - Anorexia
  - Malaise
  - Drowsiness
  - Headache
  - Insomnia
  - Altered color vision
  - Arrhythmia
- Almost all known cardiac arrhythmias may be caused by digitalis toxicity
- Toxicity is facilitated by hypokalemia
  - Severe digoxin toxicity causes hyperkalemia secondary to paralysis of Na^+/K^+ exchange pump
- Diuretics cause hypokalemia and thus facilitate digitalis toxicity
- Other drugs, such as amiodarone and verapamil, increase digitalis serum levels

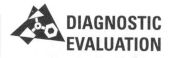 **CLINICAL PRESENTATION**

SYMPTOMS AND SIGNS

- Nausea, vomiting, diarrhea, anorexia
- Drowsiness, malaise, headache, altered color vision
- Palpitation

PHYSICAL EXAM FINDINGS

- Bradycardia is common
- Tachycardia can occur

DIFFERENTIAL DIAGNOSIS

- Arrhythmias secondary to underlying heart disease
- Gastrointestinal disorders
- Central nervous system disorders

DIAGNOSTIC EVALUATION

LABORATORY TESTS

- Low potassium (common)
- Reduced renal function—may contribute
- Creatinine level: elevated
- Digoxin level: outside therapeutic range

ELECTROCARDIOGRAPHY

- Premature ventricular contractions
- First-, second-, and third-degree heart block
- Atrial tachycardia with 2:1 block
- Alternating ventricular tachycardia
- Junctional tachycardia, often with atrial fibrillation

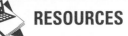

 TREATMENT

CARDIOLOGY REFERRAL

- Suspected digoxin toxicity
- Serious ventricular arrhythmias
- Symptomatic bradycardia

HOSPITALIZATION CRITERIA

- Serious ventricular arrhythmias
- Second- or third-degree heart block
- Need for digoxin antibody therapy

MEDICATIONS

- Reversal of symptoms or cessation of arrhythmia occurs after withdrawal of digoxin for 48 hours
- Ventricular arrhythmia may require phenytoin or lidocaine 100 mg IV
- Antidigoxin immunotherapy may be used, particularly if hyperkalemia is present

MONITORING

- ECG monitoring in hospital

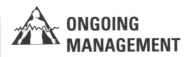 **ONGOING MANAGEMENT**

HOSPITAL DISCHARGE CRITERIA

- Resolution of problem
- Digoxin level in therapeutic range

FOLLOW-UP

- Serum digoxin level and ECG 10–14 days after new dosage

COMPLICATIONS

- Cardiac arrest
- Syncope

PROGNOSIS

- Excellent with appropriate treatment

PREVENTION

- Serum digoxin level 10–14 days after starting therapy
- Reduce digoxin dose when starting drugs that interact with it and recheck digoxin levels in 2 weeks

RESOURCES

PRACTICE GUIDELINES

- The safest way to initiate digoxin therapy is with the expected dialysis maintenance dose
- Because of the long half-life of digoxin, it takes 10–14 days to reach a steady state
- The usual maintenance dosage is 0.25 mg PO daily (0.125–0.5); lower doses should be given for renal insufficiency or small lean body mass
- If more rapid action is required to control rapid atrial fibrillation, for example, 1.0 mg can be given over 24 hours in divided doses 4–6 hours apart

REFERENCE

- Rathore SS et al: Association of serum digoxin concentration and outcomes in patients with heart failure. JAMA 2003;289:871.

INFORMATION FOR PATIENTS

- www.nlm.nih.gov/medlineplus/ency/article/000165.htm

WEB SITE

- www.emedicine.com/med/topic568.htm

Ebstein Anomaly

 KEY FEATURES

ESSENTIALS OF DIAGNOSIS

- History of dyspnea, atypical chest pain, or intermittent cyanosis
- Palpitations associated with supraventricular arrhythmias and preexcitation syndrome (Wolff-Parkinson-White [WPW])
- Right parasternal lift, widely split S_1, systolic clicks, and systolic murmur of tricuspid regurgitation (without inspiratory accentuation)
- Right atrial enlargement, right bundle branch block, posteriorly directed delta waves with accessory pathway by ECG; frequent first-degree atrioventricular block
- Normal or reduced pulmonary vascularity without pulmonary artery enlargement, right atrial enlargement, normal left-sided cardiac silhouette on chest radiograph
- Apical displacement of septal tricuspid valve leaflet, variable degrees of tricuspid regurgitation originating from apical portion of right ventricle, and enlarged right atrium on echocardiography

GENERAL CONSIDERATIONS

- Ebstein's anomaly is characterized by deformity of the tricuspid valve with apical displacement of the septal and posterior leaflets
- A variable degree of tricuspid regurgitation is present and is dependent on the extent of apical displacement and maladaptation of the tricuspid leaflets
- Right ventricular pump function may be inadequate if the proportion of right ventricle proximal to the leaflets (atrialized right ventricle) is substantial and the remaining right ventricle is inadequate
- Cyanosis may be present as a result of right-to-left shunting across a patent foramen ovale in the presence of significant tricuspid regurgitation or elevated right atrial pressures
- Atrial septal defect is the most common associated anomaly
- Twenty-five–30% of patients have an accessory pathway with preexcitation (WPW) and a tendency for supraventricular tachyarrhythmias

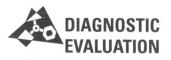 **CLINICAL PRESENTATION**

SYMPTOMS AND SIGNS

- Tremendous variability in clinical presentation exists, depending on the morphology and physiologic consequences of the tricuspid valve disorder and associated anomalies
- Dyspnea
- Arrhythmias, including WPW syndrome
- Decreased exercise tolerance

PHYSICAL EXAM FINDINGS

- Variable cyanosis
- Right parasternal lift
- Widely split S_1
- Systolic clicks from delayed tricuspid valve closure
- Systolic murmur of tricuspid regurgitation that does not increase in intensity during inspiration owing to the inability of the right ventricle to accept an increase in venous return
- S_3 and S_4 gallops may be present
- An early diastolic snap may be present from the opening of an elongated anterior tricuspid leaflet

DIFFERENTIAL DIAGNOSIS

- Other causes of tricuspid regurgitation
- Other causes of exertional dyspnea, chest pressure, and intermittent cyanosis
- Other causes of supraventricular arrhythmias
- Other causes of congestive heart failure

DIAGNOSTIC EVALUATION

ELECTROCARDIOGRAPHY

- Right atrial enlargement
- Right bundle branch block
- PR interval may be prolonged, except in the presence of an accessory pathway
- WPW syndrome
- Atrial fibrillation may be present in older patients

IMAGING STUDIES

- Chest x-ray:
  - Normal or reduced pulmonary vasculature without pulmonary artery enlargement
  - Right atrial enlargement, normal left atrium and left ventricle size
- Echocardiography:
  - Elongated anterior tricuspid leaflet with increased excursion and delayed closure
  - Abnormal apical displacement of the septal tricuspid valve leaflet
  - Enlarged right atrium
  - Reduced right ventricle size (variable)
  - Variable degrees of tricuspid regurgitation
  - Pulmonary artery systolic pressure is usually normal
  - Atrial septal defect or patent foramen ovale may be present and visualized by two-dimensional color flow and/or saline contrast injection

DIAGNOSTIC PROCEDURES

- Cardiac catheterization: simultaneous recordings of a right ventricle electrogram and right atrial pressure tracing with a catheter in the atrialized right ventricle is considered pathognomonic of Ebstein's anomaly

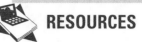

TREATMENT

CARDIOLOGY REFERRAL

- Signs or symptoms of right heart failure
- History of syncope
- Suspected arrhythmia

HOSPITALIZATION CRITERIA

- Right heart failure
- Supraventricular tachycardia
- Syncope

MEDICATIONS

- Diuretics as needed for right heart failure
- Atrioventricular nodal blockers (eg, calcium channel blockers or beta blockers) for narrow complex tachycardias and/or antiarrhythmic drugs
- Avoid atrioventricular nodal blockers with atrial fibrillation in patient with WPW

THERAPEUTIC PROCEDURES

- Catheter ablation of bypass tracts and other foci of supraventricular arrhythmia
- Device closure of an atrial septal defect in certain patients with exercise-induced cyanosis

SURGERY

- Tricuspid valve repair or replacement
- Fontan procedure (connection of systemic venous drainage to the pulmonary artery) in certain patients with inadequate right ventricular size and function

MONITORING

- Event monitoring for suspected supraventricular tachyarrhythmias in patients with palpitations and/or dizziness or syncope

DIET AND ACTIVITY

- Low-sodium diet for patients with right heart failure
- Avoidance of cardiac stimulants
- In the absence of severe Ebstein's anomaly and arrhythmias, patients may participate in competitive sports

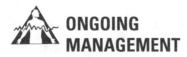

ONGOING MANAGEMENT

HOSPITAL DISCHARGE CRITERIA

- After stabilization of cardiac rhythm disturbances
- After successful surgery or catheter-based procedures

FOLLOW-UP

- Visit with cardiologist within 2 weeks of hospital discharge

COMPLICATIONS

- Recurrent supraventricular arrhythmias due to bypass tracts or right atrial enlargement
- Progressive right heart failure or tricuspid regurgitation

PROGNOSIS

- Fifty percent survival to age 50 years
- Survival depends on the degree of anatomic and physiologic abnormalities

PREVENTION

- Prevention of supraventricular arrhythmias with catheter ablation of bypass tracts

RESOURCES

PRACTICE GUIDELINES

- ECG, chest x-ray, echocardiogram, pulse oximetry at rest and/or during exercise, electrophysiology study (if documented or suspected atrial arrhythmia) every 1–3 years
- Surgery is indicated for patients with congestive heart failure/deteriorating exercise capacity, progressive cyanosis at rest or with exercise, progressive cardiac enlargement, systemic embolization despite anticoagulation, NYHA Class II symptoms with repairable valve, atrial fibrillation

REFERENCES

- DiRusso GB et al: Ebstein's anomaly: Indications for repair and surgical technique. In: Spray TL et al, eds: Semin Thorac Cardiovasc Surg Pediatr Card Surg Annu 1999.

INFORMATION FOR PATIENTS

- www.achaheart.org

WEB SITES

- www.americanheart.org
- www.pediheart.org

Effort Syncope

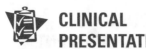 KEY FEATURES

ESSENTIALS OF DIAGNOSIS

- Sudden transient loss of consciousness during exercise, especially unaccustomed exercise, with rapid spontaneous recovery
- Absence of prodromal symptoms
- History of heart disease, heart murmurs, or other cardiac symptoms

GENERAL CONSIDERATIONS

- Usually secondary to a hemodynamic abnormality
- Stenotic valvular heart disease and left ventricular outflow tract abnormality are the most frequent hemodynamic causes
- Once experienced, patients usually avoid the same type of exertion
- Exercised-induced ventricular tachycardia (VT) is uncommon
- Exercised-related VT is more likely to be idiopathic
- Intracardiac tumors such as atrial myxoma are a rare cause of effort syncope

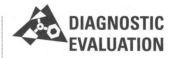 CLINICAL PRESENTATION

SYMPTOMS AND SIGNS

- Effort syncope
- Other symptoms depend on the underlying cause for effort syncope
- History of avoiding the exertion that precipitated syncope
- Dyspnea may be present in patients with significant valvular heart disease
- Chest pain in some patients

PHYSICAL EXAM FINDINGS

- Depends on the underlying cause
- Auscultation:
  - Ejection murmur in aortic stenosis and hypertrophic cardiomyopathy, the most common causes
  - *Tumor plop* during early diastole in left atrial myxoma
- Clinical examination may be normal if the precipitating cause is an arrhythmia or ischemia

DIFFERENTIAL DIAGNOSIS

- Severe aortic stenosis
- Hypertrophic obstructive cardiomyopathy
- Discrete subaortic stenosis or supravalvular aortic stenosis
- Severe mitral stenosis
- Severe pulmonic stenosis
- Severe pulmonary hypertension
- Intracardiac tumors
- Arrhythmia-induced syncope
- Transient myocardial ischemia
- Severe left ventricular dysfunction

DIAGNOSTIC EVALUATION

LABORATORY TESTS

- CBC, brain natriuretic peptide

ELECTROCARDIOGRAPHY

- ECG: abnormality noted depends on the underlying cause
- Exercise treadmill ECG in patients with structurally normal heart and effort syncope to identify arrhythmogenic causes

IMAGING STUDIES

- Echocardiogram to identify and quantify valvular heart disease, myocardial disease, cardiac tumor, and left ventricular function

DIAGNOSTIC PROCEDURES

- Coronary angiogram if transient severe ischemia is the leading suspicion for the effort syncope
- Rarely electrophysiologic study may be required (generally not very helpful)

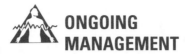

TREATMENT

CARDIOLOGY REFERRAL

• All patients should be evaluated by a cardiologist

HOSPITALIZATION CRITERIA

• Most patients require an in-hospital evaluation unless an echocardiogram is completely normal

MEDICATIONS

• Treat the underlying condition
• Avoid unaccustomed exertion

THERAPEUTIC PROCEDURES

• Depends on the underlying cause

SURGERY

• Depends on the underlying cause

MONITORING

• Depends on the underlying cause

DIET AND ACTIVITY

• Depends on the underlying cause

ONGOING MANAGEMENT

HOSPITAL DISCHARGE CRITERIA

• After adequate treatment of underlying cause

FOLLOW-UP

• Depends on the underlying cause

COMPLICATIONS

• Depends on the underlying cause

PROGNOSIS

• Depends on the underlying cause

PREVENTION

• Depends on the underlying cause

RESOURCES

PRACTICE GUIDELINES

• Effort syncope is associated with organic heart disease
• Investigations must be done for the first episode

REFERENCES

• Haner KE: Discovering the cause of syncope. A guide to the focused evaluation. Postgrad Med 2003;113:31.
• O'Connor FG, Oriscello RG, Levine BD: Exercise-related syncope in the young athlete: reassurance, restriction or referral? Am Fam Physician 1999;60:2001.

INFORMATION FOR PATIENTS

• www.drpen.com/hd424.1
• www.nlm.nih.gov/medlineplus/arrhythmia.html

WEB SITES

• www.acc.org
• www.hrsonline.org

Eisenmenger Syndrome

KEY FEATURES

ESSENTIALS OF DIAGNOSIS

- History of murmur or cyanosis in infancy
- Symptoms of dyspnea and exercise intolerance since childhood
- Hemoptysis, chest pain, and syncope in the adult
- Clubbing, cyanosis, and prominent pulmonic component of S_2
- Compensatory erythrocytosis, iron deficiency, and hyperuricemia
- Right ventricular hypertrophy; large central pulmonary arteries with peripheral pruning on chest radiograph
- Severe right ventricular hypertrophy and right atrial enlargement and elevated pulmonary artery pressures
- Detection of a bidirectional shunt by echocardiography or cardiac catheterization

GENERAL CONSIDERATIONS

- Defined as pulmonary hypertension and shunt reversal in the presence of a congenital defect such as ventricular septal defect, atrial septal defect, atrioventricular canal defect, aortopulmonary window, or patent ductus arteriosus
- Pulmonary hypertension usually develops before puberty, the exception being the patient with ostium secundum atrial septal defect who acquires pulmonary vascular disease after puberty
- Hemoptysis is occasionally due to bronchitis or pneumonia, although pulmonary infarction and pulmonary arteriolar rupture are potentially fatal complications that must be excluded
- Pregnancy is contraindicated because of an unacceptably high rate of maternal and fetal mortality
- Patients with marked secondary polycythemia may develop symptoms and signs of hyperviscosity syndrome, especially with hematocrit levels above 70%

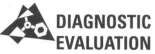 CLINICAL PRESENTATION

SYMPTOMS AND SIGNS

- Murmur or cyanosis during infancy
- Exertional dyspnea is most common symptom
- Chest pain, hemoptysis, and presyncope are less common
- Transient bacteremias can lead to brain abscesses because of right-to-left shunting

PHYSICAL EXAM FINDINGS

- Cyanosis (more pronounced in the lower extremities when associated with a patent ductus arteriosus)
- Right ventricular parasternal heave
- Accentuated P_2
- Jugular venous pressure may be elevated in right ventricular failure and the *a* wave may be prominent
- Systolic murmur of the tricuspid regurgitation may be present
- High-pitched diastolic murmur of the pulmonic regurgitation (Graham Steele murmur) is common
- Hepatomegaly, ascites, and peripheral edema may be present

DIFFERENTIAL DIAGNOSIS

- Pulmonary emboli
- Other causes of hemoptysis, chest pain, and syncope
- Other causes of cyanosis

DIAGNOSTIC EVALUATION

LABORATORY TESTS

- Elevated hematocrit with an increase in red blood cell mass
- Iron deficiency is common after injudicious phlebotomies
- Hyperuricemia caused by an increase in red cell turnover may be present

ELECTROCARDIOGRAPHY

- Right atrial enlargement
- Right ventricular hypertrophy with right-axis deviation
- A leftward or superior axis suggests an ostium primum atrial septal defect or atrioventricular canal defect as underlying cause

IMAGING STUDIES

- Chest x-ray: right atrial enlargement, right ventricular enlargement, prominent proximal pulmonary arteries with pruning of the peripheral pulmonary vessels and pulmonary oligemia
- Echocardiography:
  - Severe right atrial enlargement and right ventricular hypertrophy
  - Variable right ventricular dysfunction
  - Small underfilled left ventricle
  - Deviated septum toward the left ventricle
  - Pulmonary and tricuspid insufficiency
  - The level of the shunt can be aided by color-flow Doppler and saline contrast injection
  - The peak right ventricular systolic pressure can be estimated from the peak tricuspid regurgitant velocity
  - Mitral regurgitation is present with an ostium primum atrial septal defect

DIAGNOSTIC PROCEDURES

- Cardiac catheterization: elevated pulmonary artery pressure, increased pulmonary vascular resistance, and right-to-left shunting
  - Oxygen, nitric oxide, or other pulmonary vasodilators is administered to determine whether pulmonary vascular reactivity persists
  - The degree of left-to-right shunting is calculated

TREATMENT

CARDIOLOGY REFERRAL

- Patients with exertional presyncope, syncope, worsened dyspnea, or cyanosis
- Signs and symptoms of right heart failure

HOSPITALIZATION CRITERIA

- Hemoptysis
- Symptomatic hypotension
- Syncope
- Signs or symptoms of endocarditis or brain abscess
- Decompensated right heart failure

MEDICATIONS

- Digoxin and diuretics for right heart failure
- Pulmonary vasodilator therapy may improve symptoms in these patients

THERAPEUTIC PROCEDURES

- Phlebotomy when hematocrit > 65%
- Intravenous saline should be administered in a volume equal to that phlebotomized

SURGERY

- Once pulmonary vascular resistance is fixed (no response to oxygen or nitric oxide), surgical correction of the underlying shunt is contraindicated
- Heart-lung transplantation

MONITORING

- Telemetry
- Intakes and outflows, daily weights
- Serum hematocrit

DIET AND ACTIVITY

- Encourage oral fluid intake
- Activity as tolerated

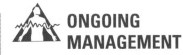

ONGOING MANAGEMENT

HOSPITAL DISCHARGE CRITERIA

- Stable medications

FOLLOW-UP

- See cardiologist within 2 weeks of discharge
- For patients with severe polycythemia, regular follow-up serum hematocrit levels with phlebotomy as needed

COMPLICATIONS

- Hyperviscosity syndrome
- Gout
- Bleeding diathesis
- Pulmonary infarction or pulmonary arteriolar rupture

PROGNOSIS

- In patients who are severely symptomatic and undergo transplantation, survival with heart and lung transplantations appears to be better than with double lung transplantation, especially in patients with ventricular septal defect or multiple congenital anomalies
- Most patients die from progressive heart failure, sudden cardiac death, or intrapulmonary hemorrhage

PREVENTION

- Early surgical repair of congenital left-to-right shunts is key to preventing pulmonary vascular disease

RESOURCES

PRACTICE GUIDELINES

- Pulmonary vasodilator therapy may improve hemodynamics and the quality of life in some patients
- Avoidance of high-risk situations, such as pregnancy, high altitude, volume depletion, and exercise is important
- Extreme caution should be taken when noncardiac surgery is considered because even relatively minor surgery is potentially life-threatening
- Heart and lung or lung transplantation with repair of the cardiac defect may be appropriate in some patients with severe disease

REFERENCE

- Waddell TK et al: Heart-lung or lung transplantation for Eisenmenger syndrome. J Heart Lung Transplant 2002;21:731.

INFORMATION FOR PATIENTS

- www.achaheart.org

WEB SITES

- www.americanheart.org
- www.pediheart.org

Endocarditis, Infective

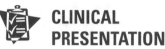 KEY FEATURES

ESSENTIALS OF DIAGNOSIS

- Major criteria:
  - ≥ Two positive blood cultures with a typical microbe
  - New murmur or echocardiogram finding of oscillating mass, abscess, or prosthetic valve dehiscence
- Minor criteria:
  - Predisposing cardiac condition or IV drug use
  - Fever ≥ 38 ° Celsius
  - Vascular phenomena, such as Osler's nodes, Janeway lesions
  - Immunologic phenomena, such as splenomegaly
  - Echocardiogram consistent with endocarditis, but not meeting major criteria
  - Positive blood culture, but not meeting major criteria, or positive serology for a combatable microbe
- Definite diagnosis:
  - Positive histology or positive culture from a vegetation
  - Two major criteria
  - One major and three minor criteria
  - All six minor criteria
- Diagnosis rejected:
  - Alternative diagnosis established
  - Resolution of illness after ≤ 4 days of antibiotics
- Possible diagnosis:
  - Neither definite nor rejected

GENERAL CONSIDERATIONS

- Infective endocarditis represents an endothelial infection that usually occurs at sites of endothelial damage, with the superimposed thrombus serving as the nidus
- For the nidus to become infected, bacteria must enter the bloodstream in sufficient numbers from a break in the epidermal or mucosal surfaces of the body
- As the vegetation grows, regurgitation of the affected valve almost always occurs due to destruction, scarring, or retraction of the leaflet
- Occasionally, chordal involvement results in rupture, causing sudden severe atrioventricular valve regurgitation
- Very large vegetations rarely can obstruct the valve orifice

- Embolization of vegetations can result in damage to other organs from ischemia or remote infection
- Invasion of the valve annulus by the organisms can lead to abscesses and fistulas
- Infection of arterial walls due to vegetation embolization can lead to aneurysm formation and rupture, which can be devastating in the central nervous system

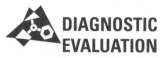 CLINICAL PRESENTATION

SYMPTOMS AND SIGNS

- Malaise, weight loss, fatigue, night sweats, fever, chills, arthralgias, myalgias
- Specific symptoms due to sites of damage, such as dyspnea with heart failure due to severe valvular regurgitation

PHYSICAL EXAM FINDINGS

- Osler's node, Janeway lesion, petechiae, splinter hemorrhages, Roth spots, blue toe syndrome
- Fever
- Regurgitant heart murmurs, especially new or worsening
- Signs of heart failure
- Signs of stroke
- Splenomegaly

DIFFERENTIAL DIAGNOSIS

- Fever due to other causes
- Sepsis not due to infective endocarditis
- Valvular lesions on echocardiography that resemble vegetations (eg, myxomatous valves)

DIAGNOSTIC EVALUATION

LABORATORY TESTS

- Blood cultures: three from separate venipunctures over 24 hours
- Serologic testing for organisms such as *Histoplasma*, Q fever, *Brucella*
- Rheumatoid factor may be falsely positive
- Leukocytosis, elevated gamma globulins, elevated erythrocyte sedimentation rate, anemia

ELECTROCARDIOGRAPHY

- Aortic valve abscess formation can lead to first-, second-, or third-degree heart block
- Increased QRS voltage in acute aortic or mitral regurgitation owing to left ventricular volume increase

IMAGING STUDIES

- Chest x-ray: may show cardiomegaly, pulmonary edema, or septic pulmonary emboli (right-sided endocarditis)
- Echocardiography
  - Transesophageal echocardiography is the preferred diagnostic technique because of its high sensitivity and specificity compared with transthoracic echocardiography
  - Findings that are almost certainly endocarditis include (major criteria) oscillating low-density masses, abscess, fistulas, prosthetic valve dehiscence
  - Probable endocarditis findings include localized leaflet thickening, nonmobile valve-related masses, chordal rupture, aortic leaflet prolapse, paraprosthetic valve regurgitation (minor criteria)
  - Possible endocarditis findings include valve lesions such as diffuse thickening, which could be a substrate for endocarditis, but specific findings are not seen
  - A negative echocardiographic study does not completely rule out endocarditis, but makes it less likely
  - If clinical suspicion remains high, a repeat study should be done in 5 days

DIAGNOSTIC PROCEDURES

- Rarely, cardiac catheterization is done to draw blood cultures in proximity of the valve lesions

TREATMENT

CARDIOLOGY REFERRAL

- Suspected endocarditis
- Heart failure
- Myo-pericarditis

HOSPITALIZATION CRITERIA

- Suspected endocarditis

MEDICATIONS

- Appropriate antibiotic therapy

SURGERY

- Cardiac surgery, usually to replace the infected valve(s)

MONITORING

- ECG and blood pressure monitoring as appropriate in the hospital
- Repeat blood cultures to assess response to therapy

DIET AND ACTIVITY

- Restricted activity
- Low-salt diet

ONGOING MANAGEMENT

HOSPITAL DISCHARGE CRITERIA

- Resolution of problem
- Sufficient IV therapy to warrant oral antibiotics
- Successful surgery

FOLLOW-UP

- After course of antibiotics, repeat blood cultures and echocardiogram in 2–4 weeks; then careful clinical follow-up at 3-, 6-, then 12-month intervals

COMPLICATIONS

- Heart failure, pulmonary edema
- Pericarditis/myocarditis
- Myocardial infarction
- Heart block
- Stroke
- Brain abscess
- Renal failure
- Sudden death

PROGNOSIS

- Despite modern antibiotics and improved surgical techniques, mortality rate for patients with infective endocarditis is almost 40%

PREVENTION

- Antibiotic prophylaxis for invasive procedures/surgery in naturally colonized places such as the mouth, and gastrointestinal tract in patients with the substrate for endocarditis, such as rheumatic valvular disease, audible heart murmurs, or cyanotic congenital heart disease

RESOURCES

PRACTICE GUIDELINES

- Absolute indications for valve surgery in endocarditis:
  - Intracardiac abscess or fistula
  - Left heart failure
  - Endocarditis due to fungi or gram-negative organisms
  - New prosthetic valve paravalve regurgitation, fistula, abscess, or dehiscence

REFERENCE

- Li JS et al: Proposed modifications to the Duke criterion for the diagnosis of infective endocarditis. Clin Infect Dis 2000;30:633.

INFORMATION FOR PATIENTS

- www.nlm.nih.gov/medlineplus/ency/article/001098.htm

WEB SITE

- www.emedicine.com/med/topic671.htm

Friedreich's Ataxia, Cardiac Manifestations

 ## KEY FEATURES

ESSENTIALS OF DIAGNOSIS

- Neurologic symptoms usually precede cardiac symptoms
- Frequently associated with concentric hypertrophic cardiomyopathy
- Echocardiography shows left ventricular hypertrophy
- ECG may not show changes of hypertrophy despite echocardiographic evidence
- Widespread T-wave inversion is detected on ECG

GENERAL CONSIDERATIONS

- An autosomal recessive disorder, Friedreich's ataxia is characterized by ataxia, areflexia, and extremity muscle weakness due to degeneration of the spinocerebellar tracts
- Almost all Friedreich's patients have cardiac involvement
- Cardiac hypertrophy is the most common heart manifestation and may lead to sudden death
- Cardiac manifestations appear with or up to 20 years after neurologic symptoms

CLINICAL PRESENTATION

SYMPTOMS AND SIGNS

- Dyspnea
- Palpitation

PHYSICAL EXAM FINDINGS

- Left ventricular lift
- S_4
- Harsh systolic outflow tract murmur

DIFFERENTIAL DIAGNOSIS

- Hypertrophic cardiomyopathy (asymmetric septal hypertrophy may occur, but myocardial fiber disarray as described in genetic hypertrophic cardiomyopathy is rare)

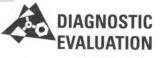 ## DIAGNOSTIC EVALUATION

ELECTROCARDIOGRAPHY

- Almost all patients have ECG abnormalities; the most common in order of prevalence are:
  - ST-T–wave changes
  - Right axis deviation
  - Short PR interval
  - Tall R in V1
  - Inferolateral Q waves

IMAGING STUDIES

- Echocardiogram may show:
  - Concentric left ventricular hypertrophy
  - Asymmetric septal hypertrophy
  - Global hypokinesis
  - Diastolic dysfunction

TREATMENT

CARDIOLOGY REFERRAL

- Suspected cardiac disease

HOSPITALIZATION CRITERIA

- Heart failure
- Syncope
- Rapid tachyarrhythmias

MEDICATIONS

- Symptomatic management of arrhythmias with drugs
- Pharmacologic management of heart failure
- Antioxidants have helped some patients

THERAPEUTIC PROCEDURES

- Automatic implanted cardioverter-defibrillator in selected patients

MONITORING

- ECG monitoring in hospital patients as appropriate

DIET AND ACTIVITY

- Low-sodium diet if heart failure is present
- Restricted activity as appropriate for cardiac disease

ONGOING MANAGEMENT

HOSPITAL DISCHARGE CRITERIA

- Resolution of heart failure
- Successful device placement

FOLLOW-UP

- As appropriate for cardiac condition

COMPLICATIONS

- Heart failure
- Syncope
- Progressive neuromuscular debilitation

PROGNOSIS

- Because the neuromuscular disease cannot be arrested, it usually causes death; however, a few patients develop a malignant form of dilated cardiomyopathy

PREVENTION

- This is an inherited disease

RESOURCES

PRACTICE GUIDELINES

- Heart transplantation is usually not indicated because the neuromuscular disease is progressive

REFERENCES

- Blamire AM et al: Antioxidant treatment improves in vivo cardiac and skeletal muscle bioenergetics in patients with Friedreich's ataxia. Ann Neurol 2001;49:560.
- Weidemann F et al: Quantification of regional right and left ventricular function by ultrasonic strain rate and strain indexes in Friedreich's ataxia. Am J Cardiol 2003;91:622.

INFORMATION FOR PATIENTS

- www.nlm.nih.gov/medlineplus/ency/article/001411.htm

WEB SITE

- www.emedicine.com/neuro/topic265.htm

Heart Disease in Pregnancy

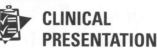

KEY FEATURES

ESSENTIALS OF DIAGNOSIS

- Pregnancy
- History of heart disease
- Symptoms, signs, and echocardiographic evidence of heart disease

GENERAL CONSIDERATIONS

- Heart disease occurs in < 5% of pregnancies
- Congenital heart disease and valvular disease are most common
- Hemodynamic changes of normal pregnancy challenge the diagnosis and management of heart disease
- Risks to mother and fetus need to be considered
- Relative contraindications to pregnancy:
  - Occlusive pulmonary vascular disease
  - Severe pulmonary hypertension
  - Marfan syndrome with dilated aorta
  - Severe aortic stenosis
  - Severe left ventricular dysfunction
  - Cyanotic congenital heart disease

CLINICAL PRESENTATION

SYMPTOMS AND SIGNS

- Atrial septal defect: usually well tolerated unless significant anemia or atrial arrhythmias develop
- Pulmonic stenosis: mild to moderate stenosis is well tolerated; severe stenosis may result in congestive heart failure
- Coarctation of the aorta: major risks are fetal underdevelopment and maternal hypertension
- Tetralogy of Fallot: increased cyanosis, syncope, and sudden death
- Mitral stenosis: dyspnea, fatigue, orthopnea, and syncope
- Mitral valve prolapse with mitral regurgitation: usually well tolerated unless regurgitation is severe
- Aortic valve disease: mild to moderate disease well tolerated
- Peripartum cardiomyopathy: symptoms of left heart failure must be distinguished from symptoms and signs of normal pregnancy
- Hypertrophic cardiomyopathy: usually well tolerated if asymptomatic before pregnancy
- Coronary artery disease: angina most common presentation; myocardial infarction can occur
- Symptomatic arrhythmias often due to underlying cardiac disease
- Primary pulmonary hypertension: dyspnea, fatigue, chest pain, palpitation, and syncope

PHYSICAL EXAM FINDINGS

- Findings normal to pregnancy include: increased resting heart rate, wide pulse pressure, jugular venous distention, edema, increased amplitude of left ventricular impulse, loud split S_1 and S_2, S_3, and innocent flow murmur:
- Cervical venous hum (decreases with sitting) and mammary soufflé may be confused with pathologic findings
- Pregnancy augments the murmurs of aortic, mitral, and pulmonic stenosis, but decreases the murmurs of aortic and mitral regurgitation and hypertrophic obstructive cardiomyopathy
- The midsystolic click and murmur of mitral valve prolapse are less prominent during pregnancy

DIFFERENTIAL DIAGNOSIS

- Symptoms from increased cardiac output in normal pregnancy, such as fatigue, dyspnea on exertion, and reduced exercise tolerance
- Symptoms from reduced peripheral resistance in normal pregnancy, such as orthostatic intolerance
- Symptoms from compression of the inferior vena cava by the gravid uterus, such as orthopnea
- Signs of increased blood volume in normal pregnancy, such as systolic ejection murmur at the left sternal border

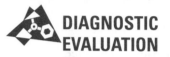

DIAGNOSTIC EVALUATION

LABORATORY TESTS

- Positive pregnancy test
- CBC may show mild dilutional anemia

ELECTROCARDIOGRAPHY

- Sinus tachycardia
- Leftward axis shift
- Nonspecific ST-T changes

IMAGING STUDIES

- Chest x-ray (only if necessary), with abdominopelvic shielding
  - Elevated diaphragm and horizontal heart position not to be interpreted as evidence of cardiopulmonary disease
- Echocardiography: safe and highly desirable test for most heart diseases suspected during pregnancy; normal physiologic changes include increased chamber sizes and increased stroke volume
  - Evidence of mitral valve prolapse may disappear as well as Doppler left ventricular outflow tract gradients in hypertrophic cardiomyopathy

TREATMENT

CARDIOLOGY REFERRAL

- History of significant cardiac disease
- Symptoms out of proportion to pregnancy
- Signs of cardiac disease
- Abnormal echocardiogram

HOSPITALIZATION CRITERIA

- Heart rates > 120 bpm
- Heart failure
- Syncope
- Evidence of myocardial ischemia
- New or worsening cynanosis

MEDICATIONS

- Avoid unnecessary drug treatment of cardiac conditions, especially in first trimester. Unsafe drugs include angiotensin-converting enzyme inhibitors, angiotensin-receptor blockers, amiodarone, calcium channel blockers, and warfarin
- Heart failure can be treated with digoxin, hydralazine, diuretics, and nitrates
- Arrhythmias can be treated with digoxin, adenosine, quinidine, procainamide, lidocaine, and beta blockers
- Necessary anticoagulation for patients with prosthetic valves: heparin for the first trimester, then warfarin until 36–38 weeks, then heparin again until 4–6 hours after delivery
- Primary pulmonary hypertension can be safely treated with prostacyclin infusions, but premature labor may occur

THERAPEUTIC PROCEDURES

- Vaginal delivery with regional anesthesia; antibiotic prophylaxis given when indicated
- Cardioversion appropriate for hemodynamic compromise due to tachyarrhythmia
- Primary pulmonary hypertension: vaginal delivery with epidural anesthesia is safe
- Percutaneous valvuloplasty (mitral or pulmonic) is feasible during pregnancy

SURGERY

- Cardiac surgery is feasible during pregnancy, but heart-lung bypass often causes fetal wastage

MONITORING

- ECG monitoring during labor and delivery for those with heart disease or arrhythmias
- Hemodynamic monitoring with a right heart catheter during labor and delivery up to 48 hours for pregnant patients with symptomatic heart disease

DIET AND ACTIVITY

- For heart failure during pregnancy: salt and activity restrictions, but maintaining adequate volume is important to avoid decreased uterine blood flow

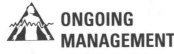

ONGOING MANAGEMENT

HOSPITAL DISCHARGE CRITERIA

- Resolution of tachyarrhythmias
- Resolution of heart failure

FOLLOW-UP

- Problems during pregnancy due to increased intravascular volume may persist during lactation
- Baseline evaluation or tests should be delayed until after lactation if possible

COMPLICATIONS

- Peripartum hemorrhage can lead to severe problems
- Vaginal delivery is normally preferred
  - Cesarean section should be done for obstetric indications
- Pulmonary embolism: heparin can be used but thrombolytics are contraindicated
- Infective endocarditis is a rare but devastating complication

PROGNOSIS

- The greatest risk for maternal mortality (25–50%) is with:
  - Pulmonary hypertension
  - Coarctation of the aorta
  - Marfan syndrome with dilated aorta
- Pulmonary vascular disease, mitral stenosis, aortic stenosis, mechanical prosthetic valves, and uncorrected congenital heart disease carry a 5–10% maternal mortality rate
- Volume-loading conditions such as left-to-right shunts, bioprosthetic valves, and corrected congenital heart disease have a 1% maternal mortality rate

PREVENTION

- Patients with high-risk conditions should not become pregnant or should consider an early therapeutic abortion
- Endocarditis prophylaxis is not recommended for uncomplicated labor and delivery
- Urinary or vaginal infections or complicated deliveries: antibiotic prophylaxis for mechanical heart valves, congenital heart disease (except atrial septal defect), hypertrophic cardiomyopathy, and mitral valve prolapse with mitral regurgitation

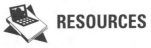

RESOURCES

PRACTICE GUIDELINES

- Depends on specific condition

REFERENCES

- Colman JM, Sermer M, Seaward PG et al: Congenital heart disease in pregnancy. Cardiol Rev 2000;8:166.
- Elkayam U, Tummala PT, Rao K et al: Maternal and fetal outcomes of subsequent pregnancies in women with peripartum cardiomyopathy. N Engl J Med 2001;344:1567.
- Joglar JA, Page RI: Antiarrhythmic drugs in pregnancy. Curr Opin Cardiol 2001;16:40.
- Mauri L, O'Gara PT: Valvular heart disease in the pregnant patient. Curr Treat Options Cardiovasc Med 2001;3:7.
- Stewart R, Tuazon D, Olson G et al: Pregnancy and primary pulmonary hypertension: successful outcome with epoprostenol therapy. Chest 2001;119:973.

INFORMATION FOR PATIENTS

- www.americanheart.org/presenter .jhtml?identifier=4688

WEB SITE

- www.merck.com/mrkshared/mmanual/ section18/chapter251/251b.jsp

Hemochromatosis and the Heart

KEY FEATURES

ESSENTIALS OF DIAGNOSIS

- Fasting transferrin saturation > 50–60% is a sensitive screening test
- Conduction abnormalities, arrhythmias, and heart failure
- History of severe anemia with repeated blood transfusion
- Bronze skin, diabetes, and liver cirrhosis

GENERAL CONSIDERATIONS

- Autosomal recessive iron storage disease that involves the heart, as well as the pancreas, skin, liver, and gonads
- Usually causes dilated cardiomyopathy, but may cause restrictive cardiomyopathy
- Conduction abnormalities and supraventricular and ventricular arrhythmias occur in one third of patients
- Primary iron overload is due to inappropriately increased iron absorption from the gut
- Secondary iron overload is due to repeated blood transfusions for severe anemia often due to thalassemia

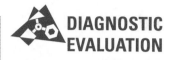

CLINICAL PRESENTATION

SYMPTOMS AND SIGNS

- Dyspnea, fatigue, edema
- Diabetes
- Hepatic cirrhosis, liver failure or hepatoma
- Pituitary failure

PHYSICAL EXAM FINDINGS

- Irregular pulse, bradycardia, or tachycardia
- Signs of congestive heart failure
- Bronze skin

DIFFERENTIAL DIAGNOSIS

- Idiopathic dilated cardiomyopathy
- Idiopathic restrictive cardiomyopathy

DIAGNOSTIC EVALUATION

LABORATORY TESTS

- Fasting transferrin saturation > 50%

ELECTROCARDIOGRAPHY

- Conduction disturbances
- Supraventricular or ventricular tachycardia

IMAGING STUDIES

- Echocardiography: may show a dilated cardiomyopathy or a restrictive cardiomyopathy

DIAGNOSTIC PROCEDURES

- Myocardial biopsy may be required in some cases to establish the cause of cardiomyopathy

TREATMENT

CARDIOLOGY REFERRAL

- Significant arrhythmias
- Heart failure

HOSPITALIZATION CRITERIA

- Severe heart failure
- Heart block
- Hemodynamically significant cardiac arrhythmias

MEDICATIONS

- Iron chelation with desferrioxamine

THERAPEUTIC PROCEDURES

- Phlebotomy (cardiomyopathy may show dramatic recovery)

SURGERY

- Cardiac transplantation in advanced cases

MONITORING

- ECG monitoring in hospital as appropriate

ONGOING MANAGEMENT

HOSPITAL DISCHARGE CRITERIA

- Resolution of problem

FOLLOW-UP

- Frequent and throughout long

COMPLICATIONS

- Heart block
- Syncope
- Cardiogenic shock
- Sudden death

PROGNOSIS

- Cardiac disease causes death in about one third of hemachromatosis patients

PREVENTION

- Aggressive iron chelation therapy reduces the progression of myocardial dysfunction and mortality

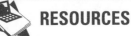

RESOURCES

PRACTICE GUIDELINES

- Phlebotomy is effective for removing iron and improving myocardial function in primary hemachromatosis
- Iron chelation therapy is more effective than phlebotomy in chronic anemia cases

REFERENCE

- Mahon NG et al: Haemochromatosis gene mutations in idiopathic dilated cardiomyopathy. Heart 2000;84:541.

INFORMATION FOR PATIENTS

- www.drpen.com/425.7

WEB SITE

- www.emedicine.com/med/topic289.htm

High-Altitude Pulmonary Edema

KEY FEATURES

ESSENTIALS OF DIAGNOSIS

- Rapid ascent to altitude over 7200 feet
- Symptoms and signs of pulmonary edema
- Likelihood increased by higher elevations, vigorous physical activity, alcohol consumption, cold exposure, and a history of altitude sickness

GENERAL CONSIDERATIONS

- High-altitude pulmonary edema (HAPE) is potentially life threatening
- HAPE is a form of noncardiac pulmonary edema that typically affects healthy individuals who ascend rapidly to high altitudes
- Typically, HAPE appears after 6–24 hours of exposure to high altitude
- HAPE rarely occurs below 8000 feet (2440 meters), and most occur at > 10,000 feet (3050 meters)
- The altitude at which one sleeps is as important as the altitude where activity takes place
- In addition to pulmonary edema, HAPE leads to in situ pulmonary artery thrombosis and right heart strain
- The pathophysiology of HAPE is poorly understood

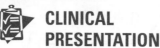 CLINICAL PRESENTATION

SYMPTOMS AND SIGNS

- Dyspnea, orthopnea, cough, hemoptysis (pink frothy sputum)
- Chest pressure
- Headache, fatigue, nausea

PHYSICAL EXAM FINDINGS

- Tachycardia
- Tachydyspnea
- Low-grade fever
- Edema
- Anoxia, cyanosis
- Pulmonary rales, wheezes

DIFFERENTIAL DIAGNOSIS

- Acute myocardial infarction
- Exacerbation of preexisting heart condition
- Pulmonary embolus
- Pneumonia

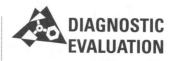 DIAGNOSTIC EVALUATION

LABORATORY TESTS

- Increased hematocrit

ELECTROCARDIOGRAPHY

- Acute right heart strain pattern

IMAGING STUDIES

- Chest x-ray: pulmonary congestion with normal heart size
- Echocardiogram: right heart enlargement with Doppler evidence of pulmonary hypertension

TREATMENT

CARDIOLOGY REFERRAL

- Suspected coronary artery disease

HOSPITALIZATION CRITERIA

- All patients with HAPE

MEDICATIONS

Treatment

- Descend to a lower altitude as soon as possible
- Oxygen
- Nifedipine 20 mg every 8 hours to lower pulmonary pressure
- Nitric oxide inhalation (40 ppm)

THERAPEUTIC PROCEDURES

- Hyperbaric pressure bag

MONITORING

- ECG in hospital

DIET AND ACTIVITY

- Low-sodium diet
- Restrict activity

ONGOING MANAGEMENT

HOSPITAL DISCHARGE CRITERIA

- Resolution of HAPE

FOLLOW-UP

- None necessary because cardiac function is usually normal

COMPLICATIONS

- Death
- High-altitude cerebral edema
- Hypotension
- Pulmonary emboli
- Arrhythmias

PROGNOSIS

- Excellent with prompt, effective treatment

PREVENTION

- Avoid exertion for 24 hours
- Avoid alcohol for 24 hours
- "Climb high, sleep low" (eg, sleep at a lower altitude than one climbs during the day)
- Avoid dehydration
- Salmeterol may prevent HAPE

RESOURCES

PRACTICE GUIDELINES

- Prevention is the best strategy and acclimation before exertion at high altitude is the cornerstone

REFERENCES

- Sartori C et al: Salmeterol for the prevention of high-altitude pulmonary edema. N Engl J Med 2002;346:1631.
- Swenson ER et al: Pathogenesis of high-altitude pulmonary edema: inflammation is not an etiologic factor. JAMA 2002;287:2228.

INFORMATION FOR PATIENTS

- www.nlm.nih.gov/medlineplus/ency/article/000133.htm

High-Output Heart Failure

KEY FEATURES

ESSENTIALS OF DIAGNOSIS

- Symptoms and signs of congestive heart failure
- Echocardiographic or right-heart catheterization evidence of high cardiac output and normal systolic function
- Presence of a stimulus for high cardiac demands (eg, severe anemia, thyrotoxicosis, Paget's disease, arteriovenous fistula, beriberi, following-liver transplantation)

GENERAL CONSIDERATIONS

- High demand for cardiac output may not be adequately met, leading to:
  - Reduced organ perfusion and compensatory mechanisms, such as salt and water retention
  - Congestion despite normal or elevated cardiac output
- Left ventricular systolic and diastolic function are usually normal, but may be reduced if increased demand is incessant

CLINICAL PRESENTATION

SYMPTOMS AND SIGNS

- Dyspnea, fatigue, edema

PHYSICAL EXAM FINDINGS

- Typical findings of congestive heart failure
- Sinus tachycardia frequent

DIFFERENTIAL DIAGNOSIS

- Diastolic heart failure: normal systolic function, but low cardiac output
- Systolic dysfunction heart failure
- Fluid overload, usually iatrogenic

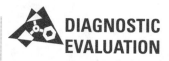 DIAGNOSTIC EVALUATION

LABORATORY TESTS

- Tests of underlying problem: hemoglobin, thyroid hormones, and others

ELECTROCARDIOGRAPHY

- Increased voltage may be present

IMAGING STUDIES

- Echocardiography
  - Mild chamber enlargement
  - Doppler evidence of high cardiac output

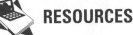

 TREATMENT

CARDIOLOGY REFERRAL

• Heart failure

HOSPITALIZATION CRITERIA

• Depends on underlying disease since heart failure is usually mild

MEDICATIONS

• Eliminate the underlying cause
• Give diuretics to relieve congestion

MONITORING

• ECG monitoring in hospital as appropriate

DIET AND ACTIVITY

• Low-sodium diet
• Restricted activities

ONGOING MANAGEMENT

HOSPITAL DISCHARGE CRITERIA

• Resolution of problem

FOLLOW-UP

• Depends on underlying problem

COMPLICATIONS

• Eventual systolic dysfunction

PROGNOSIS

• Excellent with relief of underlying problem

PREVENTION

• Avoid conditions that excessively increase cardiac demand

RESOURCES

PRACTICE GUIDELINES

• Echocardiography: indicated for all new cases of congestive heart failure and identifies this subtype

REFERENCE

• Pfitzmann R et al: Liver transplantation for treatment of intrahepatic Osler's disease: first experiences. Transplantation 2001;72:237.

INFORMATION FOR PATIENTS

• www.drpen.com/428

WEB SITE

• www.emedicine.com/med/topic3552.htm

Hibernating and Stunned Myocardium

KEY FEATURES

ESSENTIALS OF DIAGNOSIS

- Stunned: prolonged myocardial contractile dysfunction after a brief period of absent or reduced blood flow
- Hibernating: myocardial contractile dysfunction associated with reduced blood flow that reverses with revascularization
- Imaging evidence of myocardial viability in areas of reduced myocardial contractility:
  - Delayed thallium uptake
  - Wall motion response to dobutamine infusion
  - Metabolic activity on positron emission tomography scan

GENERAL CONSIDERATIONS

- Affects both systolic and diastolic function
- Stunned myocardium recognized by persistent wall motion abnormalities even after chest pain, ST-segment deviation and regional perfusion have recovered
- Lack of recovery after a few weeks suggestive of true infarction or scar formation
- Intracellular calcium overload has a significant role in stunning
- Hibernating myocardium is recognized by improvement of left ventricular function after revascularization of chronic ischemia
- Hibernation may be related to dedifferentiation with altered mitochondrial function and reduced adenosine triphosphate utilization
- Recovery of function may occur over days to weeks in both situations
- Transient improvement occurs in both situations with inotopic stimulation

CLINICAL PRESENTATION

SYMPTOMS AND SIGNS

- Stunned myocardium:
  - Persistent shortness of breath after an infarction despite evidence of reperfusion
  - A similar situation may occur with cardioplegia during cardiopulmonary bypass (lack of recovery after a few weeks suggests true infarction)
- Hibernation:
  - Persistent dyspnea in chronic coronary artery disease

PHYSICAL EXAM FINDINGS

- Hypotension may be present
- S_3 may be present
- Occasionally S_4

DIFFERENTIAL DIAGNOSIS

- Stunned: acute ischemia with compromised blood flow
- Hibernating: infarcted myocardium

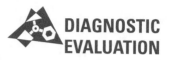 DIAGNOSTIC EVALUATION

LABORATORY TESTS

- CBC, brain natriuretic peptide

ELECTROCARDIOGRAPHY

- ECG may show infarction or ischemia

IMAGING STUDIES

- Resting echocardiogram to evaluate left ventricular function after adequate revascularization or reperfusion
- Thallium-201 imaging: unimpaired thallium extraction at areas of regional wall motion with late uptake on delayed imaging
- Dobutamine echocardiogram:
  - Improvement of function at areas of resting regional wall motion (biphasic response with hibernation)
  - Improvement with low-dose dobutamine and deterioration with higher dose

DIAGNOSTIC PROCEDURES

- Coronary angiography to define anatomy in hibernation before revascularization

TREATMENT

CARDIOLOGY REFERRAL

- All patients must be evaluated by a cardiologist

HOSPITALIZATION CRITERIA

- Stunned myocardium is usually seen in a hospitalized setting
- Hibernation:
  - Most patients undergo evaluation in a hospitalized setting before revascularization
  - This can be done in stable patients on outpatient basis

MEDICATIONS

- Stunned: calcium channel blockers, angiotensin-converting enzyme inhibitors, positive inotropic agents, circulatory support (see cardiogenic shock)
- Hibernating: coronary artery revascularization

THERAPEUTIC PROCEDURES

- Percutaneous coronary intervention (PCI) for hibernating myocardium

SURGERY

- Coronary artery bypass graft for hibernating myocardium

MONITORING

- ECG and hemodynamic monitoring in the hospital

DIET AND ACTIVITY

- Same as for coronary artery disease

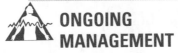

ONGOING MANAGEMENT

HOSPITAL DISCHARGE CRITERIA

- After revascularization, when clinically stable

FOLLOW-UP

- Follow-up for coronary artery disease

COMPLICATIONS

- Persistent heart failure if stunning does not recover
- Persistent left ventricular dysfunction in hibernation if revascularization is inadequate

PROGNOSIS

- Depends on extent and duration of hibernation
- Long-term prognosis depends on left ventricular function after recovery from hibernating myocardium

PREVENTION

- Similar to that for any atherosclerosis
- Low-fat diet
- Aerobic exercise
- Statins

RESOURCES

PRACTICE GUIDELINES

- Reassess left ventricular function 3 months after myocardial infarction (MI) if the ejection fraction soon after the MI is low
- Consider evaluation for hibernating myocardium if there is low ejection fraction and a fixed defect on nuclear stress study
- Revascularization improves left ventricular function and prognosis if there is hibernating myocardium

REFERENCES

- Galasko GI, Lahiri A: The non-invasive assessment of hibernating myocardium in ischaemic cardiomyopathy: a myriad of techniques. Eur J Heart Fail 2003;5(3):217.
- Schinkel AF et al: Dobutamine-induced contractile reserve in stunned, hibernating, and scarred myocardium in patients with ischemic cardiomyopathy. J Nucl Med 2003;44:127.

INFORMATION FOR PATIENTS

- www.nhlbi.nih.gov/health/dci/Diseases/Cad/CAD_WhatIs.html

WEB SITE

- www.americanheart.org

Hyperaldosteronism, Primary

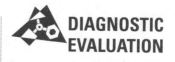

KEY FEATURES

ESSENTIALS OF DIAGNOSIS

- Hypertension due to sodium and water retention
- Hypokalemia and alkalosis
- Suppressed plasma renin and elevated aldosterone
- Imaging results showing adrenal adenoma or hyperplasia

GENERAL CONSIDERATIONS

- Increased autonomous production of aldosterone by the adrenal gland
- This causes sodium retention, plasma volume expansion, and hypertension
- Renal loss of potassium and bicarbonate cause hypokalemia and alkalosis
  - Patients usually identified because of hypertension and hypokalemia

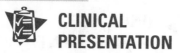

CLINICAL PRESENTATION

SYMPTOMS AND SIGNS

- Usually asymptomatic

PHYSICAL EXAM FINDINGS

- Hypertension, rarely severe

DIFFERENTIAL DIAGNOSIS

- Other causes of hypertension (primary aldosteronism accounts for 10–20% of hypertensive patients referred to hypertension clinics)
- Other causes of hypokalemia

DIAGNOSTIC EVALUATION

LABORATORY TESTS

- Serum potassium reduced
  - Hypokalemia
  - Reduced plasma renin activity
  - Elevated plasma aldosterone

ELECTROCARDIOGRAPHY

- Occasionally left ventricular hypertrophy or left atrial abnormality is seen

IMAGING STUDIES

- CT scan distinguishes adrenal hyperplasia from adenoma

DIAGNOSTIC PROCEDURES

- Aldosterone suppression test
- Adrenal vein aldosterone levels in selected cases

TREATMENT

CARDIOLOGY REFERRAL

- Suspected cardiac disease

HOSPITALIZATION CRITERIA

- Planned surgery

MEDICATIONS

- Aldosterone antagonists for adrenal hyperplasia: spironolactone 100–400 mg/day PO or eplerenone 50–100 mg/day
- Calcium channel blockers

SURGERY

- Surgical resection of adenoma

DIET AND ACTIVITY

- Low-sodium diet

ONGOING MANAGEMENT

HOSPITAL DISCHARGE CRITERIA

- Successful surgery

FOLLOW-UP

- Depends on situation

COMPLICATIONS

- Those of systemic hypertension

PROGNOSIS

- Excellent with early recognition and management

PREVENTION

- Serum potassium off diuretics should be part of every hypertension evaluation

RESOURCES

PRACTICE GUIDELINES

- This diagnosis should be considered:
  - Inpatients with hypertension and spontaneous hypokalemia, resistant hypertension, incidental adrenal masses on imaging studies
  - In patients suspected of having secondary hypertension

REFERENCE

- Young WF Jr: Primary aldosteronism: a common and curable form of hypertension. Cardiol Rev 1999;7:2107.

INFORMATION FOR PATIENTS

- www.drpen.com/276.8

WEB SITE

- www.emedicine.com/med/topic432.htm

Hyperlipidemia (Lipid Disorders)

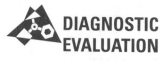

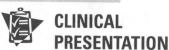

KEY FEATURES

ESSENTIALS OF DIAGNOSIS

- Total serum cholesterol > 200 mg/dL in two samples at least 2 weeks apart
- Low-density lipoprotein (LDL) cholesterol > 100 mg/dL
- High-density lipoprotein (HDL) cholesterol < 40 mg/dL
- Triglycerides > 150 mg/dL

GENERAL CONSIDERATIONS

- Elevated total and LDL cholesterol are risk factors for coronary artery disease
- Oxidation of LDL leads to rapid uptake by foam cells lining the arterial wall leading to cholesterol plaque
- The liver plays a role in removing LDL from the blood via the LDL receptor
- HDL cholesterol exerts a protective effect by removing cholesterol from the circulation and returning it to the liver
- Hyperlipidemia may be primary or the result of other diseases such as diabetes, hypothyroidism, renal failure, or alcoholism

CLINICAL PRESENTATION

SYMPTOMS AND SIGNS

- Usually asymptomatic

PHYSICAL EXAM FINDINGS

- Eruptive xanthomas are present if triglycerides are high
- Tendon xanthomas and tuberous xanthomas are characteristic of familial hypercholesterolemia
- Palmer and tuboeruptive xanthomas are seen in familial dyes–beta-lipoproteinemia
- Xanthelasmas are nonspecific and can be found in persons with normal lipids

DIFFERENTIAL DIAGNOSIS

- Hypothyroidism increases LDL cholesterol
- Nonfasting state increases triglycerides
- Diabetes increases triglycerides, reduces HDL cholesterol
- Alcohol increases triglycerides
- Oral contraceptives increase triglycerides
- Nephrotic syndrome increases LDL cholesterol and triglycerides
- Renal failure increases LDL cholesterol and triglycerides
- Primary biliary cirrhosis increases LDL cholesterol
- Acute hepatitis increases triglycerides
- Obesity increases triglycerides

DIAGNOSTIC EVALUATION

LABORATORY TESTS

- Total cholesterol, LDL and HDL cholesterol, triglycerides, liver function tests, creatinine kinase

TREATMENT

CARDIOLOGY REFERRAL

• Suspected cardiovascular disease

MEDICATIONS

• Bile acid sequestrants: cholestyramine, colestipol, colesevelam
• Intestinal endothelium blockers: ezetimibe 10 mg/day PO
• Fibric acid derivatives: gemfibrozil, clofibrate, fenofibrate
• Nicotinic acid 500–2000 mg/day PO
• Hepatic 3-methylglutaryl coenzyme A reductase inhibitors: atorvastatin, pravastatin, simvastatin, lovastatin, rosuvastatin, fluvastatin

MONITORING

• Lipid profile yearly in adults with normal values
• Lipid profile every 3 months during lifestyle modification until stable; then yearly
• Lipid profile monthly during drug therapy titration until stable; then every 6 months
• Liver function tests and creatinine kinase should be measured once after stable, then repeated only if symptoms develop

DIET AND ACTIVITY

• Exercise, weight loss, low-fat diet (cholesterol < 200 mg/day, fat < 30% of total calories, saturated fat < 7% of total calories), and high-fiber diet

ONGOING MANAGEMENT

FOLLOW-UP

• Every 6–12 months

COMPLICATIONS

• Atherosclerosis and its complications
• Side effects of drugs
  – Rhabdomyolysis with statins is most serious, though rare

PROGNOSIS

• Excellent, if lipid values can be normalized by diet or drugs

PREVENTION

• Effective lipid lowering reduces cardiovascular event rates

RESOURCES

PRACTICE GUIDELINES

• Lipid goals are based on the Framingham Study risks of a cardiovascular event
• LDL goals
  – Coronary artery disease or risk equivalents < 100 mg/dL
  – 2+ risk factors, 10-year risk < 20% <130 mg/dL
  – 0–1 risk factor, 10-year risk < 10% < 160 mg/dL
• HDL goals
  – Men > 40 mg/dL
  – Women >50 mg/dL
• Triglyceride goals < 150 mg/dL

REFERENCE

• Expert Panel on Detection, Evaluation, and Treatment of High Blood Cholesterol in Adults: executive summary of the Third Report of the National Cholesterol Education Program (NCEP) Expert Panel on Detection, Evaluation, and Treatment of High Blood Cholesterol in Adults (Adult Treatment Panel III). JAMA 2001;285:2486.

INFORMATION FOR PATIENTS

• www.drpen.com/272.0
• www.drpen.com/272.4

WEB SITES

• www.emedicine.com/med/topic1072.htm
• www.emedicine.com/med/topic1073.htm

Hyperparathyroidism and the Heart

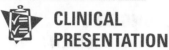 **KEY FEATURES**

ESSENTIALS OF DIAGNOSIS

- Elevated serum calcium due to parathyroid hormone excess
- Valvular sclerosis and left ventricular hypertrophy
- Shortened ST segment and reduced QT interval on ECG
- Acute hypercalcemia can cause hypertension, bradycardia, and heart block

GENERAL CONSIDERATIONS

- The most common cause of hyperparathyroidism is overproduction of parathyroid hormone (PTH) from a parathyroid adenoma
- Secondary hyperparathyroidism is seen with vitamin D deficiency or renal failure with chronic low calcium
- Tertiary hyperparathyroidism occurs when secondary hyperparathyroidism becomes autonomous
- Rarely PTH overproduction can occur with parathyroid hyperplasia as part of multiple endocrine neoplasms
- Secondary causes of hypercalcemia must be excluded
- Increased calcium can adversely affect the cardiovascular system and lead to hypertension, arrhythmias, and calcification of heart and vascular structures

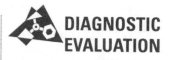 **CLINICAL PRESENTATION**

SYMPTOMS AND SIGNS

- Most patients are asymptomatic

PHYSICAL EXAM FINDINGS

- Calcium deposits in the cornea, soft tissue, and joints
- Signs of left ventricular hypertrophy or valve sclerosis
- Bradycardia and hypertension may occur with acute hypercalcemia

DIFFERENTIAL DIAGNOSIS

- Other causes of hypercalcemia without PTH excess
- Valvular sclerosis from atherosclerosis or rheumatic disease
- Other causes of hypertension and left ventricular hypertrophy

DIAGNOSTIC EVALUATION

LABORATORY TESTS

- Elevated serum calcium and ionized calcium
- Inappropriately normal or high PTH level
- Other causes of high calcium are associated with low PTH levels
- Low serum phosphate levels
- Hyperchloremic acidosis, elevated serum chloride, reduced carbon dioxide
- Elevated alkaline phosphatase levels

ELECTROCARDIOGRAPHY

- Shortened ST segment and increased QT interval
- For calcium levels > 16 mg/dL, the T wave widens prolonging the QT interval

IMAGING STUDIES

- Echocardiography: shows left ventricular hypertrophy and calcification of the aorta and aortic and mitral valves
- Chest x-ray: calcification of the coronary arteries and aorta

TREATMENT

CARDIOLOGY REFERRAL

- Suspected cardiac disease

HOSPITALIZATION CRITERIA

- Planned surgery

MEDICATIONS

- Pharmacologic treatment with biphosphates, pamidronate, risedronate, and estrogen in postmenopausal women is less effective than surgery
- Acute hypercalcemia is treated with saline infusion plus furosemide
- Thiazide diuretics are contraindicated

SURGERY

- Parathyroidectomy is the definitive treatment

DIET AND ACTIVITY

- Low-calcium diet
- Exercise is important to reduce bone loss

ONGOING MANAGEMENT

HOSPITAL DISCHARGE CRITERIA

- After successful surgery

FOLLOW-UP

- Depends on condition

COMPLICATIONS

- Systemic hypertension usually due to nephrosclerosis
- Complications of hypertension, such as stroke, heart failure
- Acute hypercalcemia can cause bradycardia
- Complications of vascular and valvular calcinosis

PROGNOSIS

- Good with early recognition and effective treatment

PREVENTION

- Serum calcium should be part of the general medical evaluation
- A short QTc interval on ECG should prompt consideration of this diagnosis

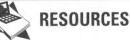

RESOURCES

PRACTICE GUIDELINES

- Despite the potential for serious cardiovascular disease, cardiovascular mortality is not increased in hyperparathyroidism

REFERENCE

- Bilezikian JP: Primary hyperparathyroidism: when to operate and when to observe. Endocrinol Metab Clin N Am 2000;29:465.

INFORMATION FOR PATIENTS

- www.drpen.com/252.0

WEB SITE

- www.emedicine.com/med/topic3200.htm

Hypertension, Gestational

 KEY FEATURES

ESSENTIALS OF DIAGNOSIS

- Occurs after 20 weeks of gestation or up to 6 weeks postpartum in previously normotensive women
- Usually diagnosed after a rise in blood pressure of ≥30/15 mm Hg to a level above 140/90 mm Hg
- May progress to preeclampsia when complicated by proteinuria, edema, or hematologic or hepatic abnormalities
- May progress to cerebral symptoms, leading to convulsions

GENERAL CONSIDERATIONS

- Preeclampsia is the combination of hypertension and proteinuria, and it accounts for 25% of low birth weight infants
  - Is a leading cause of maternal mortality
  - Is an endothelial disorder that results in placental ischemia
  - Occurs more frequently in women with hypertension predating pregnancy
- Occurs more frequently in primigravidas and in subsequent pregnancies with a different father
- The cause of gestational hypertension is not known

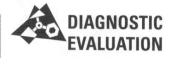 **CLINICAL PRESENTATION**

SYMPTOMS AND SIGNS

- Nonspecific symptoms are common, such as headache, nausea, visual disturbances

PHYSICAL EXAM FINDINGS

- Increased blood pressure
- Edema
- Hyperreflexia and clonus can occur

DIFFERENTIAL DIAGNOSIS

- Chronic hypertension
- Unclassified hypertension when blood pressure status before conception and during first trimester is unknown

DIAGNOSTIC EVALUATION

LABORATORY TESTS

- Urinanalysis: to check for protein
- CBC, platelets (often low)
- Uric acid: may be elevated
- Serum albumin: may be low
- Liver function tests: may be abnormal

ELECTROCARDIOGRAPHY

- No specific abnormalities

IMAGING STUDIES

- Fetal ultrasound: may show reduced size for gestational age
- Umbilical Doppler: may show flow abnormalities

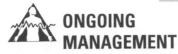

TREATMENT

CARDIOLOGY REFERRAL

- Cardiac complications of hypertension

HOSPITALIZATION CRITERIA

- Almost all with severe preeclampsia
- Complications of hypertension such as heart failure

MEDICATIONS

- Methyldopa is the primary treatment 250–1500 mg PO bid
- Nifedipine (10–20 mg PO tid) and labetalol (100–400 mg PO bid) may be used in succession for severe hypertension
- Hydralazine 10-mg boluses IV can be used every 20 minutes for acute elevations in blood pressure
- Angiotensin-converting enzyme inhibitors, angiotensin-receptor blockers, and atenolol are contraindicated
- For intrapartum management, IV magnesium prevents progression of preeclampsia to seizures

THERAPEUTIC PROCEDURES

- Termination of pregnancy when fetal or maternal crisis develops

SURGERY

- Cesarean section if indicated for fetal or maternal crisis

MONITORING

- Fetal monitoring in hospital
- ECG monitoring in hospital
- Blood pressure monitoring in hospital

DIET AND ACTIVITY

- Low-sodium diet
- Bed rest

ONGOING MANAGEMENT

HOSPITAL DISCHARGE CRITERIA

- Control of hypertension
- After pregnancy termination

FOLLOW-UP

- Close follow-up before delivery
- Routine follow-up after delivery

COMPLICATIONS

- Low birth weight infant
- Maternal mortality
- Infant mortality
- Stroke
- Pulmonary edema
- Seizures
- Renal failure
- Retinal detachment
- Disseminated intravascular coagulopathy
- Myocardial infarction

PROGNOSIS

- Excellent after delivery
- Guarded until delivery

PREVENTION

- Prompt treatment of gestational hypertension

RESOURCES

PRACTICE GUIDELINES

- Conservative management is acceptable in mild to moderate cases, but pregnancy termination is the only known 100% effective treatment for preeclampsia toxemia

REFERENCE

- Borghi C et al: The treatment of hypertension in pregnancy. J Hypertens 2002;20(suppl 2):S52.

INFORMATION FOR PATIENTS

- www.drpen.com/642.00

WEB SITE

- www.emedicine.com/med/topic3250.htm

Hypertension, Renovascular

KEY FEATURES

ESSENTIALS OF DIAGNOSIS

- Severe hypertension occurring before age 25 or after age 55
- Abdominal or flank systolic and diastolic bruits, or evidence of peripheral vascular disease
- Unilateral small kidney on any imaging study
- Hypertension resistant to three medications
- Worsening renal function after an angiotensin-converting enzyme inhibitor
- Elevated plasma renin activity with or without captopril administration
- Imaging evidence of renal artery occlusive disease

GENERAL CONSIDERATIONS

- Renal vascular disease is an unusual cause of hypertension, but is potentially curable
- Renal vascular hypertension usually results from obstruction of one main artery in one kidney
- The most common cause in women < age 25 is fibromuscular hyperplasia
- The most common cause in men > age 55 is atherosclerosis

CLINICAL PRESENTATION

SYMPTOMS AND SIGNS

- No specific symptoms or signs

PHYSICAL EXAM FINDINGS

- Advanced eye fundoscopic changes are common
- Renal bruits may be heard
- Evidence of other vascular disease

DIFFERENTIAL DIAGNOSIS

- Essential hypertension
- Renal parenchymal disease
- Other causes of secondary hypertension

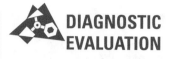 DIAGNOSTIC EVALUATION

LABORATORY TESTS

- High plasma renin activity and plasma aldosterone

ELECTROCARDIOGRAPHY

- Left heart chamber enlargement may be seen

IMAGING STUDIES

- Magnetic resonance angiography is improving and has largely replaced captopril renal scintigraphy as the first-choice noninvasive test

DIAGNOSTIC PROCEDURES

- Renal arteriogram is almost always diagnostic

TREATMENT

CARDIOLOGY REFERRAL

• Refractory hypertension
• Suspected cardiac disease
• Planned renal artery stenting

HOSPITALIZATION CRITERIA

• Complications of hypertension
• Planned procedure

MEDICATIONS

• Pharmacologic therapy if hypertension is mild or readily controlled

THERAPEUTIC PROCEDURES

• Percutaneous angioplasty with or without stenting

SURGERY

• Surgical repair or nephrectomy

MONITORING

• Blood pressure
• ECG in hospital as appropriate

DIET AND ACTIVITY

• Low-sodium diet, limited alcohol intake
• Exercise as tolerated

ONGOING MANAGEMENT

HOSPITAL DISCHARGE CRITERIA

• Resolution of problem
• Definitive procedure or surgery

FOLLOW-UP

• One month, then 3 months, 6 months, yearly after procedure or surgery

COMPLICATIONS

• Restenosis can occur after angioplasty
• Persistent hypertension may occur after successful relief of arterial obstruction

PROGNOSIS

• Excellent with correction of the vascular obstruction

PREVENTION

• Preventive measures for atherosclerosis

RESOURCES

PRACTICE GUIDELINES

• Since medical therapy can achieve normotension in most cases of renovascular hypertension, the risk-benefit of angioplasty or surgery must be carefully weighed

REFERENCES

• Safian RD, Textor SC: Renal artery stenosis. N Engl J Med 2001;344:431.

INFORMATION FOR PATIENTS

• www.mayoclinic.com/ invoke.cfm?id=HQ01345

WEB SITE

• www.emedicine.com/med/ topic2006.htm

Hypertension, Resistant or Refractory

 KEY FEATURES

ESSENTIALS OF DIAGNOSIS

- Blood pressure > 140/90 mm Hg in patients adhering to a triple-drug regimen (including a diuretic) at near-maximal doses
- In older patients, systolic blood pressure > 160 mm Hg despite adequate triple-drug therapy

GENERAL CONSIDERATIONS

- Resistant or refractory hypertension is usually due to patient factors, such as:
  - Excessive sodium, alcohol, and calories
  - Noncompliance with medications
- Occasionally, the patient ingests other substances that interfere with the effectiveness of treatment, such as:
  - Nonsteroidal anti-inflammatory drugs
  - Oral contraceptives
- Another common problem is under-dosing of medications, especially diuretics

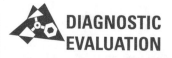 **CLINICAL PRESENTATION**

SYMPTOMS AND SIGNS

- Patient may report being under increased stress

PHYSICAL EXAM FINDINGS

- Elevated blood pressure despite multidrug therapy

DIFFERENTIAL DIAGNOSIS

- Inaccurate blood pressure measurement (eg, cuff too small)
- Stimulant exposure (eg, nasal sprays, diet pills, alcohol)
- Aggravating medical conditions (eg, sleep apnea)
- Secondary hypertension (eg, renal artery stenosis)

DIAGNOSTIC EVALUATION

ELECTROCARDIOGRAPHY

- ECG findings: left ventricular and atrial hypertrophy

DIAGNOSTIC PROCEDURES

- Ambulatory blood pressure monitoring: to confirm resistance and document temporal trends in relation to medication ingestion

TREATMENT

CARDIOLOGY REFERRAL

- Suspected cardiac disease
- Refractory hypertension

HOSPITALIZATION CRITERIA

- Severe hypertension (>220/120 mm Hg)
- Heart failure
- Stroke
- Myocardial infarction
- Aortic dissection
- Renal failure

MEDICATIONS

- Maximize medications, especially diuretics
- Use the most efficacious combinations of drugs first (eg, a diuretic, an angiotensin-converting enzyme inhibitor, and a calcium channel blocker), then add either a beta blocker or a central alpha$_2$-receptor agonist such as clonidine, or a combined adrenergic inhibitor such as labetalol

MONITORING

- ECG and blood pressure in hospital

DIET AND ACTIVITY

- Intensify lifestyle modifications (eg, low-salt diet or DASH diet, exercise)
- Restrict activities as appropriate

ONGOING MANAGEMENT

HOSPITAL DISCHARGE CRITERIA

- Blood pressure control
- Resolution of complications

FOLLOW-UP

- Two weeks, 4 weeks, 3 months, then every 6 months if stable

COMPLICATIONS

- Heart failure
- Stroke
- Renal failure
- Aortic dissections
- Myocardial infarction

PROGNOSIS

- Resistant hypertension can usually be brought under control if patients are compliant with their medications

PREVENTION

- Adequate pharmacotherapy
- Patient cooperation with lifestyle changes

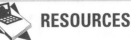

RESOURCES

PRACTICE GUIDELINES

- Inadequately controlled hypertension is common, but truly refractory hypertension is rare
- Most resistant hypertension can be controlled by increased patient cooperation and an adequate medical regimen

REFERENCE

- Ouzan J et al: The role of spiranolactone in the treatment of patients with refractory hypertension. Am J Hypertens 2002;15:333.

INFORMATION FOR PATIENTS

- www.drpen.com/401.0

WEB SITE

- www.emedicine.com/med/topic1106.htm

Hypertension, Systemic

 KEY FEATURES

ESSENTIALS OF DIAGNOSIS

- Diastolic pressure > 90 mm Hg, systolic pressure >140 mm Hg, or both on three separate occasions
- In diabetic patients: diastolic pressure > 80 mm Hg, systolic pressure > 130 mm Hg, or both on three separate occasions

GENERAL CONSIDERATIONS

- Systemic hypertension is associated with insulin resistance, glucose intolerance, hyperlipidemia, and truncal obesity
- Systemic hypertension often leads to left ventricular hypertrophy, altered diastolic filling, and eventually heart failure
- The major complications are stroke, myocardial infarction, and heart and renal failure
- Treatment of even moderate hypertension lowers the risk of these complications
- African Americans have a greater prevalence of hypertension than do whites, and they have a higher incidence of severe hypertension

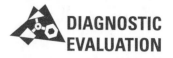 **CLINICAL PRESENTATION**

SYMPTOMS AND SIGNS

- Most are asymptomatic
- Headache, nosebleeds, and other symptoms are nonspecific

PHYSICAL EXAM FINDINGS

- Elevated blood pressure using an appropriate-sized cuff, after at least 5 minutes in the sitting position on three occasions
- Signs of secondary causes should be sought:
  - Flank bruits (renovascular)
  - Diminished femoral pulses (coarctation of the aorta)
- Eye fundus exam for signs of vascular damage
- Cardiac exam for signs of left ventricular hypertrophy or dysfunction
- Neurologic exam for signs of stroke

DIFFERENTIAL DIAGNOSIS

- Pseudo- or white-coat hypertension
- High-output state (eg, marked aortic regurgitation)
- Secondary causes:
  - Steroid therapy (eg, oral contraceptives, prednisone)
  - Pheochromocytoma
  - Coarctation of the aorta
  - Renal artery stenosis
  - Cushing's syndrome
  - Primary hyperaldosteronism
  - Chronic alcohol use

DIAGNOSTIC EVALUATION

LABORATORY TESTS

- CBC, urine analysis, electrolytes, creatine, blood urea nitrogen, glucose, lipids, calcium and uric acid

ELECTROCARDIOGRAPHY

- Left ventricular hypertrophy
- Left atrial abnormality

IMAGING STUDIES

- Echocardiogram may show left ventricular hypertrophy, left atrial enlargement
- Doppler echo may show diastolic dysfunction
- Chest x-ray is no longer indicated as a screening study for hypertension

TREATMENT

CARDIOLOGY REFERRAL

• Suspected cardiac disease
• Unresponsive or difficult to control hypertension

HOSPITALIZATION CRITERIA

• Severe hypertension > 220/120 mm Hg
• Acute myocardial infarction
• Stroke
• Heart failure
• Aortic dissection

MEDICATIONS

• Nonpharmacologic therapy: lose weight, get regular exercise, reduce alcohol consumption, restrict sodium intake, reduce stress levels
• Pharmacologic therapy: alpha-adrenergic blockers, beta-adrenergic blockers, angiotensin-converting enzyme (ACE) inhibitors, angiotensin-receptor blockers (ARBs), calcium channel blockers, diuretics, central nervous system agents, and direct peripheral vasodilators
• Multiple drug regimens are often necessary for blood pressure control; the starting drug depends on age and ethnicity:
  – Young white: ACEI/ARB or beta blocker
  – Older white: calcium channel blocker or beta blocker
  – Young black: calcium channel blocker
  – Older black: diuretic

MONITORING

• Ambulatory blood pressure monitoring is useful to exclude white-coat hypertension and design treatment regimens for difficult to control patients

DIET AND ACTIVITY

• Low-sodium diet, American Heart Association DASH diet
• Aerobic exercise encouraged

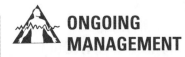 **ONGOING MANAGEMENT**

HOSPITAL DISCHARGE CRITERIA

• Control of blood pressure
• Resolution of complications

FOLLOW-UP

• Two to 4 weeks, then 3 months; every 6 months if stable

COMPLICATIONS

• Stroke
• Myocardial infarction
• Heart failure
• Renal failure
• Aortic dissection

PROGNOSIS

• Even modest reductions in blood pressure decrease the risk of complications, but attention must be paid to co-morbidities such as high cholesterol levels for maximum benefits

PREVENTION

• Maintaining ideal weight, adequate aerobic exercise, moderate alcohol and sodium intake, and reductions in stress, can often prevent hypertension in susceptible individuals

RESOURCES

PRACTICE GUIDELINES

• Choice of antihypertension agents also must take into consideration concomitant diseases:
  – Coronary disease: beta-blocker, ACE inhibitor/ARB, diuretic
  – Heart failure: ACE inhibitor, ARB, beta blockers, diuretic
  – Renal insufficiency: beta blocker, calcium channel blocker, diuretic, clonidine
  – Diabetes: ACE inhibitor, beta blocker, ARB, diuretic

REFERENCE

• MacMahon S: Blood pressure and the risk of cardiovascular disease. N Engl J Med 2000;342:50.

INFORMATION FOR PATIENTS

• www.drpen.com/401.1

WEB SITE

• www.emedicine.com/med/topic3432.htm

Hypertensive Emergencies

KEY FEATURES

ESSENTIALS OF DIAGNOSIS

- Blood pressure > 220/120 mm Hg
- Symptoms and signs of encephalopathy, acute myocardial ischemia, stroke, pulmonary edema, or aortic dissection

GENERAL CONSIDERATIONS

- Hypertensive emergencies:
  - Can be the first presentation of hypertension or can occur in patients known to have hypertension
  - Are more common in African-American men
- Hypertensive urgencies are described as the same severely elevated blood pressure levels as in hypertensive emergencies, but without symptoms or signs of target organ damage

CLINICAL PRESENTATION

SYMPTOMS AND SIGNS

- Symptoms of the target organ problem, such as headache and lethargy with encephalopathy

PHYSICAL EXAM FINDINGS

- Findings of the target organ problem, such as localizing neurologic findings in stroke

DIFFERENTIAL DIAGNOSIS

- Increased intracranial pressure—lowering blood pressure contraindicated
- Acute drug-induced pressure elevation (eg, cocaine)

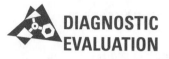 DIAGNOSTIC EVALUATION

LABORATORY TESTS

- Serum catecholamines: to check for pheochromocytoma
- Toxic drug screen

ELECTROCARDIOGRAPHY

- ECG findings:
  - Signs of acute myocardial ischemia or infarction
  - Nonspecific ST-T–wave changes
  - Left atrial and ventricular hypertrophy

IMAGING STUDIES

- As indicated for organ problem, such as echocardiography for heart failure

DIAGNOSTIC PROCEDURES

- As indicated for organ problem, such as coronary angiography for acute ST-elevation myocardial infarction

TREATMENT

CARDIOLOGY REFERRAL

- Myocardial infarction
- Heart failure

HOSPITALIZATION CRITERIA

- Encephalopathy
- Acute myocardial ischemia/infarction
- Heart failure
- Stroke
- Aortic dissection

MEDICATIONS

- Nitroprusside 0.25–10 µg/kg/min
- Fenoldopam 0.1 µg/kg/min; increase by 0.05 µg/kg/min
- Labetalol 20–40 mg IV every 10 minutes to 300 mg
- Esmolol 500 µg/kg over 1 minute, then 25–200 µg/kg/min
- Clonidine 0.1–0.2 mg PO, 0.05–0.1 mg every hour to 0.8 mg
- Captopril 6.24–50 mg PO every 6–8 hours

THERAPEUTIC PROCEDURES

- For specific organ problems as indicated, such as angioplasty for acute ST-elevation myocardial infarction

SURGERY

- As indicated for organ problem, such as surgical repair of aortic dissection

MONITORING

- ECG and blood pressure in hospital
- Neurologic signs

DIET AND ACTIVITY

- Low-sodium diet
- Restricted activity as indicated for the problem

ONGOING MANAGEMENT

HOSPITAL DISCHARGE CRITERIA

- Control of blood pressure
- Resolution of organ problem

FOLLOW-UP

- Two weeks, 4 weeks, 3 months, then every 6 months if stable

COMPLICATIONS

- Myocardial infarction
- Stroke
- Heart failure
- Aortic dissection

PROGNOSIS

- Depends on severity of target organ damage

PREVENTION

- Periodic home blood pressure measurements, which can reveal increasing blood pressure and prompt medical consultation for better control or elimination of aggravating factors before a hypertensive emergency occurs

RESOURCES

PRACTICE GUIDELINES

- Patients with severely elevated blood pressure with or without target organ damage should have their blood pressure rapidly reduced to appropriate levels while avoiding hypotension
- The target blood pressure depends on the organ damage
  - In aortic dissection, blood pressure should be as low as tolerated
  - For certain types of strokes, higher pressures are desirable
- Immediately lowering the blood pressure to 160–80 mm Hg systolic is usually safe until appropriate targets can be determined

REFERENCE

- Lip GYH et al: Do patients with de novo hypertension differ from patients with previously known hypertension when malignant phase hypertension occurs? Am J Hypertens 2000;13:934.

INFORMATION FOR PATIENTS

- www.drpen.com/401.0

WEB SITE

- www.emedicine.com/med/topic667.htm

Hypertensive Nephrosclerosis

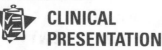 KEY FEATURES

ESSENTIALS OF DIAGNOSIS

- Chronic systemic hypertension before the onset of proteinuria
- Declining renal function; proteinuria
- Renal biopsy evidence of hyaline arteriolar sclerosis (afferent), myointimal hypertrophy/hyperplasia, and fibrinoid necrosis

GENERAL CONSIDERATIONS

- The cause of hypertensive nephrosclerosis is still unknown and is not always prevented by the treatment of hypertension
- Thus, there is debate about optimal blood pressure levels to prevent this complication
- Hypertensive nephrosclerosis is one of the most common causes of end-stage renal disease
- Once initiated, the condition is progressive
- It is more common in males of African origin
- Once renal disease ensues, it can cause hypertension

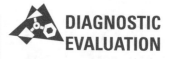 CLINICAL PRESENTATION

SYMPTOMS AND SIGNS

- Typically nonspecific symptoms of hypertension

PHYSICAL EXAM FINDINGS

- Elevated blood pressure without a nocturnal dip
- Retinopathy may be seen
- Left ventricular lift or heave

DIFFERENTIAL DIAGNOSIS

- Because renal biopsy is rarely performed, hypertensive nephrosclerosis is usually a diagnosis of exclusion
- Parenchymal renal disease
- Renovascular hypertension with renal insufficiency

DIAGNOSTIC EVALUATION

LABORATORY TESTS

- Urinalysis: hyaline and granular casts, microalbuminuria
- Elevated serum creatinine, uric acid

ELECTROCARDIOGRAPHY

- Left ventricular and atrial hypertrophy

IMAGING STUDIES

- Renal ultrasound may show small kidneys with cortical thinning

DIAGNOSTIC PROCEDURES

- Renal biopsy is diagnostic

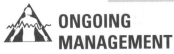

 TREATMENT

CARDIOLOGY REFERRAL

- Hypertension that is difficult to control
- Suspected cardiac disease

HOSPITALIZATION CRITERIA

- Renal failure

MEDICATIONS

- Twenty-four-hour blood pressure < 130/85 mm Hg with multiple drugs as necessary
- Sodium restriction and diuretics
- Angiotensin-converting enzyme (ACE) inhibitors or angiotensin-receptor blockers are best first therapy

THERAPEUTIC PROCEDURES

- Renal dialysis if necessary

MONITORING

- ECG and blood pressure in hospital

ONGOING MANAGEMENT

FOLLOW-UP

- Depends on blood pressure control

COMPLICATIONS

- End-stage renal disease

PROGNOSIS

- When serum creatinine is > 1.7 mg/dL, mortality is increased threefold
- The most common cause of death is cardiovascular disease

PREVENTION

- Adequate blood pressure control; optimal blood pressure levels have not been determined, but < 135/85 mm Hg is recommended

RESOURCES

PRACTICE GUIDELINES

- Although ACE inhibitors are considered the preferred treatment, monotherapy rarely controls the blood pressure adequately
- The choice of other agents depends on the volume status of the patient. If there is edema, loop diuretics should be added, then other agents

REFERENCE

- Moore MA et al: Current strategies for management of hypertensive renal disease. Arch Intern Med 1999;159:23.

INFORMATION FOR PATIENTS

- www.nkdep.nih.gov/patientspublic/index.htm

WEB SITE

- www.nkdep.nih.gov/healthprofessionals/index.htm

Hyperthyroid Heart Disease

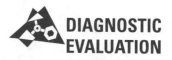 KEY FEATURES

ESSENTIALS OF DIAGNOSIS

- Palpitations, dyspnea, and chest pain
- Atrial fibrillation, tachycardia
- Hyperreflexia, tremor
- Stare, lid lag, and lid retraction due to high catecholamines
- Depressed thyroid-stimulating hormone (TSH) and high thyroxine levels
- Goiter and exophthalmos in Graves' disease

GENERAL CONSIDERATIONS

- Hyperthyroidism increases levels of T_3, which enhances myocardial systolic and diastolic function
- Beta catecholamine receptor responsiveness is increased, also leading to effects mimicking sympathetic nervous system activation such as increased heart rate
- Although cardiac performance is augmented, the heart functions at near capacity in hyperthyroidism, with little reserve
- Hyperthyroidism can be caused by:
  - Diseases of the thyroid gland such as Graves' disease
  - Exogenous agents such as amiodarone
  - *Rare* thyroid hormone-producing tumors such as struma ovarii
- In apathetic hyperthyroidism of the elderly, atrial fibrillation may be the only manifestation

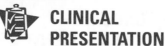 CLINICAL PRESENTATION

SYMPTOMS AND SIGNS

- Weight loss despite increased appetite
- Nervousness, anxiety, insomnia
- Heat intolerance, diaphoresis, diarrhea
- Proximal muscle weakness
- Palpitations, dyspnea, chest pain

PHYSICAL EXAM FINDINGS

- Stare, lid retraction and lag
- Exophthalmos in Graves' disease
- Goiter
- Tachycardia, loud heart sounds, flow murmurs
- Hyperreflexia
- Pretibial myxedema

DIFFERENTIAL DIAGNOSIS

- Anxiety disorder
- Factitious or iatrogenic thyrotoxicosis
- Angina, atrial fibrillation, and other signs without thyrotoxicosis

DIAGNOSTIC EVALUATION

LABORATORY TESTS

- Reduced TSH, elevated free T_4 and T_3

ELECTROCARDIOGRAPHY

- Sinus tachycardia in many
- Atrial fibrillation in some

IMAGING STUDIES

- Echocardiography:
  - Hypercontractile state
  - Left ventricular hypertrophy
  - Left atrial enlargement in some patients

DIAGNOSTIC PROCEDURES

- Radioactive iodine thyroid uptake may be increased or decreased, depending on the cause of hyperthyroidism

TREATMENT

CARDIOLOGY REFERRAL

- Atrial fibrillation
- Heart failure
- Acute coronary syndromes

HOSPITALIZATION CRITERIA

- Atrial fibrillation
- Heart failure
- Acute coronary syndromes

MEDICATIONS

- Beta blockers to reduce heart rate and improve symptoms
  - Propranolol is preferred because it blocks peripheral conversion of T_4 to T_3
- Thionamides to block thyroid hormone release and prevent synthesis

THERAPEUTIC PROCEDURES

- Radioactive iodine ablation

SURGERY

- Subtotal thyroidectomy in selected cases

MONITORING

- ECG monitoring in hospital as appropriate
- TSH monitoring during treatment

DIET AND ACTIVITY

- Restricted activity until thyroid controlled

ONGOING MANAGEMENT

HOSPITAL DISCHARGE CRITERIA

- Control or cessation of atrial fibrillation
- Resolution of problem

FOLLOW-UP

- Depends on degree and severity of cardiac abnormalities

COMPLICATIONS

- Rapid atrial fibrillation
- Stroke
- Heart failure
- Acute coronary syndromes

PROGNOSIS

- Excellent in most cases with treatment

RESOURCES

PRACTICE GUIDELINES

- Most patients who develop heart failure or serious ventricular tachyarrhythmias have underlying cardiac disease
- High-output heart failure is rare
- Hyperthyroidism, by increasing myocardial oxygen demand, can cause an exacerbation of coronary artery disease
- Angina is common and improves with treatment of the thyrotoxicosis
  - Myocardial infarction is rare

REFERENCE

- Klein I, Ojamaa K: Thyroid hormone and the cardiovascular system. N Engl J Med 2001;344:501.

INFORMATION FOR PATIENTS

- www.drpen.com/242.9

WEB SITE

- www.emedicine.com/med/topic1109.htm

Hypotension Complicating Hemodialysis

 ## KEY FEATURES

ESSENTIALS OF DIAGNOSIS

- Marked decrease (>30 mm Hg systolic) in blood pressure during dialysis
- Symptoms of decreased cerebral perfusion

GENERAL CONSIDERATIONS

- More common in those with diabetes, atherosclerosis, and hypertension
- Hypotension limits the achievement of diuresis during dialysis

CLINICAL PRESENTATION

SYMPTOMS AND SIGNS

- Symptoms of decreased cerebral perfusion:
  - Somnolence
  - Dizziness
  - Syncope

PHYSICAL EXAM FINDINGS

- Systolic blood pressure drop of > 30 mm Hg

DIFFERENTIAL DIAGNOSIS

- Pericardial effusion due to uremia or other causes
- Left ventricular diastolic dysfunction due to hypertrophy
- Autonomic dysfunction, often due to diabetes
- Myocardial ischemia (may be produced by hypotension also)
- Overzealous use of antihypertensive agents
- Cardiac arrhythmias
- Severe left ventricular systolic dysfunction
- Low dry weight of patient
- Decreased plasma osmolarity
- Splanchnic vasodilation due to a large meal
- Characteristics of the dialysate (eg, acetate)

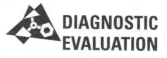 ## DIAGNOSTIC EVALUATION

LABORATORY TESTS

- CBC: Anemia frequently a contributing factor

ELECTROCARDIOGRAPHY

- Left chamber enlargement signs

IMAGING STUDIES

- Echocardiography:
  - Usually shows left ventricular hypertrophy and left atrial enlargement
  - Reduced systolic left ventricular function may be present

TREATMENT

CARDIOLOGY REFERRAL

- When simple measures do not correct the problem
- Suspected cardiac disease

HOSPITALIZATION CRITERIA

- Inability to safely dialyze

MEDICATIONS

- Identify and treat myocardial ischemia
- Carefully adjust antihypertensive medications
- Prevent cardiac arrhythmias
- Treat heart failure
- Administer vasoconstrictors in refractory cases

THERAPEUTIC PROCEDURES

- Identify and remove pericardial fluid

MONITORING

- Blood pressure during dialysis
- ECG as appropriate in hospital

DIET AND ACTIVITY

- Renal disease diet
- Low-fat diet
- Activity as tolerated

ONGOING MANAGEMENT

HOSPITAL DISCHARGE CRITERIA

- Resolution of problem

FOLLOW-UP

- According to dialysis routine
- As appropriate for underlying diseases

COMPLICATIONS

- Myocardial infarction
- Stroke

PROGNOSIS

- In general, hypotension during dialysis is a poor prognostic sign

PREVENTION

- Decrease fluid removal in patients with low dry weight
- Adjust sodium in dialysate to > 135 mmol/L to prevent hypo-osmolarity
- Use cooled bicarbonate dialysate

RESOURCES

PRACTICE GUIDELINES

- Hypotension complicating hemodialysis is a common problem, the causes of which are often multifactorial
- The problem can usually be eliminated with careful attention to:
  - Comorbidities
  - Drug therapy
  - Dialysis techniques

REFERENCE

- Schreiber MJ Jr: Clinical case-based approach to understanding intradialytic hypotension. Am J Kidney Dis 2001;38:S37.

INFORMATION FOR PATIENTS

- http://kidney.niddk.nih.gov/kudiseases/pubs/hemodyalysis/index.htm

Hypothyroid Heart Disease

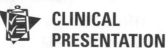

KEY FEATURES

ESSENTIALS OF DIAGNOSIS

- Weakness, weight gain, cold intolerance
- Reduced exercise tolerance, dyspnea on exertion
- Pleural and pericardial effusions, edema, anasarca
- Bradycardia, hypothermia, mild hypertension
- Goiter, delayed reflexes, myxedema coma
- Elevated thyroid-stimulating hormone and reduced thyroxine levels
- Hyperlipidemia and premature atherosclerosis

GENERAL CONSIDERATIONS

- Hypothyroidism is caused by thyroid hormone insufficiency
- Myxedema refers to profound hypothyroidism resulting in severe hypothermia, hypoventilation, and hypotension with signs of neurologic impairment
- Hypothyroidism accelerates atherosclerosis, but angina and myocardial infarction are rare until thyroid hormone is replaced because of the reduced metabolic demands of the hypothyroid state
- Hypothyroidism can be caused by:
  - Thyroid disease
  - Congenital abnormalities
  - Iodine deficiency
  - Drugs such as lithium

CLINICAL PRESENTATION

SYMPTOMS AND SIGNS

- Weight gain, weakness, lethargy, cold intolerance, dry skin, and coarse hair
- Amenorrhea or impotence
- Dyspnea on exertion

PHYSICAL EXAM FINDINGS

- Bradycardia
- Hypotension
- Pleural effusion
- Hypothermia
- Goiter in some
- Distant heart sounds
- Delayed reflexes
- Nonpitting edema

DIFFERENTIAL DIAGNOSIS

- Congestive heart failure due to other causes
- Other causes of effusions and edema
- Hyperlipidemia and atherosclerosis without hypothyroidism

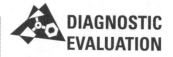

DIAGNOSTIC EVALUATION

LABORATORY TESTS

- Elevated thyroid-stimulating hormone (TSH), reduced T_4 and T_3
- Hyperlipidemia is common
- Anemia

ELECTROCARDIOGRAPHY

- Sinus bradycardia
- Increased PR and QT intervals

IMAGING STUDIES

- Echocardiography:
  - Pericardial effusion common, but signs of tamponade unusual
  - Reduced cardiac performance
  - Asymptomatic septal hypertrophy with obstruction in many

DIAGNOSTIC PROCEDURES

- Coronary angiography may be necessary

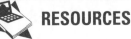

 TREATMENT

CARDIOLOGY REFERRAL

- Suspected cardiac disease

HOSPITALIZATION CRITERIA

- Heart failure symptoms and signs

MEDICATIONS

- Thyroid hormone replacement, which must be given slowly to older patients or those suspected of having coronary artery disease, to prevent exacerbation of angina and precipitation of myocardial infarction

THERAPEUTIC PROCEDURES

- Coronary revascularization should be considered before thyroid replacement therapy in high-risk patients

MONITORING

- ECG monitoring in hospital as appropriate
- TSH levels during treatment

DIET AND ACTIVITY

- Low-fat diet
- Reduced activity until condition improves

ONGOING MANAGEMENT

HOSPITAL DISCHARGE CRITERIA

- Resolution of problem

FOLLOW-UP

- As appropriate for condition

COMPLICATIONS

- Heart failure
- Angina or myocardial infarction during treatment

PROGNOSIS

- Excellent in the absence of heart disease

PREVENTION

- Continue thyroid hormone replacement lifelong
- Adequate iodine in diet

RESOURCES

PRACTICE GUIDELINES

- Because hypothyroidism and adrenal insufficiency may coexist, thyroid hormone replacement may precipitate adrenal crisis

REFERENCE

- Tielens ET et al: Changes in cardiac function at rest before and after treatment in primary hypothyroidism. Am J Cardiol 2000;85:376.

INFORMATION FOR PATIENTS

- www.drpen.com/244.9

WEB SITE

- www.emedicine.com/med/topic1145.htm

Implantable Cardioverter-Defibrillator, Frequent Discharges

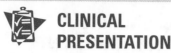 KEY FEATURES

ESSENTIALS OF DIAGNOSIS

- Appropriate therapy for recurrent ventricular arrhythmia
- Supraventricular arrhythmia including sinus tachycardia and atrial fibrillation with rapid ventricular response
- Frequent and inappropriate discharges of implantable cardioverter-defibrillator (ICD)

GENERAL CONSIDERATIONS

- Inappropriate programming is a rare cause of frequent discharge
- Conductor fracture can lead to oversensing and multiple inappropriate shocks
- Device–device interaction is becoming infrequent because almost all modern ICDs have intrinsic pacing feature
- Dual-chamber ICD has refined programming choices to avoid inappropriate interpretation of supraventricular arrhythmia and therapy; the complexity has theoretical potential to increase interpretation errors
- In patients with frequent appropriate shock therapy, investigate for the following:
  - Progression of heart disease
  - Ischemia
  - Metabolic disturbance
  - Thyroid dysfunction
  - Medication interaction
- If shocks are inappropriate and frequent in a hospitalized setting, a magnet can be placed over the device to eliminate sensing function and thereby eliminate inappropriate shocks until definitive therapy is accomplished

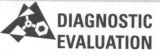 CLINICAL PRESENTATION

SYMPTOMS AND SIGNS

- Frequent shocks

PHYSICAL EXAM FINDINGS

- Clinical symptoms point to worsening of underlying heart condition

DIFFERENTIAL DIAGNOSIS

- T-wave or P-wave oversensing
- Double counting of intrinsic wide QRS complex in biventricular defibrillator
- Myopotential oversensing (eg, diaphragm)
- Device–device interaction (sensing of pacemaker stimuli)
- Device malfunction
- Electromagnetic interference

DIAGNOSTIC EVALUATION

LABORATORY TESTS

- CBC, metabolic panel to evaluate serum potassium
- Serum thyroid-stimulating hormone to assess thyroid function

ELECTROCARDIOGRAPHY

- Device interrogation with the programmer will reveal the appropriateness and the reason for shocks
- ECG, if obtained during a shock, may be helpful

IMAGING STUDIES

- Echocardiogram to evaluate change in left ventricular function and regional wall motion if the shocks are appropriate
- Chest x-ray may identify lead fracture

DIAGNOSTIC PROCEDURES

- Device interrogation with the programmer
- Coronary angiogram if ischemia is considered a cause of appropriate shocks

TREATMENT

CARDIOLOGY REFERRAL

- All patients should be evaluated by a cardiac electrophysiologist

HOSPITALIZATION CRITERIA

- If there are more than two shocks within 24 hours patients must be hospitalized for an evaluation

MEDICATIONS

- If appropriate, consider altering the substrate for arrhythmias with antiarrhythmic drugs
- Exclude or treat precipitating factors such as:
  - Metabolic derangement
  - Ischemia
  - Thyroid dysfunction

THERAPEUTIC PROCEDURES

- If the cause is rhythm misinterpretation or device malfunction, manage appropriately with electrophysiology consultation, which may involve device reprogramming, change to a new device or ventricular tachycardia ablation

SURGERY

- Occasionally may involve surgical ventricular tachycardia ablation

MONITORING

- ECG monitoring in hospital

DIET AND ACTIVITY

- Usual cardiac diet
- If sinus tachycardia secondary to exercise is a cause for inappropriate shock, the device should be reprogrammed rather than restricting exercise

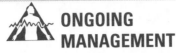

ONGOING MANAGEMENT

HOSPITAL DISCHARGE CRITERIA

- No shocks for 24 hours and the underlying problem is adequately addressed

FOLLOW-UP

- One week after discharge or change in programming

COMPLICATIONS

- Patient may become very apprehensive of shocks
- Psychological counseling may be required

PROGNOSIS

- Almost all problems can be resolved, and the prognosis is related to the underlying condition

PREVENTION

- Appropriate device programming by an electrophysiologist
- Monitoring of the device every 3 months at an experienced electrophysiology clinic
- Follow-up with a cardiologist every 3 months to evaluate the progression and management of underlying heart disease

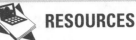

RESOURCES

PRACTICE GUIDELINES

- If the patient is hospitalized and inappropriate shocks are noted, place a magnet over the device until definite reprogramming
- Electrophysiology consultation is essential for management

REFERENCES

- Gollob MH, Seger JJ: Current status of the implantable cardioverter-defibrillator. Chest 2001;119:1210
- Srivathsan K, Bazzell JL, Lee RW: Biventricular implantable cardioverter defibrillator and inappropriate shocks. J Cardiovasc Electrophysiol 2003;14:88.

INFORMATION FOR PATIENTS

- www.nlm.nih.gov/medlineplus/ arrhythmia.html

WEB SITE

- www.hrsonline.org

Inherited Neuromuscular Disease and the Heart

KEY FEATURES

ESSENTIALS OF DIAGNOSIS

- Evidence of progressive muscle wasting and weakness
- Dilated cardiomyopathy
- Conduction abnormalities
- Arrhythmias
- Nonspecific ECG abnormalities
- Specific genetic diagnosis of a muscular dystrophy

GENERAL CONSIDERATIONS

- Cardiac manifestations of inherited neuromuscular diseases can range from incidental findings on ECG to severe cardiomyopathy
- Duchenne's muscular dystrophy:
  - The most common type (3/100,000 population) of inherited neuromuscular disease
  - Mainly seen in males (X-linked recessive)
  - Causes cardiomyopathy
- Becker's muscular dystrophy:
  - Also sex linked, but with a delayed onset and slower progression than Duchenne's
  - The cardiomyopathy is often more severe
- Myotonic dystrophy (Steinert's disease):
  - Autosomal dominant
  - Associated with myotonia, frontal balding, gonadal dysfunction, and cataracts
  - Seen in 3–5/100,000 population
  - Usually manifests as conduction disturbances and tachyarrhythmias
- Emery-Dreifuss disease or X-linked humeroperoneal dystrophy:
  - An autosomal recessive or X-linked disease
  - Usually causes conduction system disease, but can cause cardiomyopathy
- Peroneal muscular atrophy (Charcot-Marie-Tooth syndrome):
  - An autosomal dominant disease
  - Can cause conduction abnormalities and cardiomyopathy
- Facioscapulohumeral dystrophy (Landovzy-Dejerine disease):
  - A rare autosomal dominant disease
  - Often causes atrial standstill
- Limb-girdle dystrophy of Erb:
  - An autosomal recessive condition

- Can cause brady-tachycardia syndromes
- Kearns-Sayre syndrome:
  - A mitochondrial disease
  - Causes heart block in about 50% of cases

CLINICAL PRESENTATION

SYMPTOMS AND SIGNS

- Weakness of the affected skeletal muscles or dystonia
- Dyspnea
- Syncope
- Palpitation

PHYSICAL EXAM FINDINGS

- Signs of congestive heart failure
- Murmur of mitral regurgitation

DIFFERENTIAL DIAGNOSIS

- Cardiomyopathy from other causes with muscle atrophy and weakness from inactivity (cardiac cachexia)
- Conduction, rhythm, and ECG abnormalities from other causes

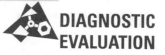

DIAGNOSTIC EVALUATION

LABORATORY TESTS

- Atrial and brain natriuretic peptides: elevated
- Specific genetic analyses

ELECTROCARDIOGRAPHY

- Conduction abnormalities
- Ventricular hypertrophy signs
- Repolarization abnormalities
- Arrhythmias

IMAGING STUDIES

- Echocardiography may show dilated cardiomyopathy, pulmonary hypertension, and mitral regurgitation by Doppler
- Myocardial perfusion defects by single positron emission computed tomography or positron emission tomography imaging
- MRI may show fatty deposits in the right ventricle of myotonic dystrophy patients

TREATMENT

CARDIOLOGY REFERRAL

- Suspected cardiac disease
- Syncope

HOSPITALIZATION CRITERIA

- Syncope
- Heart failure

MEDICATIONS

- Therapy as indicated for heart failure
- Antiarrhythmic drug therapy as appropriate

THERAPEUTIC PROCEDURES

- Pacemaker or implantable cardioverter-defibrillator as indicated

SURGERY

- Cardiac transplantation in selected cases

MONITORING

- ECG monitoring in hospital as appropriate

DIET AND ACTIVITY

- Low-sodium diet if heart failure

ONGOING MANAGEMENT

HOSPITAL DISCHARGE CRITERIA

- Resolution of problem
- Successful procedure

FOLLOW-UP

- As appropriate for the cardiac problem

COMPLICATIONS

- Sudden death due to arrhythmias
- Heart failure
- Syncope

PROGNOSIS

- Depends on the severity of the heart disease
- Duchenne's muscular dystrophy has a poor prognosis with death by the third decade
- Becker's and Emery-Dreifuss have near-normal life expectancy, so cardiac transplantation is a viable option

PREVENTION

- These are inherited diseases

RESOURCES

PRACTICE GUIDELINES

- Modern pharmacologic treatment of heart failure and pacemaker/implantable cardioverter defibrillators have greatly improved the prognosis in these patients with regard to their heart disease

REFERENCES

- Antonini G et al: Natural history of cardiac involvement in myotonic dystrophy: correlation with CTG repeats. Neurology 2000;55:1207.
- Emery AEH: The muscular dystrophies. Lancet 2002;359:687.

INFORMATION FOR PATIENTS

- www.nlm.nih.gov/medlineplus/ency/article/001190.htm

WEB SITE

- www.thedoctorsdoctor.com/diseases/mitochondrial_myopathy.htm

In-Stent Restenosis

KEY FEATURES

ESSENTIALS OF DIAGNOSIS

- Focal or diffuse intimal proliferation inside the stent or at the edges, resulting in restenosis
- Late luminal loss of ≥ 50% compared with acute luminal gain is generally considered in-stent restenosis (ISR)
- Recurrent angina or detection on routine stress tests, confirmed at angiography

GENERAL CONSIDERATIONS

- Stimulation of smooth muscle cells followed by proliferation and migration leads to neointimal thickening
- Prior to stents (balloon angioplasty), ISR was 30–50
  - After the bare metal stents, the ISR rate was between 20% and 30%
  - With the advent of coated stents (sirolimus coated) the ISR rate is between 0% and 9%, depending on the complexity of the cases studied
- Patient factors that increase the risk of restenosis:
  - Diabetes mellitus
  - Smoking
  - Male gender
  - Severe angina before stent placement
- Anatomic risk factors that increase the risk of ISR:
  - Chronic total occlusion
  - Sapahenous vein grafts
  - Long lesions
  - Left anterior descending artery location
  - Multivessel stents
- Procedural variables that increase the risk of ISR:
  - Greater residual stenosis
  - Severe dissection
  - Absence of an intimal tear
  - Presence of thrombus and choice of inappropriate balloon size
- Peak incidence is between 3–6 months

CLINICAL PRESENTATION

SYMPTOMS AND SIGNS

- May be asymptomatic
- Angina at rest or on exertion, sometimes worse than before intervention
- Dyspnea, leg edema may occur secondary to heart failure from ischemia
- Palpitations and syncope may occur as a consequence of arrhythmias

PHYSICAL EXAM FINDINGS

- Elevated jugular venous distention if heart failure present
- S_3 and S_4
- Bilteral lung rales if heart failure present

DIFFERENTIAL DIAGNOSIS

- Symptoms early after stenting (< 1 month) usually mean in-stent thrombosis
- Symptoms late after stenting (> 9 months) usually mean progressive disease in nonstented segments
- Other causes of chest pain or positive stress tests may be found

DIAGNOSTIC EVALUATION

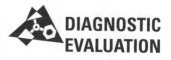

LABORATORY TESTS

- CBC, brain natriuretic peptide test

ELECTROCARDIOGRAPHY

- ECG may show ischemic changes

IMAGING STUDIES

- Stress or vasodilator perfusion nuclear imaging
- Stress or dobutamine echocardiogram

DIAGNOSTIC PROCEDURES

- Coronary angiogram

TREATMENT

CARDIOLOGY REFERRAL

- All patients should be evaluated by a cardiologist

HOSPITALIZATION CRITERIA

- If the presentation is unstable angina or heart failure, hospitalization is required
- Following percutaneous coronary intervention (PCI) of ISR

MEDICATIONS

- Antianginal medications if re-revascularization not feasible

THERAPEUTIC PROCEDURES

- Balloon angioplasty, especially for focal lesions
- Repeat stenting, especially with drug-eluting stents
- Catheter-delivered radiation (brachytherapy), usually as an adjunct to repeat angioplasty or stenting

SURGERY

- Coronary artery bypass surgery (CABG)
  – ISR within 3 months at a site previously treated for ISR leads to very high rate of recurrence and CABG is preferred in those circumstances

MONITORING

- ECG monitoring in hospital

DIET AND ACTIVITY

- Same as for coronary artery disease

ONGOING MANAGEMENT

HOSPITAL DISCHARGE CRITERIA

- After adequate revascularization either with PCI or CABG

FOLLOW-UP

- Stress or pharmacologic perfusion study (alternatively stress or dobutamine echocardiogram) 3 months after PCI

COMPLICATIONS

- Myocardial infarction
- Left ventricular dysfunction

PROGNOSIS

- Generally good, but if there is a second recurrence then the failure rate is high

PREVENTION

- Use of coated stent during the first PCI

RESOURCES

PRACTICE GUIDELINES

- Use coated stent when feasible
- Recurrent angina in 3–6 months after PCI must be investigated expeditiously, preferably with an angiogram

REFERENCES

- McPherson JA et al: Angiographic findings in patients undergoing catheterization for recurrent symptoms within 30 days of successful coronary intervention. Am J Cardiol 1999;84:589.
- Sarembock IJ: Stent restenosis and the use of drug-eluting stents in patients with diabetes mellitus. Curr Diab Rep 2004;4:13.

INFORMATION FOR PATIENTS

- www.nhlbi.nih.gov/health/dci/Diseases/Cad/CAD_WhatIs.html

WEB SITES

- www.theheart.org
- www.americanheart.org

Intra-atrial Reentrant Tachycardia

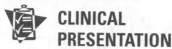

KEY FEATURES

ESSENTIALS OF DIAGNOSIS

- Atrial rate of 120–240 bpm
- P waves different from sinus P wave
- Structural heart disease in most cases

GENERAL CONSIDERATIONS

- Occurs with supraventricular tachycardia in 6% of the population
- P-wave morphology is different from sinus P-wave morphology and differentiates it from sinus node reentry and inappropriate sinus tachycardia
- May follow atrial surgery for congenital heart disease in children
- Occurs in paroxysms that are frequently sustained, responding to vagal maneuvers only 25% of the time
- Precipitated by closely coupled atrial depolarization and does not exhibit warm-up phase
- The substrate that facilitates reentry is inhomogeneity of atrial conduction, refractoriness, or both

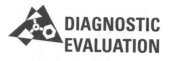

CLINICAL PRESENTATION

SYMPTOMS AND SIGNS

- Palpitations
- Dyspnea

PHYSICAL EXAM FINDINGS

- Usually findings of underlying structural heart disease
- Many patients have features of heart failure such as S_3, elevated jugular venous distention, and rales in the lung fields

DIFFERENTIAL DIAGNOSIS

- Automatic atrial tachycardia
- Atypical atrioventricular (AV) nodal reentrant tachycardia

DIAGNOSTIC EVALUATION

LABORATORY TESTS

- CBC, basic metabolic panel

ELECTROCARDIOGRAPHY

- ECG: may document rhythm disturbance or point to underlying heart disease
- Holter monitoring to detect rhythm disturbance

IMAGING STUDIES

- Echocardiogram to evaluate structural heart disease

DIAGNOSTIC PROCEDURES

- Invasive electrophysiologic study to assess rhythm mechanism

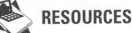

 TREATMENT

CARDIOLOGY REFERRAL

• All patients should be evaluated by a cardiac electrophysiologist

HOSPITALIZATION CRITERIA

• If the patient has active heart failure or is hemodynamically unstable

MEDICATIONS

• Beta blockers or calcium channel blockers with negative chronotropic properties (verapamil or diltiazem)
• Amiodarone, class IC, class IA, and other class III drugs are alternates when this arrhythmia is difficult to control

THERAPEUTIC PROCEDURES

• Radiofrequency ablation of the slow conduction area that facilitates reentry
• AV nodal ablation followed by permanent pacemaker implantation if the arrhythmia cannot be ablated

SURGERY

• Generally not required

MONITORING

• ECG monitoring in hospital

DIET AND ACTIVITY

• Depends on underlying cause

ONGOING MANAGEMENT

HOSPITAL DISCHARGE CRITERIA

• After radiofrequency ablation or adequate rate control on medications

FOLLOW-UP

• Two weeks after discharge from hospital; thereafter, depends on clinical situation

COMPLICATIONS

• Uncontrolled tachycardia may worsen cardiomyopathy
• Atrial fibrillation is common secondary to diseased and dilated atria

PROGNOSIS

• Although tachycardia may be controlled, overall prognosis depends on advanced state of the underlying heart disease

PREVENTION

• Early treatment of valvular heart disease
• Adequate treatment of hypertension

RESOURCES

PRACTICE GUIDELINES

• If frequent heart failure episodes are precipitated by the tachycardia, refer for radiofrequency ablation
• Atrial tachycardia may be a harbinger of atrial fibrillation; aggressive management of heart failure is recommended

REFERENCE

• Kirsh JA, Walsh EP, Triedman JK: Prevalence of and risk factors for atrial fibrillation and intra-atrial reentrant tachycardia among patients with congenital heart disease. Am J Cardiol 2002;90:338.

INFORMATION FOR PATIENTS

• www.nlm.nih.gov/medlineplus/arrhythmia.html

WEB SITE

• www.hrsonline.org

Ischemic Heart Disease, Chronic

KEY FEATURES

ESSENTIALS OF DIAGNOSIS

- Typical exertional angina pectoris or its equivalents
- Objective evidence of myocardial ischemia by ECG, myocardial imaging, or myocardial perfusion scanning
- Likely occlusive coronary artery disease (CAD) because of history and objective evidence of prior myocardial infarction
- Known CAD demonstrated by coronary angiography

GENERAL CONSIDERATIONS

- Some patients are asymptomatic despite objective evidence of CAD
- Coronary atherosclerosis is the most common cause
- In older patients, vasculitides are not uncommon
- In young patients with angina pectoris, coronary anomalies should be considered
- Myocardial bridges may be a causative factor in some patients
- Coronary vasospasm without underlying atherosclerosis is a rare cause for angina in United States

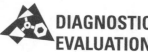 CLINICAL PRESENTATION

SYMPTOMS AND SIGNS

- Angina pectoris
- Usually precipitated by exertion or emotional upset and relieved by rest
- The discomfort usually subsides within 30 minutes
- If pain lasts longer than 30 minutes, myocardial infarction should be suspected
- The discomfort may typically radiate to the arms, neck, or jaw
- The pain may have higher intensity at the radiating site than in the chest
- Dyspnea may present as an anginal equivalent
- Palpitations and syncope secondary to arrhythmia may occur

PHYSICAL EXAM FINDINGS

- Often not helpful
- S_4 (not specific)
- S_3 and transient mitral regurgitation murmur may be heard but are not specific
- A diagonal earlobe crease may be seen in younger patients with CAD
- Tendon xanthoma and xanthelasma increase the likelihood that CAD is the cause of chest pain

DIFFERENTIAL DIAGNOSIS

- Other causes of chest pain, such as:
  - Esophageal reflux
  - Costochondritis
- False-positive evidence of ischemia, such as:
  - Cardiomyopathy
  - Technical shortcomings of tests
- Cholecystitis
- Peptic ulcer disease
- Cervical radiculopathy

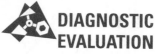 DIAGNOSTIC EVALUATION

LABORATORY TESTS

- Complete white blood cell count to exclude anemia and thrombocytosis as aggravating causes
- Metabolic panel:
  - To assess renal function
  - Renal failure patients have a higher chance of developing CAD
  - May also help to plan angiography depending on serum creatinine
- Serum thyroid-stimulating hormone:
  - To evaluate hypo- and hyperthyroidism; both may play a role in causing angina
- Prothrombin time and partial thromboplastin time:
  - To assess coagulation cascade
  - To help plan intervention and use of antiplatelet and anticoagulation therapy
- Further tests depend on other comorbidities

ELECTROCARDIOGRAPHY

- 12-lead ECG
- Exercise ECG
- Holter monitoring

IMAGING STUDIES

- Stress echocardiogram
- Nuclear stress test
- Coronary CT calcium score

DIAGNOSTIC PROCEDURES

- Coronary angiogram

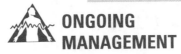

 TREATMENT

CARDIOLOGY REFERRAL

- When medical therapy is not controlling symptoms
- Left ventricular dysfunction
- Accelerating angina

HOSPITALIZATION CRITERIA

- High-risk predictors on noninvasive stress test: > 2 mm ST depression, ST elevation, large burden of ischemia or left ventricular dilatation on stress
- Unstable angina
- After angiography, either for percutaneous coronary intervention (PCI) or coronary artery bypass graft (CABG)

MEDICATIONS

- Treat reversible risk factors for CAD such as: smoking, hypertension, hypercholesterolemia, hyperglycemia, inflammation
- Eliminate factors that aggravate myocardial oxygen supply/demand imbalance such as tachyarrhythmias, thyrotoxicosis, anemia, hypoxia, heart failure, catecholamine analogs
- Pharmacologic therapy: sublingual nitroglycerin for acute angina episodes
- Prophylactic therapy: aspirin 325 mg/day, long-acting nitrates 60 mg/day, beta blockers (eg, metoprolol, usual dose 200 mg/day), calcium blocker (amlopidine, maximum dose 10 mg/day)

THERAPEUTIC PROCEDURES

- Revascularization for persistently symptomatic patients
- Percutaneous coronary intervention (angioplasty, stenting) for suitable coronary anatomy

SURGERY

- CABG favored for left main disease and 2- or 3-vessel disease with involvement of the left anterior descending coronary artery, reduced left ventricular function, or diabetes

MONITORING

- ECG monitoring in hospitalized patients

DIET AND ACTIVITY

- Cardiac low-fat diet
- Exercise regimen; objective evaluation may be done with a stress test

ONGOING MANAGEMENT

HOSPITAL DISCHARGE CRITERIA

- Symptom-free
- Postrevascularization

FOLLOW-UP

- Two weeks after revascularization
- If medications are adjusted, reevaluation recommended within 4 weeks
- Annual visit in well-compensated patients
- Stress test in asymptomatic patients postrevascularization controversial but frequently done

COMPLICATIONS

- Acute myocardial infarction
- Unstable angina
- Postrevascularization complications

PROGNOSIS

- Depends on Canadian functional class: the higher the Canadian class, the worse the prognosis
- Excellent prognosis for patients who can do more than 9 minutes on a Bruce protocol
- Duke treadmill score useful in predicting outcome
- Worse prognosis for left ventricular dysfunction
- Coronary anatomy used for prognosis but revascularization in asymptomatic patients has not been shown to influence outcome

PREVENTION

- Low-fat diet
- Aerobic exercise
- Control diabetes, hypertension
- Smoking cessation
- Statin when appropriate

RESOURCES

PRACTICE GUIDELINES

- Indications for revascularization:
  - Left main disease
  - Three-vessel disease with depressed left ventricular function (ejection fraction < 0.50, two- or three-vessel disease with proximal left anterior descending disease
- Percutaneous coronary intervention (PCI) of single-vessel disease
- PCI of vein grafts from prior CABG

REFERENCES

- Bales AC: Medical management of chronic ischemic heart disease. Selecting specific drug therapies, modifying risk factors. Postgrad Med 2004;115:39.
- Thadani U: Management of stable angina pectoris. Prog Cardiovasc Dis 1999;14:349.

INFORMATION FOR PATIENTS

- www.nhlbi.nih.gov/health/dci/ Diseases/Angina/Angina_WhatIs.html

WEB SITES

- www.amercanheart.org
- www.acc.org

Kawasaki Disease

KEY FEATURES

ESSENTIALS OF DIAGNOSIS

- Fever lasting 5 or more days with at least four of the following:
  - Bilateral nonexudative conjunctival injection
  - Injected lips or pharynx, or "strawberry tongue"
  - Acute nonsuppurative cervical lymphadenopathy
  - Erythema of the palms and soles, or edema of the hands and feet
  - Polymorphous exanthem
- Exclusion of common bacterial and viral infections
- Coronary artery aneurysms, myocarditis, and valve regurgitation

GENERAL CONSIDERATIONS

- Also called mucocutaneous lymph node syndrome
- Acute vasculitis of unknown etiology, which occurs mostly in infants and children
- One of the most common vasculitides of childhood
- Heart failure may rarely complicate the acute phase of illness due to myocarditis
- Routine treatment with intravenous immune globulin (IVIG) and aspirin usually results in rapid clinical improvement
- Myocardial dysfunction during or after the second week of illness may suggest coronary artery aneurysm and resultant ischemia or infarction
- In severe cases, coronary or peripheral artery occlusions may occur and children may experience myocardial infarction, arrhythmias, or sudden death

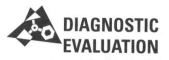

CLINICAL PRESENTATION

SYMPTOMS AND SIGNS

- Unexplained fever in an infant or child
- Skin rash
- Heart failure symptoms in patients with myocarditis in the first week of illness
- Chest pain, arrhythmias, or sudden death in patients

PHYSICAL EXAM FINDINGS

- Bilateral conjunctival injection
- Oral mucous membrane changes, including injected or fissured lips, injected pharynx, or "strawberry tongue"
- Palmar or solar erythema or edema
- Periungual desquamation
- Polymorphous rash
- Cervical lymphadenopathy
- Tachycardia out of proportion to the degree of fever
- Cardiac gallop sounds and muffled heart tones
- In severe cases, palpable brachial artery aneurysms; cold, pale, cyanotic or rarely gangrenous digits

DIFFERENTIAL DIAGNOSIS

- Streptococcal and staphylococcal infections
- Measles, enterovirus, and adenovirus infections
- Systemic allergic reactions to medications

DIAGNOSTIC EVALUATION

LABORATORY TESTS

- Acute-phase reactants (C-reactive protein, erythrocyte sedimentation rate, and alpha$_1$-antitrypsin) elevation
- White blood count: leukocytosis and left-shift in white blood count
- Reactive thrombocytosis
- Normocytic, normochronic anemia
- Pyuria of urethral origin (may be missed by bladder tap or catheterization)
- Elevated liver transaminase levels or hyperbilirubinemia due to intrahepatic congestion
- Mononuclear pleocytosis without low glucose or elevated protein in cerebrospinal fluid

ELECTROCARDIOGRAPHY

- Low R-wave voltages
- T-wave flattening
- Findings of acute myocardial infarction in rare cases

IMAGING STUDIES

- Echocardiography: small pericardial effusion, mild left ventricular dilatation, reduced left ventricular systolic function, mitral regurgitation, aortic root dilation, mild aortic regurgitation, diffuse dilation of coronary artery lumen or coronary artery aneurysms
  - Limited usefulness for measurement of coronary aneurysms after the acute phase of the illness

DIAGNOSTIC PROCEDURES

- Coronary angiography: can detect and quantify coronary artery aneurysms, stenosis, occlusion, and collateral circulation
- Stress testing: primarily indicated to detect myocardial ischemia
- Magnetic resonance angiography: may accurately identify coronary aneurysms and/or ectasia

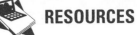

 TREATMENT

CARDIOLOGY REFERRAL

- Any child or infant with unexplained fever, difficulty in breathing, or suspected Kawasaki disease

HOSPITALIZATION CRITERIA

- Patients who fulfill the criteria for diagnosis are hospitalized for treatment

MEDICATIONS

- Aspirin 81 mg/kg/day in four divided doses; once fever subsides 3–5 mg/kg/day for 6–8 weeks
- Intravenous immune globulin (IVIG) 2 g/kg in a single infusion, preferably within 10 days of onset of symptoms
- Use of corticosteroids remains controversial
- If coronary aneurysms develop, long-term antiplatelet therapy with aspirin or clopidogrel
- For giant aneurysms, anticoagulants are recommended
- Persistent fever after IVIG indicates ongoing vasculitis and higher risk of coronary artery aneurysms
  - These patients are retreated with IVIG or salvage therapy with corticosteroids, pentoxifylline, plasmapheresis, or immunosuppression
- Vasodilators for coronary or peripheral arterial vasospasm
- Thrombolytics for acute myocardial infarction

THERAPEUTIC PROCEDURES

- Percutaneous coronary revascularization may be considered for selected patients with residual coronary artery stenosis

SURGERY

- Coronary artery stenosis may be treated with bypass surgery

MONITORING

- ECG monitoring in the hospital

DIET AND ACTIVITY

- Restricted activity for patients with unstable coronary syndromes or heart failure

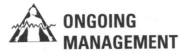 **ONGOING MANAGEMENT**

HOSPITAL DISCHARGE CRITERIA

- After successful, medical, procedural, or surgical treatment

FOLLOW-UP

- Serial dobutamine stress echocardiography or myocardial perfusion imaging
- Coronary angiography if there is any new evidence of myocardial ischemia
- Echocardiography in 6–8 weeks
- Repeated physical examinations during the first 2 months to detect arrhythmias, heart failure, or valvular insufficiency

COMPLICATIONS

- Acute myocardial infarction is the main cause of death, with most occurring in the first year
- Heart failure due to myocarditis
- Coronary artery aneurysms may regress, thrombose and recanalize, form localized stenosis, cause a myocardial infarction, or rupture (rare)
- Later, coronary artery obstruction due to internal fibrosis, ongoing inflammation, calcification, and thrombosis
- Peripheral artery occlusions may lead to strokes, limb ischemia, or gangrene

PROGNOSIS

- Coronary artery aneurysms < 8 mm usually regress over time; most smaller aneurysms fully resolve
- Twenty to 25% of untreated patients develop coronary artery aneurysms in the first 2 weeks
- Less than 1% mortality rate with early detection and prompt treatment
- Five percent of treated patients develop coronary artery aneurysms

PREVENTION

- Early detection and treatment within the first 10 days of illness with aspirin and IVIG may help prevent coronary artery aneurysms
- In severe cases, long-term aspirin is recommended for prevention of myocardial infarction

RESOURCES

PRACTICE GUIDELINES

- Aspirin and IVIG remain the mainstays of treatment
- Thrombolytics should be considered in patients with acute myocardial infarction during the acute phase of Kawasaki disease
- Serial noninvasive stress testing with dobutamine stress echocardiography or myocardial perfusion imaging are generally recommended to detect myocardial ischemia
- Coronary angiography is generally reserved for patients with abnormal stress tests or unstable coronary syndromes in the chronic phase of the disease

REFERENCES

- Beiser AS et al: A predictive instrument for coronary artery aneurysms in Kawasaki disease. US Multicenter Kawasaki Disease Study Group. Am J Cardiol 1998;81:1116.
- Sundel RP: Update on the treatment of Kawasaki disease in childhood. Curr Rheumatol Rep 2002;4:474.

INFORMATION FOR PATIENTS

- http://www.americanheart.org/presenter.jhtml?identifier=4634

WEB SITE

- http://www.emedicine.com/radio/topic878.htm

Left Atrial Myxoma

KEY FEATURES

ESSENTIALS OF DIAGNOSIS

- Symptoms of valvular dysfunction such as dyspnea
- Thromboemboli
- Constitutional symptoms (eg, fever, arthralgias, weight loss)
- Tumor plop sound in early diastole
- Mitral systolic or diastolic murmurs
- Echocardiographic evidence of characteristic cardiac mass

GENERAL CONSIDERATIONS

- Primary cardiac tumors are rare but left atrial myxoma is the most common in adults and is usually benign
- Mean age at discovery of left atrial myxoma is 50 years—more common in women
- About 10% of left atrial myxoma are familial in an autosomal dominant pattern and present earlier (mean age 25 years)
- Carney's syndrome includes:
  - Multiple cardiac myxoma
  - Lentigines
  - Breast fibroadenomas
  - Pituitary and testicular tumors
  - Primary pigmented nodular adrenocortical disease
- About 75% of all cardiac myxomas occur in the left atrium, 20% in the right atrium, and 5% in the ventricles
- Left atrial myxomas usually are attached by a stalk near the fossa ovalis

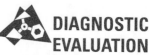

CLINICAL PRESENTATION

SYMPTOMS AND SIGNS

- Patients may present with the classic triad of constitutional, systemic embolic and mitral valve obstruction symptoms, but more often they have one or two of these manifestations
- Constitutional symptoms:
  - Weight loss
  - Fatigue
  - Fever
  - Arthralgias
- Dyspnea from mitral valve obstruction or regurgitation

PHYSICAL EXAM FINDINGS

- Signs of pulmonary congestion—pulmonary rales, wheezing
- Auscultation:
  - Loud S_1 due to delayed mitral closure
  - Early diastolic tumor plop
  - Mitral diastolic rumble
  - Mitral regurgitation murmur
  - Loud pulmonary component of S_2 if pulmonary hypertension present
  - Occasionally signs of right heart failure

DIFFERENTIAL DIAGNOSIS

- Cardiac thrombus
- Vegetations
- Flail or prolapsing leaflets
- Rheumatic mitral valve disease
- Connective tissue disease
- Other causes of stroke
- Other febrile illnesses

DIAGNOSTIC EVALUATION

LABORATORY TESTS

- Normochronic, normocytic, or low-grade hemolytic anemia
- Polycythemia, thrombocytosis, leukocytosis
- Elevated sedimentation rate and immunoglobulins

ELECTROCARDIOGRAPHY

- May show signs of left atrial enlargement
- Occasionally, atrial fibrillation

IMAGING STUDIES

- Chest x-ray:
  - Enlarged left atrium
- Echocardiography is the imaging procedure of choice because of its ability to distinguish the tumor mass from the left atrial cavity into which it protrudes
  - The stalk attached to the atrial septum and the mobile mass that moves toward or through the mitral valve in diastole and pops back into the atrium in systole is characteristic
  - Transesophageal echo can provide more detailed anatomic information that may be needed in some cases to plan surgery

DIAGNOSTIC PROCEDURES

- Cardiac catheterization may be required in older patients to define coronary anatomy prior to surgery

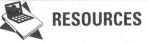

 TREATMENT

CARDIOLOGY REFERRAL

- Any suspected left atrial myxoma

HOSPITALIZATION CRITERIA

- Heart failure
- Atrial fibrillation
- Stroke
- Planned surgery

MEDICATIONS

- Anticoagulation is not beneficial because emboli are due to the friable tumor material

THERAPEUTIC PROCEDURES

- Transcatheter ensnarement and extraction of small myxomas may be feasible via a retrograde arterial approach, but the risk of leaving tumor behind would be high and embolization of the friable tissue would be likely

SURGERY

- Surgical removal is the treatment of choice
- Occasionally damage to the mitral valve requires repair or replacement
- Complete removal of the stalk often creates an atrial septal defect that has to be repaired
- Cardiac transplantation in rare cases

MONITORING

- ECG monitoring in hospitalized patients as appropriate

DIET AND ACTIVITY

- Low-sodium diet, restricted fluids in heart failure
- Avoidance of vigorous exercise until tumor is removed

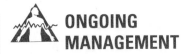 **ONGOING MANAGEMENT**

HOSPITAL DISCHARGE CRITERIA

- After successful surgery

FOLLOW-UP

- Follow-up echocardiography is recommended because of a small recurrence rate (1–2% for benign myxoma, 10–20% for familial ones)
- Baseline echo at 3 months after surgery, then yearly for 10–15 years

COMPLICATIONS

- Atrial fibrillation
- Stroke
- Heart failure
- Extremity or abdominal organ ischemia/infarction from embolus

PROGNOSIS

- Excellent after surgical removal
- Strokes due to myxoma emboli usually clear completely without significant residual defects

PREVENTION

- Familial variety is autosomal dominant, which would deter procreation

RESOURCES

PRACTICE GUIDELINES

- Left atrial myxoma should be removed promptly once the diagnosis is made

REFERENCES

- Keeling IM et al: Cardiac myxomas: 24 years of experience in 49 patients. Eur J Cardiothorac Surg 2002;22:971.
- Schaff HV, Mullany CJ: Surgery for cardiac myxomas. Semin Thorac Cardiovasc Surg 2000;12:77.
- Selkane C et al: Changing management of cardiac myxoma based on a series of 40 cases with long-term follow-up. Ann Thorac Surg 2003;76:1935.

INFORMATION FOR PATIENTS

- www.nlm.nih.gov/medlineplus/ency/article/000196.htm

WEB SITES

- www.emedicine.com/med/topic2999.htm
- www.emedicine.com/med/topic186.htm

Left Ventricular Aneurysm

 ## KEY FEATURES

ESSENTIALS OF DIAGNOSIS

- True aneurysm:
  - Echocardiographic evidence of thinned, scarred myocardium that deforms the diastolic silhouette of the left ventricle with systolic akinesis or dyskinesis
- False aneurysm:
  - Echocardiographic evidence of a thin-walled sac communicating with an infarcted segment of the left ventricle by a narrow neck
  - Systolic expansion of the sac is often observed
  - Color flow imaging shows flow in and out of the sac

GENERAL CONSIDERATIONS

- True left ventricular (LV) aneurysms develop in less than 5% of all patients with acute myocardial infarction (MI)
- Intraventricular pressure stretches the infarcted noncontractile segment, leading to aneurysm formation
- Over time, dense fibrous tissue replaces infarcted myocardium, but systolic expansion of the segment can be visualized on echocardiogram
- Aneurysms are more likely to occur after an anterior MI, particularly at the apex
- Aneurysms rarely occur with multivessel disease (poor contraction of the nonaffected segments)
- Rupture is rare, unlike in pseudoaneurysm
- High incidence of ventricular arrhythmias is major cause of increased mortality
- Calcification of the scar may occur eventually and may be visible on chest x-ray
- Thrombus formation in the aneurysm is common
- In pseudoaneurysm, the wall is made up of thrombus and pericardium, and the risk of rupture is high

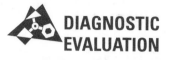 ## CLINICAL PRESENTATION

SYMPTOMS AND SIGNS

- Dyspnea secondary to LV dysfunction
- Chest pain may be present if there is associated pericarditis

PHYSICAL EXAM FINDINGS

- Enlarged and sustained precordial impulse (most often in the third intercostal space at the midclavicular line)

DIFFERENTIAL DIAGNOSIS

- Akinetic or dyskinetic segments without diastolic deformity
- Pericardial cyst or loculated effusion

DIAGNOSTIC EVALUATION

LABORATORY TESTS

- CBC, brain natriuretic peptide test

ELECTROCARDIOGRAPHY

- ECG: persistent ST elevation with Q waves most common

IMAGING STUDIES

- Echocardiogram shows:
  - Systolic expansion of a thin-walled segment of the LV and often the presence of thrombus (laminated or fresh)
  - The size of the neck of the aneurysm compared with the fundus of the LV is useful for distinguishing true aneurysm from pseudoaneurysm
  - In pseudoaneurysm, the neck is small (< 50% of diameter of fundus)
- Cardiac MRI can also be used to identify LV aneurysms and may be useful if echocardiography is not diagnostic

DIAGNOSTIC PROCEDURES

- Left ventriculography can also demonstrate aneurysms and should be done if coronary angiography is done

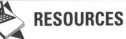

Left Ventricular Aneurysm

TREATMENT

CARDIOLOGY REFERRAL

- Heart failure
- Ventricular arrhythmias
- Persistent angina
- Systemic emboli or visible thrombus

HOSPITALIZATION CRITERIA

- Pulmonary edema
- Unstable angina
- Symptomatic ventricular arrhythmias
- Stroke or peripheral arterial occlusion

MEDICATIONS

- Heart failure medications as needed
- Anti-arrhythmic medications as indicated
- Anticoagulation for true aneurysms
- Antianginal medications as needed

THERAPEUTIC PROCEDURES

- Automatic inplantable cardioverter-defibrillator indicated if serious ventricular arrhythmias or reduced LV function

SURGERY

- True aneurysm: aneurysmectomy for intractable heart failure, recurrent arrhythmias and repeated emboli on therapy
- Pseudoaneurysm: surgical correction to prevent rupture
- Concomitant coronary artery bypass graft if needed

MONITORING

- ECG monitoring in hospital
- INR monitoring for those on warfarin

DIET AND ACTIVITY

- Same as for coronary artery disease (CAD)

ONGOING MANAGEMENT

HOSPITAL DISCHARGE CRITERIA

- Pseudoaneurysm: after surgical correction
- True aneurysm: when anticoagulation is adequate and patient is clinically stable

FOLLOW-UP

- Two weeks after discharge and periodically after that, depending on clinical symptoms

COMPLICATIONS

- True aneurysm:
  - Embolic manifestations
  - LV dysfunction
  - Life-threatening ventricular arrhythmia
- Pseudoaneurysm: rupture

PROGNOSIS

- Sudden cardiac death is more common in CAD patients with LV aneurysm and this risk persists after aneurysmectomy, but is reduced by about 50%
- Heart failure symptoms may be persistent after aneurysmectomy depending on the contractile state of the remaining myocardium
- After resection, often a residual, but smaller aneurysm persists and may be a source of systemic emboli

PREVENTION

- Prevention of MI

RESOURCES

PRACTICE GUIDELINES

- The major indications for LV aneurysmectomy with coronary bypass surgery are pump failure or intractable ventricular arrhythmias unresponsive to medical and catheter-based therapy

REFERENCES

- Khairy P, Thibault B, Talajic M et al: Prognostic significance of ventricular arrhythmias post-myocardial infarction. Can J Cardiol 2003;19:1393.
- Pasini S et al: Early and late results after surgical therapy of postinfarction left ventricular aneurysm. J Cardiovasc Surg 1998;39:209.

INFORMATION FOR PATIENTS

- www.nhlbi.nih.gov/health/dci/ Diseases/Cad/CAD_WhatIs.html

WEB SITES

- www.acc.org
- www.americanheart.org

Left Ventricular Free Wall Rupture, Acute

KEY FEATURES

ESSENTIALS OF DIAGNOSIS

- Sudden marked bradycardia and hypotension up to 2 weeks after acute myocardial infarction (MI)
- Cardiac arrest with electromechanical dissociation after acute MI
- Acute cardiac tamponade:
  - Elevated jugular venous pressure
  - Hypotension after acute MI

GENERAL CONSIDERATIONS

- Rupture of the free wall, interventricular septum, and papillary muscle may account for 15% of all deaths after an MI
- Delay in seeking treatment after MI is seen in these patients
- Sustained physical activity after an MI may precipitate this condition
- Role of prior use of corticosteroids and nonsteroidal anti-inflammatory drugs in promoting free wall rupture is controversial
- Common in elderly and women
- History of hypertension is common in affected patients
- Terminal branches of left anterior descending coronary artery disease seem to cause this problem
- Rupture usually involves anterior or lateral walls
- Usually involves a large infarct (> 20% of left ventricle [LV])
- Most common between 1 and 4 days after acute MI but may occur up to 3 weeks after MI
- Uncommon with thick ventricle
- Uncommon in patients with prior infarction and poor LV function
- Rupture leads to hemopericardium, cardiac tamponade, and death
- Survival depends on early recognition and emergent surgery
- Most common in LV; right ventricular rupture is uncommon; atrial rupture is rare
- Thrombolytics and percutaneous intervention have reduced the frequency of this complication

CLINICAL PRESENTATION

SYMPTOMS AND SIGNS

- Acute rupture: immediate death
- Subacute rupture:
  - Nausea, diaphoresis
  - Sharp chest pain secondary to pericardial irritation
  - Shortness of breath

PHYSICAL EXAM FINDINGS

- Severe hypotension
- Tachycardia
- Soft heart sounds
- Pulmonary rales and dyspnea

DIFFERENTIAL DIAGNOSIS

- Acute ventricular septal rupture
- Acute mitral regurgitation
- Massive recurrent myocardial infarction
- Arrhythmic cardiac arrest

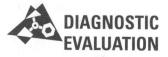 DIAGNOSTIC EVALUATION

LABORATORY TESTS

- CBC
- Arterial blood gases
- Cardiac biomarkers
- Type and crossmatch for blood transfusion

ELECTROCARDIOGRAPHY

- ECG shows evolving MI pattern usually without acute changes

IMAGING STUDIES

- Emergency bedside transthoracic echocardiogram demonstrates ruptured wall and pericardial blood

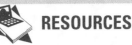

TREATMENT

CARDIOLOGY REFERRAL

- Immediate referral to a cardiologist

HOSPITALIZATION CRITERIA

- All patients should be transferred to a coronary care unit before transfer to the operating room

DIAGNOSTIC PROCEDURES

- Percutaneous cardiopulmonary bypass in preparation for surgery

THERAPEUTIC PROCEDURES

- Immediate pericardiocentesis followed by emergency corrective surgery
- Intra-aortic balloon counterpulsation to stabilize the patient for cardiac catheterization, if feasible

SURGERY

- Surgical repair: techniques to repair the ventricle include direct suture or patch to cover the ventricular perforation
- Cyanoacrylate glue may be used to hold the patch in place over the site of rupture
- Coronary artery bypass graft as needed

MONITORING

- Monitor ECG, oxygen saturation, and blood pressure with an intra-arterial line

DIET AND ACTIVITY

- Nothing by mouth until improvement after surgery
- Bed rest
- After recovery, low-fat diet
- Gradual ambulation as tolerated

ONGOING MANAGEMENT

HOSPITAL DISCHARGE CRITERIA

- Stable symptoms and hemodynamic stability
- Able to ambulate

FOLLOW-UP

- Two weeks after hospital discharge
- Subsequently 3 months after dismissal and annual visit with a stress test
- Individual patients may require more frequent visits

COMPLICATIONS

- Death
- Postsurgical death
- Postsurgical complications including infection

PROGNOSIS

- Generally poor
- Survival is low in acute massive rupture even with prompt aggressive treatment
- Subacute rupture has a better chance of survival

PREVENTION

- Early and prompt revascularization
- Public awareness to seek medical care soon after the onset of chest pain

RESOURCES

PRACTICE GUIDELINES

- Should be considered for surgical repair unless further care is futile
- Coronary artery bypass graft should be undertaken at the same time

REFERENCES

- Flajsig I: Surgical treatment of left ventricular free wall rupture after myocardial infarction: case series. Croat Med J 2002;43:643.
- Harpaz D, Kriwisky M, Cohen AJ et al: Unusual form of cardiac rupture: sealed subacute left ventricular free wall rupture, evolving to intramyocardial dissecting hematoma and to pseudoaneurysm formation—a case report and review of the literature J Am Soc Echocardiogr 2001;14:219.

INFORMATION FOR PATIENTS

- www.drpen.com/410.9
- www.drpen.com/785.5

WEB SITE

- www.americanheart.org

Localized Lymphedema

 ## KEY FEATURES

ESSENTIALS OF DIAGNOSIS

- Isolated swollen extremity secondary to lymph vessel damage from surgery, radiation, disease, or trauma, or as a primary developmental abnormality
- No evidence of heart failure, renal disease, malabsorption, or other edema-producing conditions

GENERAL CONSIDERATIONS

- Secondary lymphatic obstruction:
  - Usually caused by damage to the lymphatic vessels or enlarged lymph nodes, particularly from neoplasm
  - More common in older persons in whom diseases that obstruct the lymph vessels are more common
- Primary lymphedema:
  - A developmental abnormality that occurs in younger individual
  - Much less common than secondary lymphedema
- Lymphedema praecox (most common form of primary lymphedema):
  - More common in women (10:1)
  - Often starts after menarche or the first pregnancy
  - Often runs in families

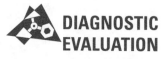 ## CLINICAL PRESENTATION

SYMPTOMS AND SIGNS

- Painless swelling of an extremity extending to the digits

PHYSICAL EXAM FINDINGS

- Nonpitting edema of an extremity
- Thickened skin in affected limb with peau d'orange appearance
- Yellow nail syndrome

DIFFERENTIAL DIAGNOSIS

- Angioneurotic edema
- Infectious lymphangitis
- Venous insufficiency
- Thrombophlebitis
- Other causes of edema such as heart failure

DIAGNOSTIC EVALUATION

IMAGING STUDIES

- Duplex Doppler echocardiography demonstrates normal arteries and veins in the affected limb
- Lymphoscintigraphy shows:
  - Reduced deep lymphatic vessels and prominent superficial lymphatics in lymphedema praecox
  - Generally reduced lymphatics in postradiation or lymphangitis
  - Obstructed dilated lymphatics with enlarged lymph nodes, filariasis or postsurgical (eg, mastectomy)

DIAGNOSTIC PROCEDURES

- Venography to exclude venous disease

TREATMENT

CARDIOLOGY REFERRAL

- Suspected heart failure

HOSPITALIZATION CRITERIA

- Thrombophlebitis
- Heart failure
- Suspected neoplasm

MEDICATIONS

- Physiotherapy and massage

THERAPEUTIC PROCEDURES

- Elevation of the limb and compressive stockings

SURGERY

- In extreme cases, surgery to reduce the amount of subcutaneous tissue can be considered (Charles operation)

DIET AND ACTIVITY

- A low-sodium diet may help reduce swelling
- Exercise can help reduce swelling

ONGOING MANAGEMENT

HOSPITAL DISCHARGE CRITERIA

- Resolution of problem
- After surgery

FOLLOW-UP

- Yearly in stable patients

COMPLICATIONS

- Thrombophlebitis
- Cellulitis

PROGNOSIS

- Excellent if infection is prevented

PREVENTION

- Meticulous skin care to prevent infections

RESOURCES

PRACTICE GUIDELINES

- In older persons, neoplasm must be excluded

REFERENCES

- Campisi C et al: Microsurgical techniques for lymphedema treatment: derivative lymphatic-venous microsurgery. World J Surg 2004;28:609.
- Kim DI et al: Excisional surgery for chronic advanced lymphedema. Surg Today 2004;34:134.

INFORMATION FOR PATIENTS

- www.nlm.nih.gov/medlineplus/ency/article/001117.htm

WEB SITE

- www.emedicine.com/med/topic2722.htm

Long QT Syndrome

KEY FEATURES

ESSENTIALS OF DIAGNOSIS

- Clinical constellation of congenital deafness, prolongation of the QT interval (QTc > 480 ms), syncope, and sudden death
- Family history of sudden death
- Characteristic arrhythmia is torsades de pointes
- The fundamental abnormality is prolongation of action potential secondary to abnormality of transmembrane ion transport
- Emotion seems to trigger cardiac events, particularly in patients with *KvLQT1*

GENERAL CONSIDERATIONS

- Family history of sudden cardiac death (SCD), QT prolongation on the ECG, and bilateral neural deafness with autosomal recessive pattern of inheritance affecting several children in a family was first reported by Jervell and Lange-Nielsen
- Family history of SCD, QT prolongation, and autosomal dominant pattern of inheritance was subsequently identified (Romano-Ward syndrome)
- Romano-Ward syndrome is more common than Jervell and Lange-Nielsen syndrome
- Deafness is not a manifestation of Romano-Ward syndrome
- Mutations in seven *LQTS* genes have thus for been identified
- Repolarization (potassium) currents are affected in most of the disorders except in *LQT3* and *LQT4,* where the sodium current is affected
- Family members with identical gene mutations may experience wide variations in clinical symptoms (variable penetrance) from asymptomatic to recurrent syncope
- *SCDLQT1* (43%) and *LQT2* (45%) account for most of the recognized patients

CLINICAL PRESENTATION

SYMPTOMS AND SIGNS

- SCD or syncope
- Incidental finding of prolonged QT interval or during family screening
- Syncope with stress
- Congenital deafness
- Symptoms usually present during adolescence
- Males are affected during adolescence and females during adulthood
- *LQT1* patients experience symptoms during exercise, and *LQT2* patients during acute arousal
- Once clinical symptoms occur, risk of recurrence is high

PHYSICAL EXAM FINDINGS

- Bilateral nerve deafness
- Otherwise clinical examination is normal

DIFFERENTIAL DIAGNOSIS

- Metabolic abnormalities with prolongation of QT
- Drug-induced long QT
- Idiopathic ventricular arrhythmia
- Central nervous system disorder, which prolongs QT

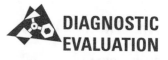 DIAGNOSTIC EVALUATION

LABORATORY TESTS

- Metabolic panel to exclude hypokalemia and hyomagnesemia
- Genetic testing may be helpful, but the test results may take too long to influence clinical decision making
  - A negative test is not helpful unless testing is performed to identify a mutation that is already known within the family

ELECTROCARDIOGRAPHY

- QTc > 480 ms
- Holter monitoring may uncover asymptomatic torsades de pointes
- Exercise ECG may be helpful if activity precipitates arrhythmia, or QT-interval prolongation occurs during recovery if there is no prior diagnosis of long QT syndrome
- Usefulness of Holter monitoring and exercise stress test, although frequently used, are supported by very few studies

IMAGING STUDIES

- Echocardiogram may be used to establish structurally normal heart
- Depending on clinical situation, exclude central nervous system disorder with imaging

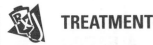

TREATMENT

CARDIOLOGY REFERRAL

- When the condition is suspected, cardiac electrophysiology referral is indicated

HOSPITALIZATION CRITERIA

- After syncope or resuscitation from SCD

MEDICATIONS

- Beta blockers
- Sympathetic denervation

THERAPEUTIC PROCEDURES

- Pacemaker to support rate during aggressive beta-blocker therapy
- Implantation of cardioverter-defibrillator:
  - In those with syncope or cardiac arrest during adrenergic modulation (beta blockers and sympathectomy)
  - When the first event is a documented cardiac arrest

SURGERY

- Left cardiothoracic ganglionectomy is considered adjuvant therapy since the introduction of beta blockers

MONITORING

- ECG monitoring in the hospital

DIET AND ACTIVITY

- Increased potassium or magnesium in the diet is not backed by sufficient data
- Competitive athletics should be prohibited
- Vigorous exercise may precipitate cardiac events in patients with *LQT1*

ONGOING MANAGEMENT

HOSPITAL DISCHARGE CRITERIA

- Once hospitalized for life-threatening ventricular arrhythmia, patients may be discharged after implantation of an implantable cardioverter-defibrillator (ICD)

FOLLOW-UP

- Asymptomatic patients should be followed up periodically or at first onset of symptoms
- Patients with devices may be followed up in the device clinic with a physician follow-up once a year

COMPLICATIONS

- SCD in undiagnosed patients or patients without an ICD

PROGNOSIS

- In untreated patients, prognosis is poor
- Prior to common use of beta-blocker therapy, mortality rate was 20% in the first year after syncope and 50% in 15 years
- In recent registry data, mortality rate is much lower
- Benefit of beta-blocker therapy has not been proved in a randomized trial

PREVENTION

- Family screening

RESOURCES

PRACTICE GUIDELINES

- Indications for an ICD:
  - Recurrent syncope
  - Sustained ventricular arrhythmias
  - SCD episode despite medical therapy
  - A strong family history of SCD
  - Noncompliance or intolerance to drugs

REFERENCES

- Moss AJ: Long QT syndrome. JAMA 2003;289:204.
- Passman R et al: Polymorphic ventricular tachycardia, long Q-T syndrome, and torsades de pointes. Med Clin North Am 2001;85:321.

INFORMATION FOR PATIENTS

- www.nlm.nih.gov/medlineplus/arrhythmia.html

WEB SITE

- www.hrsonline.org

Lutembacher Syndrome

KEY FEATURES

ESSENTIALS OF DIAGNOSIS

- Congenital atrial septal defect plus rheumatic mitral stenosis

GENERAL CONSIDERATIONS

- Atrial septal defect (ASD) is a common congenital heart disease that often escapes notice in early childhood if small
- In parts of the world where rheumatic heart disease is also common, occasionally ASD and mitral stenosis (Lutembacher's syndrome) occur together
- What makes this coincidence of special importance is the physiologic interaction between the two conditions
- Mitral stenosis increases the pressure in the left atrium and increases the left-to-right shunt at the atrial level
- An ASD allows some decompression of left atrial pressure at the expense of reduced transatrial flow into the left ventricle
- Iatrogenic Lutembacher's syndrome occurs when balloon mitral valvuloplasty for mitral stenosis is attempted by the transatrial septal approach and stenosis relief is incomplete
  - The persistently high left atrial pressure in this situation prevents atrial septal healing and results in a persistent ASD

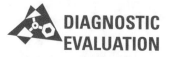

CLINICAL PRESENTATION

SYMPTOMS AND SIGNS

- Fatigue
- Dyspnea
- Signs of right heart failure

PHYSICAL EXAM FINDINGS

- Right ventricle lift
- Loud S_1
- Fixed split S_2
- Opening snap
- Pulmonary flow murmur
- Diastolic mitral rumble

DIFFERENTIAL DIAGNOSIS

- Mitral stenosis with the opening snap mistaken for a wide fixed split S_2 and another systolic murmur (eg, innocent flow, mild mitral, or tricuspid regurgitation) mistaken for a pulmonary outflow murmur
- ASD with the wide fixed split S_2 mistaken for an opening snap and a tricuspid flow rumble mistaken for the murmur of mitral stenosis
- Ebstein's anomaly of the tricuspid valve and an ASD

DIAGNOSTIC EVALUATION

ELECTROCARDIOGRAPHY

- Right ventricular hypertrophy
- Right and left atrial abnormality
- Atrial fibrillation

IMAGING STUDIES

- Echocardiography: demonstrates the thickened stenosed mitral valve and the ASD
- Doppler echocardiography: can quantitate the mitral valve area and shunt fraction across the ASD

DIAGNOSTIC PROCEDURES

- Transesophageal echocardiography: may be needed to define the atrial septal anatomy and the location of the ASD
- Cardiac catheterization: may be necessary to confirm the severity of mitral stenosis and the magnitude of the shunt

TREATMENT

CARDIOLOGY REFERRAL

- Symptoms with signs of valvular or congenital heart disease
- Atrial fibrillation
- Heart failure
- Paradoxical embolism
- Suspected endocarditis

HOSPITALIZATION CRITERIA

- Heart failure
- Atrial fibrillation with rapid ventricular response
- Stroke
- Suspected endocarditis

MEDICATIONS

- Rate control of atrial fibrillation
- Anticoagulation with warfarin

THERAPEUTIC PROCEDURES

- It is possible to go through the ASD to perform catheter balloon valvuloplasty on the mitral valve and then place a percutaneous device to close the ASD, but experience is scant

SURGERY

- When the mitral valve is not suitable for a percutaneous balloon valvuloplasty, surgery is required and the ASD is repaired at the same time

MONITORING

- ECG monitoring in hospital as appropriate

DIET AND ACTIVITY

- Low-sodium diet and restricted activity if heart failure present

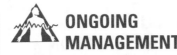

ONGOING MANAGEMENT

HOSPITAL DISCHARGE CRITERIA

- Resolution of the problem
- Successful procedure or surgery

FOLLOW-UP

- Close follow-up of symptomatic patients
- After surgery or valvuloplasty at 3, 6, 12 months, then yearly

COMPLICATIONS

- Right heart failure
- Atrial fibrillation
- Stroke due to paradoxical embolus
- Endocarditis

PROGNOSIS

- Symptoms will occur earlier than expected for either lesion alone because of their physiologic effects in combination

PREVENTION

- Rheumatic fever prophylaxis
- ASD is congenital
- Endocarditis prophylaxis

RESOURCES

PRACTICE GUIDELINES

- Correction of the defects recommended for any symptoms or evidence of a significant shunt (> 1.5:1.0)
- Percutaneous balloon valvuloplasty should not be undertaken unless the echocardiogram shows a high likelihood of success

REFERENCES

- Chau EM et al: Transcatheter treatment of a case of Lutembacher syndrome. Catheter Cardiovasc Interv 2000;50:68.
- Zanchetta M et al: Use of Amplatzer septal occluder in a case of residual atrial septal defect causing bidirectional shunting after percutaneous Inoue mitral balloon valvuloplasty. J Invasive Cardiol 2001;13:223.

INFORMATION FOR PATIENTS

- www.drpen.com/394

WEB SITE

- www.emedicine.com/med/topic3519.htm

Lyme Carditis

KEY FEATURES

ESSENTIALS OF DIAGNOSIS

- Flulike illness followed by evidence of atrioventricular block
- Diagnosis is confirmed by the association of typical clinical features with serologic testing

GENERAL CONSIDERATIONS

- Infectious disease caused by *Borrelia burgdorferi*, a tick-borne spirochete
- Male predominance 3:1 for cardiac Lyme disease
- Initial manifestations include:
  - Myalgias
  - Arthralgia
  - Fever
  - Headache
  - Erythema migrans
- Four to 10% of infected patients develop symptoms from transient cardiac involvement weeks to months after initial presentation
- The most common manifestation is conduction abnormality in the form of varying degrees of atrioventricular block
- Syncope due to complete heart block is common
- Diffuse ST-segment and T-wave changes and asymptomatic left ventricular dysfunction may be found, but congestive heart failure is rare
- Occasional patients develop symptomatic myocarditis or pericarditis

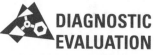 CLINICAL PRESENTATION

SYMPTOMS AND SIGNS

- Cardiac features can be coincident with other early features of Lyme disease, including erythema migrans and neurologic abnormalities or may be the only manifestation of infection
- Palpitations (common)
- Lightheadedness
- Syncope (common)
- Dyspnea
- Chest pain
- Some patients are asymptomatic

PHYSICAL EXAM FINDINGS

- Bradycardia
- Cannon *a* waves in the jugular venous pressure in patients with complete heart block
- Congestive heart failure is uncommon
- Erythema migrans
- Monoarthritis
- Cranial nerve palsy or other findings of meningoencephalitis

DIFFERENTIAL DIAGNOSIS

- Myocarditis due to other infectious agents
- Intrinsic conduction system disease

DIAGNOSTIC EVALUATION

LABORATORY TESTS

- Lyme serology with ELISA and/or Western blot analysis

ELECTROCARDIOGRAPHY

- Varying degrees of atrioventricular block, which can progress to complete heart block in a short period of time
- Bundle branch block, fascicular block
- Nonspecific ST- and T-wave changes

IMAGING STUDIES

- Chest x-ray:
  - Cardiomegaly may be present and is usually transient
- Echocardiography:
  - Mild cardiomegaly and/or mild left ventricular dysfunction
  - Pericardial effusion may be present
  - These changes are usually transient

DIAGNOSTIC PROCEDURES

- Electrophysiologic testing is rarely required; typical findings include:
  - Heart block within the atrioventricular node, although heart block may occur at other levels within the conduction systems
  - Sinus node dysfunction may also be present
- Endomyocardial biopsy (rarely indicated) but shows the following:
  - Lymphoid and plasmacytic infiltrates
  - Variable amounts of necrosis, fibrosis, and edema that is indicative of active myocarditis
  - Spirochetes have been isolated in some

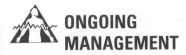

Lyme Carditis

TREATMENT

CARDIOLOGY REFERRAL

- Atrioventricular block of any type
- Evidence of myocarditis or left ventricular dysfunction

HOSPITALIZATION CRITERIA

- Symptomatic patients, including syncope
- High-grade or progressive atrioventricular block, symptomatic or asymptomatic

MEDICATIONS

- Antibiotic therapy with amoxicillin (500–875 mg PO every 12 hours) or doxycycline (100 mg PO bid) is recommended for 14–21 days in patients treated in the outpatient setting
- IV ceftriaxone (1–2 g IV every day) or cefotaxime (1–2 g IV every 6–8 hours) per day for 2–4 weeks is recommended for hospitalized patients
- Glucocorticoids (eg, prednisone 5–50 mg PO per day) may be of benefit if there is no improvement in heart block within 24–48 hours of antibiotic therapy

THERAPEUTIC PROCEDURES

- Temporary transvenous pacemaker may be required

SURGERY

- Permanent pacemaker insertion is rarely required

MONITORING

- ECG monitoring for heart block

DIET AND ACTIVITY

- Low-sodium diet for patients with heart failure (rare)
- Bed rest for patients with high-grade heart block or syncope

ONGOING MANAGEMENT

HOSPITAL DISCHARGE CRITERIA

- After stabilization of cardiac rhythm, including improvement or resolution of heart block

FOLLOW-UP

- Visit with cardiologist within 1 month or earlier depending on the clinical situation
- ECG every 2–4 weeks until changes resolve or stabilize
- Holter or event monitor if symptoms suggest intermittent high-grade atrioventricular block

COMPLICATIONS

- Progression of atrioventricular block rarely occurs beyond 6 weeks after appropriate antibiotic therapy
- Progression or the appearance of cardiomyopathy after appropriate antibiotics typically does not occur

PROGNOSIS

- Features of Lyme carditis are usually transient, including heart block and myocarditis, with a good prognosis
- Heart block usually resolves spontaneously within 3 days to 6 weeks
- A permanent pacemaker is rarely required
- Chronic cardiomyopathy is rarely the result of Lyme carditis
- Rare cases of fatal Lyme carditis have been reported

PREVENTION

- Appropriate antibiotics for erythema migrans or other features of early localized Lyme disease can prevent the development of carditis

RESOURCES

PRACTICE GUIDELINES

- The diagnosis of Lyme carditis is confirmed by serologic testing in patients with typical clinical features
- Symptomatic patients or patients with high-grade atrioventricular block are hospitalized and generally treated with IV antibiotics
- Indications for pacing are the same as in other causes of heart block

REFERENCE

- Donta ST: Late and chronic Lyme disease. Med Clin North Am 2002;86:341.

INFORMATION FOR PATIENTS

- http://www.nlm.nih.gov/medlineplus/lymedisease.html
- http://patients.uptodate.com/topic.asp?file=othr_inf/7642

WEB SITE

- http://www.emedicine.com/neuro/topic521.htm

Marfan Syndrome

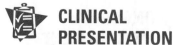 **KEY FEATURES**

ESSENTIALS OF DIAGNOSIS

- Tall stature with disproportionately long limbs
- Ectopia lentis
- Aortic aneurysms, dissection, and aortic regurgitation
- Mitral valve prolapse with regurgitation

GENERAL CONSIDERATIONS

- Autosomal dominant disorder (1 per 10,000) with multisystem involvement
- Affects the skeleton (long thin extremities), eye (ectopia lentis), and cardiovascular system (aortic aneurysms) from mutation in a gene on chromosome 15 that encodes fibrillin
- Mitral valve prolapse secondary to redundancy of the leaflets and the chordae (in 60–80%)
- Severe mitral regurgitation in 25% of patients
- Aortic root dilatation and aortic regurgitation
- Dissection of the aorta occurs with increasing frequency at a diameter of 55 mm (family history of dissection increases the risk at 50 mm)
- Pregnancy increases the risk of dissection, particularly in the third trimester
  - Low risk if root diameter is < 40 mm

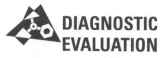 **CLINICAL PRESENTATION**

SYMPTOMS AND SIGNS

- Chest pain, back pain
- Dyspnea, fatigue
- Palpitations

PHYSICAL EXAM FINDINGS

- Diastolic murmur of aortic regurgitation
- Midsystolic click and late systolic murmur of mitral valve prolapse
- Tall stature, limbs disproportionately long, arm span > height
- Pectus excavatum and scoliosis
- Arachnodactyly
- Ratio of upper body height to lower body height < 0.93 (divided at symphysis pubis)
- High, arched palate

DIFFERENTIAL DIAGNOSIS

- Homocystinuria
- Ehlers-Danlos syndrome
- Familial aortic aneurysm

DIAGNOSTIC EVALUATION

LABORATORY TESTS

- Presence of an FNB 1 gene mutation (fibrillin gene)

ELECTROCARDIOGRAPHY

- Signs of left heart chamber enlargement

IMAGING STUDIES

- Echocardiographic findings that may be seen:
  - Aortic root dilation involving the sinuses of Valsalva
  - Aortic dissection
  - Mitral valve prolapse
  - Calcified mitral annulus
  - Dilated main pulmonary artery
  - Aortic regurgitation
- MRI or CT: ideal for imaging aortic aneurysms and dissection

DIAGNOSTIC PROCEDURES

- Slit-lamp exam of the eyes for lens dislocation

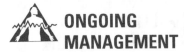

TREATMENT

CARDIOLOGY REFERRAL

- Suspected cardiovascular involvement
- Pregnancy
- Aortic dissection

HOSPITALIZATION CRITERIA

- Aortic dissection
- Heart failure
- Significant arrhythmias

MEDICATIONS

- Beta blockers to prevent or delay aortic root dilatation (recommended, but efficacy not established)
- Vasodilators for significant aortic regurgitation

SURGERY

- Surgical replacement of aorta with preservation of native aortic valve (either prophylactic at aortic root diameter of > 50 mm, or treatment for dissection)
- For pregnant women, consider surgery at 40–50 mm aortic root diameter
- Mitral valve surgery if mitral regurgitation is severe and patient has symptoms

MONITORING

- ECG monitoring in hospital as appropriate

DIET AND ACTIVITY

- Restriction from heavy weight-lifting and contact sports
- Low-sodium, low-fat diet

ONGOING MANAGEMENT

HOSPITAL DISCHARGE CRITERIA

- Resolution of problem
- After successful surgery

FOLLOW-UP

- Yearly follow-up is minimum, but depends on severity of cardiac problems

COMPLICATIONS

- Aortic dissection
- Heart failure
- Infective endocarditis
- Significant ventricular arrhythmias

PROGNOSIS

- Overall, Marfan syndrome reduces lifespan to about 70 years
- Prognosis largely depends on the severity of cardiovascular disease

PREVENTION

- Endocarditis prophylaxis
- Genetic counseling

RESOURCES

PRACTICE GUIDELINES

- Pregnancy in women with Marfan syndrome risks aortic dissection and has a 50% chance of having an affected child

REFERENCE

- Dean JC: Management of Marfan syndrome. Heart 2002;88:97.

INFORMATION FOR PATIENTS

- staff@marfan.org

WEB SITE

- www.emedicine.com/ped/topic1372.htm

Metabolic Abnormalities and Cardiovascular Disease

 KEY FEATURES

ESSENTIALS OF DIANOSIS

- Cardiac arrhythmias or dysfunction with any of the following
  - Hyponatremia
  - Hypokalemia
  - Hyperkalemia
  - Hypocalcemia
  - Hypophosphatemia
  - Hypomagnesemia

GENERAL CONSIDERATIONS

- Hyponatremia is common in advanced heart failure; diuretics may play a role
- Hypokalemia is also common with use of diuretics increases the risk of ventricular arrhythmia, particularly with digitalis toxicity
  - Extreme hypokalemia may lead to cardiac arrest
- Hyperkalemia can cause asystole
- Hypocalcemia prolongs QT interval and causes ventricular arrhythmias
- Hypocalcemia and hypophosphatemia, when prolonged, may cause cardiomyopathy
- Hypomagnesemia may cause:
  - Refractory hypokalemia and hypocalcemia
  - Ventricular arrhythmias

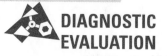 **CLINICAL PRESENTATION**

SYMPTOMS AND SIGNS

- Syncope
- Heart failure symptoms
- Palpitation
- Weakness

PHYSICAL EXAM FINDINGS

- Hypotension
- Signs of heart failure
- Edema
- Tetany with hypocalcemia
- Proximal muscle weakness with hypokalemia

DIFFERENTIAL DIAGNOSIS

- Hypokalemia and hypomagnesemia may be caused by diuretics or gastrointestinal losses
- Angiotensin-converting enzyme inhibitors and spironolactone may cause hyperkalemia

DIAGNOSTIC EVALUATION

LABORATORY TESTS

- Serum electrolytes, calcium, magnesium, phosphorus

ELECTROCARDIOGRAPHY

- Nonspecific ST-T–wave changes are common
- Hypokalemia causes prominent U waves
- Hyperkalemia causes absent P waves, peaked T waves, and eventually widened QRS, culminating in a sine-wave ventricular tachycardia or asystole
- QTc may be prolonged in hypokalemia, hypocalcemia, or hypomagnesemia
- QTc shortened by hypercalcemia

IMAGING STUDIES

- Electrocardiography: may show generalized left ventricular hypokinesis with low ejection fraction

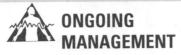

TREATMENT

CARDIOLOGY REFERRAL

- Significant cardiac arrhythmias
- Heart failure
- Cardiac arrest

HOSPITALIZATION CRITERIA

- Significant arrhythmias
- Heart failure
- Cardiac arrest
- Syncope

MEDICATIONS

- Identify and treat the underlying cause
- For hypokalemia and hypomagnesemia, provide IV or oral replacement
- Severe hyperkalemia is a cardiac emergency
  - IV calcium chloride or gluconate for cardioprotection
  - IV insulin/glucose and/or bicarbonate to shift the potassium into the cell
  - Sodium polystyrene sulfonate or diuretic to lower body potassium subacutely
  - Dialysis if necessary
- IV calcium for acute correction of low calcium and to correct hypomagnesemia
- High calcium:
  - Can be lowered by ambulation and fluids in mild cases
  - Can be lowered by bisphosphonates more severe elevations
- Hyponatremia is treated with fluid restriction and correction of the circulatory problem; rarely is hypertonic saline given

MONITORING

- Close monitoring of metabolic abnormalities during treatment

DIET AND ACTIVITY

- In general, dietary restriction or liberalization is useful, depending on the abnormality, except liberalizing sodium if hyponatremia is due to heart failure

ONGOING MANAGEMENT

HOSPITAL DISCHARGE CRITERIA

- Resolution of problem

FOLLOW-UP

- Depends on underlying condition

COMPLICATIONS

- Sudden death
- Heart failure
- Seizures

PROGNOSIS

- Excellent with correction of underlying problem

PREVENTION

- Calcium, magnesium and vitamin D supplementation for chronic hypocalcemia
- Avoidance of drugs that prolong QT in hypocalcemia and hypokalemia
- Avoidance of diuretics with high or low calcium levels
- Avoidance of calcium-containing antacids in hypercalcemia
- Low-potassium diet in renal insufficiency with hyperkalemia
- High-potassium diet for chronic hypokalemia

RESOURCES

PRACTICE GUIDELINES

- Metabolic alterations are an unusual cause of significant cardiac arrhythmias or dysfunction
- In patients with underlying heart disease, these alterations can exacerbate the propensity to arrhythmias and retard arrhythmia control; fortunately, they are readily correctable

REFERENCE

- Cohn JN et al: New guidelines for potassium replacement in clinical practice: a contemporary review by the National Council on Potassium in Clinical Practice. Arch Intern Med 2000;160:2429.

INFORMATION FOR PATIENTS

- www.drpen.com/275.2
- www.drpen.com/275.41
- www.drpen.com/275.42
- www.drpen.com/276.1
- www.drpen.com/276.7
- www.drpen.com/276.8

WEB SITES

- www.emedicine.com/med/topic1068.htm
- www.emedicine.com/med/topic1082.htm
- www.emedicine.com/med/topic1118.htm
- www.emedicine.com/med/topic1124.htm
- www.emedicine.com/med/topic1130.htm
- www.emedicine.com/med/topic1135.htm
- www.emedicine.com/med/topic3382.htm

Metabolic Syndrome and the Heart

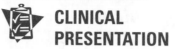 **KEY FEATURES**

ESSENTIALS OF DIAGNOSIS

- Truncal obesity
- Insulin resistance with fasting hyperglycemia
- Elevated triglycerides and reduced high-density lipoprotein (HDL) cholesterol
- Hypertension
- Hyperuricemia
- Premature coronary artery disease

GENERAL CONSIDERATIONS

- The metabolic syndrome consists of the constellation of:
  - Hypertension
  - Dyslipidemia
  - Insulin resistance
  - Obesity
- Other associated abnormalities include:
  - Microalbuminuria
  - High uric acid blood levels
  - Augmented blood clotting
  - Premature atherosclerosis
- Generally, 40% of people with hypertension also have hypercholesterolemia

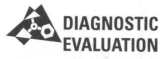 **CLINICAL PRESENTATION**

SYMPTOMS AND SIGNS

- Angina or acute coronary syndrome
- Symptoms of congestive heart failure

PHYSICAL EXAM FINDINGS

- S_4
- Signs of heart failure
- Body mass index > 30 kg/m^2

DIFFERENTIAL DIAGNOSIS

- Other causes of premature coronary artery disease
- Other causes of hypertension
- Other causes of obesity

DIAGNOSTIC EVALUATION

LABORATORY TESTS

- Fasting glucose, hemoglobin A_{1C}, lipids, uric acid

ELECTROCARDIOGRAPHY

- May show evidence of left ventricular hypertrophy or myocardial infarction

IMAGING STUDIES

- Echocardiography frequently shows:
  - Impaired diastolic function of the left ventricle
  - Left heart chamber enlargement
  - Left ventricular systolic dysfunction

DIAGNOSTIC PROCEDURES

- Coronary angiography will be necessary in some patients

TREATMENT

CARDIOLOGY REFERRAL

- Suspected cardiac disease
- Difficult to control hypertension

HOSPITALIZATION CRITERIA

- Acute coronary syndromes
- Heart failure

MEDICATIONS

- Oral hypoglycemic agents, insulin sensitizers, and insulin
- Pharmacologic treatment of hypertension with angiotensin-converting enzyme inhibitors or angiotensin-receptor blockers to < 130/80 mm Hg
- Pharmacologic lipid-lowering therapy to LDL cholesterol < 100 mg/dL
- Pharmacologic therapy to reduce triglycerides and increase HDL, eg, fenofibrate 48–145 daily PO

THERAPEUTIC PROCEDURES

- Coronary revascularization may be necessary

SURGERY

- Coronary bypass surgery may be indicated

MONITORING

- ECG monitoring in hospital as appropriate
- Monitor metabolic parameters during specific therapy

DIET AND ACTIVITY

- Low-fat, low-sodium, low-calorie diet or DASH diet
- Activity restriction if heart disease is active

ONGOING MANAGEMENT

HOSPITAL DISCHARGE CRITERIA

- Resolution of problem

FOLLOW-UP

- Depends on problem and treatment

COMPLICATIONS

- Myocardial infarction
- Heart failure
- Sudden death

PROGNOSIS

- Metabolic syndrome adversely affects survival

PREVENTION

- Aggressive risk factor modification can reduce the incidence and severity of atherosclerosis

RESOURCES

PRACTICE GUIDELINES

- Metabolic syndrome is considered a risk factor for coronary heart disease and is a precursor to type II diabetes. Thus, every effort to control or reverse this condition is warranted

REFERENCE

- Vega GL: Obesity, the metabolic syndrome, and cardiovascular disease. Am Heart J 2001;142:1108.

INFORMATION FOR PATIENTS

- www.hlm.nih.gov/medlineplus/ency/article/000313.htm

WEB SITE

- www.emedicine.com/med/topic547.htm

Mitral Regurgitation, Acute

 KEY FEATURES

ESSENTIALS OF DIAGNOSIS

- Sudden, severe orthopnea
- Evidence of pulmonary edema
- S_4
- Early systolic murmur due to rapid equilibration of left ventricular and left atrial pressures
- Doppler echocardiography establishes diagnosis, severity, and cause of mitral regurgitation

GENERAL CONSIDERATIONS

- Disruption of the mitral valve apparatus leading to severe regurgitation is uncommon, but often results in profound pulmonary edema
- Since there is insufficient time for the left ventricle and atrium to dilate, filling pressures rise dramatically back to the lung capillaries
- Forward stroke volume is markedly reduced because of the large regurgitant volume with a normal left ventricular diastolic volume, resulting in forward heart failure as well
- If not corrected quickly, acute, severe mitral regurgitation can be rapidly fatal
- The most common causes of acute, severe mitral regurgitation:
  - Acute myocardial infarction with papillary muscle rupture or dysfunction
  - Chordal rupture in mitral valve prolapse or endocarditis
  - Leaflet disruption due to trauma or endocarditis

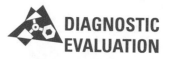 **CLINICAL PRESENTATION**

SYMPTOMS AND SIGNS

- Severe orthopnea, frank pulmonary edema (pink foam in mouth)
- Symptoms and signs of the causal event may be present, such as acute myocardial infarction, endocarditis, or trauma

PHYSICAL EXAM FINDINGS

- Low-volume, low-amplitude, and rapid pulse
- Low blood pressure may be present later in course
- Jugular venous distention may be present later in course
- Increased respiratory rate and diffuse pulmonary rales
- Pleural effusion may occur later in course
- Auscultation:
  - Owing to rapid equilibration of systolic pressure between the left ventricle and atrium, the mitral regurgitant murmur may be short and early systolic if audible at all
  - S_4 is frequently heard owing to vigorous atrial contraction because of augmented left atrial expansion during systole

DIFFERENTIAL DIAGNOSIS

- Other causes of acute pulmonary edema not associated with mitral regurgitation
- Aortic stenosis with heart failure
- Mitral stenosis with heart failure

DIAGNOSTIC EVALUATION

LABORATORY TESTS

- Tests specific to the cause of acute mitral valve disruption, such as blood cultures, may be useful

ELECTROCARDIOGRAPHY

- Signs of acute myocardial infarction may be present in cases of papillary muscle rupture

IMAGING STUDIES

- Chest x-ray:
  - Pulmonary edema without cardiomegaly is classic
  - Later, other signs of heart failure such as pleural effusions may be seen
  - Rib fractures may be present if trauma disrupted the mitral valve
- Echocardiography:
  - The detection of mitral regurgitation is the most important goal of echocardiography
  - The color flow jet may not persist throughout systole because of the rapid equilibration between left ventricular and atrial pressures
  - Also, continuous-wave Doppler regurgitant jet may slow a rapidly decreasing velocity in midsystole, giving a dagger-shaped pattern
  - Interrogation of the valve apparatus may reveal the cause of regurgitation such as papillary muscle or chordal rupture with flail leaflet
  - The velocity of the tricuspid regurgitant jet may show elevated right ventricular pressures later in the course

DIAGNOSTIC PROCEDURES

- Endocarditis is best excluded by transesophageal echocardiography
- Cardiac catheterization is rarely needed to make the diagnosis, but may be useful in cases caused by acute myocardial infarction or to preclude coronary artery disease before surgery

TREATMENT

CARDIOLOGY REFERRAL

- All cases of acute mitral regurgitation

HOSPITALIZATION CRITERIA

- Significant heart failure
- Significant arrhythmias
- Acute myocardial infarction suspected
- Infective endocarditis

MEDICATIONS

- Vasodilators useful to improve forward flow (eg, nitroprusside IV 0.25–10 μg/kg/min)
- Intravenous diuretics (eg, furosemide IV 5–10 mg/hour)

THERAPEUTIC PROCEDURES

- Intra-aortic balloon pump to stabilize severely compromised patients, especially acute myocardial infarction patients

SURGERY

- Mitral valve repair or replacement is the treatment of choice for all symptomatic patients with acute, severe mitral regurgitation
- In cases due to acute myocardial infarction or endocarditis, a period of medical stabilization, if feasible, may be desirable to reduce the surgical risk
- Acute, moderate mitral regurgitation can be managed medically and then reevaluated for surgery at a later point, depending on the usual indications for surgery such as symptoms, left ventricular ejection fraction < .60, atrial fibrillation or pulmonary artery systolic pressure > 50 mm Hg.

MONITORING

- Hemodynamic, oxygen saturation, and ECG monitoring in hospitalized patients
- Medically managed patients need echocardiography to assess left ventricular size and performance before discharge

DIET AND ACTIVITY

- Low-sodium diet
- Bed rest until heart failure symptoms subside

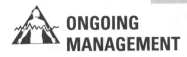 **ONGOING MANAGEMENT**

HOSPITAL DISCHARGE CRITERIA

- Resolution of symptoms
- Successful recovery from surgery

FOLLOW-UP

- In medically treated patients, visits and echocardiography should be repeated in 3 months, then 6 months, then yearly if stable

COMPLICATIONS

- Pulmonary edema
- Cardiogenic shock
- Complications of underlying disease (eg, acute myocardial infarction)
- Atrial fibrillation

PROGNOSIS

- Excellent with successful surgical repair
- Good with successful valve replacement
- Medically treated patients with moderate regurgitation are likely to need surgery within 2 years, especially if flail mitral leaflet is present

PREVENTION

- Prevention of causal events, such as myocardial infarction, trauma
- Antibiotic prophylaxis for endocarditis

RESOURCES

PRACTICE GUIDELINES

- Indications for echocardiography:
  - Anyone suspected of having acute mitral regurgitation.
- Indications for surgery:
  - The same as for mitral regurgitation, organic, chronic
  - Symptoms are the usual indication in those with severe regurgitation.

REFERENCES

- Grigioni F, Enriquez-Sarano M, Zehr KJ et al: Ischemic mitral regurgitation: long-term outcome and prognostic implications with quantitative Doppler assessment. Circulation 2001;103:1759.
- Pellizzon GG, Grines CL, Cox DA et al: Importance of mitral regurgitation in patients undergoing percutaneous coronary intervention for acute myocardial infarction: the Controlled Abciximab and Device Investigation to Lower Late Angioplasty Complications (CADIL-LAC) trial. J Am Coll Cardiol 2004;43:1368.
- Tavakoli R, Weber A, Brunner-La Rocca H et al: Results of surgery for irreversible moderate to severe mitral valve regurgitation secondary to myocardial infarction. Eur J Cardiothorac Surg 2002;21:818.
- Theleman KP, Stephan PJ, Isaacs MG et al: Late (≥ 6 years) results of combined coronary artery bypass grafting and mitral valve replacement for severe mitral regurgitation secondary to acute myocardial infarction. Am J Cardiol 2003;92:1086.
- Thompson CR, Buller CE, Sleeper LA et al: Cardiogenic shock due to acute severe mitral regurgitation complicating acute myocardial infarction: a report from the SHOCK Trial Registry. J Am Coll Cardiol 2000;36:1104.

INFORMATION FOR PATIENTS

- www.drpen.com/394

WEB SITE

- www.emedicine.com/med/CARDIOLOGY.htm

Mitral Regurgitation, Chronic Functional

 KEY FEATURES

ESSENTIALS OF DIAGNOSIS

- Major causes include ischemic heart disease and dilated cardiomyopathy
- Dyspnea or orthopnea
- Signs of left ventricular dysfunction
- Characteristic apical systolic murmur
- Doppler echocardiography shows dilated, dysfunctional left ventricle and a regurgitant jet into the left atrium

GENERAL CONSIDERATIONS

- Functional mitral regurgitation is caused by diseases of the left ventricle or atrium, which disrupt the apparatus
- Most often, the mitral regurgitation is mild to moderate and not a significant issue in overall patient management
- Occasionally, the condition is severe and alleviation or correction of the leak becomes therapeutically important
- Severe mitral regurgitation is associated with dilatation of the left heart chambers and left ventricular systolic dysfunction; it may be difficult to decide which problem occurred first

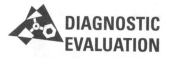 **CLINICAL PRESENTATION**

SYMPTOMS AND SIGNS

- Dyspnea on exertion, progressing to heart failure
- Fatigue
- Palpitations often from atrial fibrillation

PHYSICAL EXAM FINDINGS

- Signs of congestive heart failure
- Brisk upstroke but low-volume carotid pulse
- Enlarged apical impulse
- S_3 heart sound
- Pansystolic apical murmur that increases in intensity with handgrip exercise

DIFFERENTIAL DIAGNOSIS

- Organic mitral regurgitation
- Tricuspid regurgitation
- Aortic stenosis
- Ventricular septal defect

DIAGNOSTIC EVALUATION

LABORATORY TESTS

- Low serum sodium
- Elevated B-type natriuretic peptide

ELECTROCARDIOGRAPHY

- Atrial fibrillation may be present
- Left ventricular hypertrophy
- Left atrial abnormality if in sinus rhythm

IMAGING STUDIES

- Chest x-ray:
  - Enlarged left heart chambers
  - Normal-sized aorta
  - Possible signs of pulmonary congestion and heart failure, such as pleural effusions
- Echocardiography:
  - Evidence of left ventricular disease
  - Hypertrophic, dilated, or ischemic cardiomyopathy
  - Left atrial enlargement
  - Possibly systolic anterior motion of the mitral valve
  - Mitral valve prolapse due to papillary muscle dysfunction
- Doppler echocardiography:
  - Regurgitant jet into the left atrium during systole,
  - Estimated pulmonary artery systolic pressure from the tricuspid regurgitant velocity may be moderately elevated
  - In severe regurgitation, pulmonary venous flow may be reversed in systole

DIAGNOSTIC PROCEDURES

- Left and right heart catheterization may be useful to confirm the magnitude of left atrial and pulmonary pressures and to determine if the pulmonary pressure elevations are likely due to the regurgitation
- Coronary angiography is useful to determine the cause of functional mitral regurgitation
- Left ventriculography may be useful to confirm the presence and severity of mitral regurgitation and the degree of left ventricular disease

TREATMENT

CARDIOLOGY REFERRAL
- Moderate to severe mitral regurgitation
- Evidence of heart failure
- Any cardiovascular symptoms

HOSPITALIZATION CRITERIA
- Heart failure
- Rapid atrial fibrillation
- Unstable angina

MEDICATIONS
- Appropriate treatment of left ventricular dysfunction
- Oral anticoagulation for atrial fibrillation
- Heart rate control for atrial fibrillation

THERAPEUTIC PROCEDURES
- Percutaneous coronary revascularization in selected cases
- Interventricular septal alcohol ablation in selected cases of hypertrophic cardiomyopathy
- Cardiac resynchronization (biventricular pacing) may improve mitral regurgitation in dilated cardiomyopathy
- Percutaneous valve repair techniques are under investigation

SURGERY
- Valve repair or replacement in selected cases
- Septal myectomy in selected cases
- Coronary artery bypass graft surgery in selected cases

MONITORING
- ECG monitoring in hospital
- Weight and fluid status

DIET AND ACTIVITY
- Low-sodium diet
- Reduced activities if heart failure or its symptoms are present

ONGOING MANAGEMENT

HOSPITAL DISCHARGE CRITERIA
- Resolution of symptoms
- Resolution of heart failure
- Control or conversion of atrial fibrillation
- After successful surgery

FOLLOW-UP
- Every 3–12 months, depending on the severity of the disease
- After surgery 3, 6, and 12 months, then every 6–12 months
- Echocardiography every 6–12 months or with change of symptoms

COMPLICATIONS
- Atrial fibrillation
- Heart failure
- Stroke
- Infective endocarditis
- Ventricular tachyarrhythmias

PROGNOSIS
- Usually determined by the underlying disease; rarely is the mitral regurgitation the major issue
- Mitral regurgitation due to coronary artery disease has a worse prognosis than organic mitral regurgitation

PREVENTION
- Prevention of acquired heart disease
- Genetic counseling for hypertrophic cardiomyopathy

RESOURCES

PRACTICE GUIDELINES
- Usually, mitral regurgitation improves if underlying disease improves; occasionally, it is so severe that repair or replacement of the valve should be considered
- In hypertrophic cardiomyopathy or coronary artery disease, mitral valve repair/replacement should be considered if another operative intervention is planned, such as bypass surgery
- With dilated cardiomyopathy, mitral valve repair is rarely done

REFERENCES
- Filsoufi F et al: Current results of combined coronary artery bypass grafting and mitral annuloplasty in patients with moderate ischemic mitral regurgitation. J Heart Valve Dis 2004;13:747.
- Gummert JF et al: Mitral valve repair in patients with end stage cardiomyopathy: who benefits? Eur J Cardiothorac Surg 2003;23:1017.
- Mallidi HR et al: Late outcomes in patients with uncorrected mild to moderate mitral regurgitation at the time of isolated coronary artery bypass grafting. J Thorac Cardiovasc Surg 2004;127:636.
- Stassano P et al: Mitral valve replacement and limited myectomy for hypertrophic obstructive cardiomyopathy: a 25-year follow-up. Tex Heart Inst J 2004;31:137.
- Tahta SA et al: Outcome after mitral valve repair for functional ischemic mitral regurgitation. J Heart Valve Dis 2002;11:11.
- Tavakoli R et al: Results of surgery for irreversible moderate to severe mitral valve regurgitation secondary to myocardial infarction. Eur J Cardiothorac Surg 2002;21:818.

INFORMATION FOR PATIENTS
- www.drpen.com/394

WEB SITE
- www.emedicine.com/med/topic1485.htm

Mitral Regurgitation, Chronic Organic

KEY FEATURES

ESSENTIALS OF DIAGNOSIS

- Disease principally of the mitral valve leaflets caused by myxomatous changes, rheumatic fever, collagen vascular disease, or endocarditis
- Dyspnea or orthopnea
- Characteristic apical systolic murmur
- Doppler echocardiographic evidence of systolic regurgitation into the left atrium

GENERAL CONSIDERATIONS

- Mitral regurgitation refers to systolic leakage of blood from the left ventricle to the left atrium.
- Organic mitral regurgitation refers to diseases that involve the leaflets or their immediate supporting apparatus: chordae and the mitral annulus
- Among causes of organic mitral regurgitation, mitral valve prolapse is a unique entity (covered separately)
- Causes of chronic organic mitral regurgitation:
  - Rheumatic heart disease
  - Infective endocarditis
  - Collagen vascular diseases
  - Trauma
- Mitral regurgitation of any etiology tends to worsen over time because the volume load on the left heart results in chamber dilation, which further compromises mitral competence
- Although slowly progressive, mitral regurgitation may ultimately result in a large dysfunctional left ventricle and left atrium

CLINICAL PRESENTATION

SYMPTOMS AND SIGNS

- History of potential causal factors such as rheumatic fever and collagen vascular disease
- Progressive dyspnea
- Fatigue, orthopnea with heart failure
- Palpitation, usually due to atrial arrhythmias

PHYSICAL EXAM FINDINGS

- Tachycardia if heart failure or atrial fibrillation is present
- Brief low-amplitude carotid pulse
- Narrow pulse pressure due to reduced forward stroke volume
- Signs of congestive heart failure
- Enlarged apical impulse
- Auscultation:
  - Loud P_2 if pulmonary hypertension present
  - S_3 with or without heart failure
  - Blowing holosystolic high-pitched murmur at the apex, radiating to the axilla.
- The murmur characteristically increases in intensity with hand-grip exercise, but is unchanged in the beat after a premature beat with a compensatory pause

DIFFERENTIAL DIAGNOSIS

- Functional mitral regurgitation
- Aortic stenosis
- Ventricular septal defect
- Hypertrophic obstructive cardiomyopathy
- Other causes of dyspnea and orthopnea

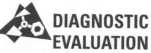 DIAGNOSTIC EVALUATION

LABORATORY TESTS

- Specific tests for the cause of mitral valve disease such as rheumatoid factor, blood cultures

ELECTROCARDIOGRAPHY

- Left atrial abnormality
- Left ventricular hypertrophy
- Atrial arrhythmias
- In severe cases, right ventricular and right atrial hypertrophy

IMAGING STUDIES

- Chest x-ray:
  - Cardiac enlargement, especially of the left heart chambers
  - Pulmonary congestion if heart failure present
- Echocardiography:
  - Left ventricular and atrial enlargement
  - Abnormalities of the leaflets, chordae, or annulus may suggest the cause
- Doppler echocardiography:
  - Color flow shows regurgitant jet through mitral valve in systole into the left atrium
  - Severity of regurgitation correlates roughly with jet size
  - Tricuspid regurgitation should be sought to estimate pulmonary pressures
  - Regurgitant flow can be calculated as the difference between mitral flow and left ventricular outflow in the absence of significant aortic valve disease

DIAGNOSTIC PROCEDURES

- Transesophageal echocardiography:
  - Useful to assess detailed valve anatomy and to assess whether surgical repair is feasible
  - Useful to assess for left atrial thrombi and infective endocarditis.
- Cardiac catheterization is rarely needed to diagnose mitral regurgitation or assess its severity, but may be useful to determine pulmonary pressures when it cannot be done by Doppler and to assess coronary anatomy before surgery

TREATMENT

CARDIOLOGY REFERRAL

- Moderate to severe regurgitation and symptoms
- Moderate to severe regurgitation with atrial arrhythmias

HOSPITALIZATION CRITERIA

- Heart failure
- Rapid atrial fibrillation

MEDICATIONS

- Rheumatic fever prophylaxis
- Endocarditis prophylaxis
- Treatment for heart failure
- Oral anticoagulation for atrial fibrillation

THERAPEUTIC PROCEDURES

- Percutaneous valvuloplasty and annuloplasty are being studied.

SURGERY

- Surgical repair or replacement:
  - Severe regurgitation with symptoms and left ventricular ejection fraction > .60 or severe regurgitation and left ventricular ejection fraction < 0.60
  - Severe regurgitation, preserved left ventricular function and atrial fibrillation, pulmonary hypertension (systolic > 50 mm Hg at rest or 60 with exercise)
  - Severe regurgitation in asymptomatic patients in whom repair is likely

MONITORING

- ECG monitoring in hospital
- Oxygen monitoring for pulmonary edema

DIET AND ACTIVITY

- Low-sodium, low-calorie diet
- Moderate noncompetitive exercise recommended

ONGOING MANAGEMENT

HOSPITAL DISCHARGE CRITERIA

- Resolution of symptoms and signs of heart failure
- Heart rate control of atrial fibrillation
- Sufficient recovery after surgery

FOLLOW-UP

- Mild regurgitation: visit and echocardiogram every 5 years
- Moderate regurgitation: visit and echocardiogram yearly
- Severe regurgitation: visit and echocardiogram every 6 months

COMPLICATIONS

- Atrial fibrillation
- Heart failure
- Chordal rupture leading to acute worsening of regurgitation and pulmonary edema
- Infective endocarditis
- Ventricular tachyarrhythmias

PROGNOSIS

- Usually slowly progressive unless chordal rupture or endocarditis supervenes
- Ten-year survival rate after valve repair is excellent
- Ten-year survival rate after valve replacement is about 50%

PREVENTION

- Treatment of any underlying diseases
- Control hypertension, which can worsen regurgitation
- Anticoagulation for those in atrial fibrillation
- Antibiotic prophylaxis for bacterial endocarditis

RESOURCES

PRACTICE GUIDELINES

- Echocardiography:
  - Baseline evaluation of severity and left ventricular function and to determine the cause of regurgitation
  - To serially assess left ventricular function in symptomatic patients with severe regurgitation or to reassess after change in symptoms
  - After valve repair or replacement for new baseline
- Surgery:
  - In symptomatic patients with severe regurgitation
  - In asymptomatic patients with severe regurgitation and left ventricular dysfunction, atrial fibrillation, pulmonary hypertension (systolic > 50 mm Hg at rest or 60 with exercise, or in whom repair is likely)

REFERENCES

- Matsumura T, Ohtaki E, Tanaka K et al: Echocardiographic prediction of left ventricular dysfunction after mitral valve repair for mitral regurgitation. J Am Coll Cardiol 2003;42:458.
- Pu M, Thomas JD, Vandervoort PM et al: Comparison of quantitative and semiquantitative methods for assessing mitral regurgitation by transesophageal endocardiography. Am J Cardiol 2001;87:66.
- Thomas L, Foster E, Julian IE et al: Prospective validation of an echocardiographic index for determining the severity of chronic mitral regurgitation. Am J Cardiol 2002;90:607.

INFORMATION FOR PATIENTS

- www.drpen.com/394

WEB SITES

- www.emedicine.com/med/CARDIOLOGY.htm
- www.acc.org/clinical/guidelines/valvular/disIndex.htm

Mitral Stenosis

 ## KEY FEATURES

ESSENTIALS OF DIAGNOSIS

- Exertional dyspnea, paroxysmal nocturnal dyspnea, orthopnea, or fatigue (later stages)
- Opening snap, loud S_1 (closing snap), diastolic rumbling murmur with pulmonary hypertension, a parasternal lift with a loud pulmonic component of the S_2
- Electrocardiographic evidence of left atrial enlargement or atrial fibrillation and right ventricular hypertrophy in later stages
- Radiographic signs of left atrial enlargement and normal left ventricular size
- Thickened mitral valve leaflets with restricted valve motion and reduced orifice area demonstrated on 2-dimensional echocardiography
- Elevated transmitral pressure gradient and prolonged pressure half-time by Doppler echocardiography

GENERAL CONSIDERATIONS

- In adults, mitral stenosis is almost always rheumatic in origin, but 50% have no history of rheumatic fever
- Affected women outnumber affected men by 2:1
- Pathology shows thickened leaflet edges with commissural fusion; thickened chordae with fusion
- The normal mitral orifice is 4–6 cm²; an elevated transmitral pressure gradient develops at < 2.5 cm²
- The elevated transmitral pressure raises left atrial pressure, which is transmitted to the lungs
- Mitral valve flow is related to heart rate and cardiac output; increases in either will increase transmitral pressure

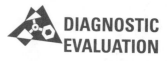 ## CLINICAL PRESENTATION

SYMPTOMS AND SIGNS

- Early patients may be asymptomatic unless they experience increases in heart rate or cardiac output such as with exercise, pregnancy, or atrial fibrillation
- Dyspnea, orthopnea, and fatigue
- Palpitation, often due to atrial fibrillation
- Stroke, usually due to atrial fibrillation
- Hoarseness due to left atrial compression of the recurrent laryngeal nerve
- Hemoptysis due to elevated bronchial venous pressure

PHYSICAL EXAM FINDINGS

- Elevated jugular venous pulse with a prominent *a* wave in sinus rhythm
- Normal left ventricular apical impulse, but palpable right ventricular lift if pulmonary pressures elevated
- S_1, P_2, and an opening snap may be palpable
- Auscultation: loud S_1; opening snap; apical diastolic rumble; murmur of mitral, pulmonic and tricuspid regurgitation may occur; loud P_2 if pulmonary hypertension present
- As the severity of mitral stenosis increases, the A_2-OS internal shortens and the diastolic rumble lengthens
- Signs of pulmonary congestion and right heart failure may be present

DIFFERENTIAL DIAGNOSIS

- Tricuspid stenosis
- Aortic regurgitation with prominent Austin Flint murmur
- Other causes of left-heart failure
- Other causes of pulmonary hypertension
- Left atrial myxoma, thrombus, vegetation
- Cor triatriatum

DIAGNOSTIC EVALUATION

LABORATORY TESTS

- Rarely, severe mitral stenosis may cause hemolytic anemia

ELECTROCARDIOGRAPHY

- Left atrial abnormality without left ventricular hypertrophy
- Signs of right ventricular hypertrophy if pulmonary hypertension present
- Atrial fibrillation

IMAGING STUDIES

- Chest x-ray: left atrial enlargement, elevated left main stem bronchus, right ventricular enlargement, calcified mitral valve, prominent upper lobe vessels, Kerley A and B lines, pulmonary edema
- Echocardiography: thickened valve leaflets, especially at the tips, thickened chordae, diastolic doming of the leaflets, reduced orifice area, occasionally left atrial thrombi
- Doppler echocardiography: elevated transmitral pressure gradient, reduced estimated mitral valve area, elevated pulmonary artery pressures

DIAGNOSTIC PROCEDURES

- Cardiac catheterization findings:
- Elevated right heart and pulmonary capillary wedge pressures
- Reduced orifice area estimates
- Given the accuracy of echocardiography, catheterization is rarely done for diagnostic purposes today

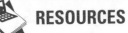

Mitral Stenosis

TREATMENT

CARDIOLOGY REFERRAL

- Typical symptoms
- Atrial fibrillation
- ECG showing right ventricular hypertrophy
- Echocardiography showing moderate to severe mitral stenosis, pulmonary hypertension, multivalve disease, or left atrial thrombi
- Chest x-ray showing pulmonary venous congestion

HOSPITALIZATION CRITERIA

- Rapid atrial fibrillation
- Congestive heart failure
- Systemic emboli
- Hemoptysis

MEDICATIONS

- Rheumatic fever prophylaxis
- Endocarditis prophylaxis
- Diuretics for heart failure; vasodilators relatively contraindicated
- Warfarin for history of systemic emboli or atrial fibrillation
- Digitalis, beta blockers, or calcium channel blockers for rate control in atrial fibrillation

THERAPEUTIC PROCEDURES

- Percutaneous mitral balloon valvuloplasty

SURGERY

- Surgical commissurotomy (open or closed)
- Mitral valve replacement

MONITORING

- ECG monitoring
- Oxygen saturation monitoring

DIET AND ACTIVITY

- Low-salt diet
- Severe and competitive exercise restricted

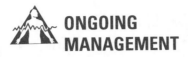

ONGOING MANAGEMENT

HOSPITAL DISCHARGE CRITERIA

- Control of atrial fibrillation rate or cardioversion
- Anticoagulation accomplished
- Resolution of congestive heart failure
- Post successful mitral valve procedure

FOLLOW-UP

- Mild (valve area 1.5–2.5): history, exam, echo every 2–3 years
- Moderate (valve area 1.0–1.4): history, exam, echo every year
- Severe (valve area < 1.0): history, exam, echo every 6 months

COMPLICATIONS

- Stroke due to left atrial thrombi, atrial fibrillation
- Congestive heart failure
- Hemoptysis, severe
- Infective endocarditis
- Sudden death

PROGNOSIS

- Mean decrease in valve area 0.09 cm^2 per year
- Mean interval between rheumatic fever and symptoms 16 ± 5 years
- Natural history: cardiac death in 85%
- Ten-year survival rate untreated after symptom onset: 20%
- Percutaneous balloon valvuloplasty mortality: 0
- Mitral valve replacement mortality rate: 5%; 10-year survival rate 85%

PREVENTION

- Prompt antibiotic treatment of streptococcal infections
- Antibiotic prophylaxis after rheumatic fever until risk of streptococcal infection is low
- Anticoagulation of atrial fibrillation
- Antibiotic prophylaxis for surgical and dental procedures

RESOURCES

PRACTICE GUIDELINES

- Indications for echocardiography: diagnosis of mitral stenosis and concomitant lesions; determination of severity of valve disease; assess valve morphology to determine suitability for percutaneous valvuloplasty; assess exercise response to mean gradient and pulmonary artery pressure when symptoms and resting hemodynamics discordant; establish presence or absence of left atrial thrombi before valvuloplasty or cardioversion
- Indications for valvuloplasty or surgery: symptomatic patients with ≥ moderate mitral stenosis (valve area < 1.5 cm^2)
- Valvuloplasty: favorable valve morphology, absence of left atrial thrombi and absence of ≥ moderate mitral regurgitation
- Asymptomatic patients who meet above criteria and have pulmonary hypertension (systolic 50 mm Hg at rest or 60 with exercise), new atrial fibrillation or recurrent embolic events on anticoagulation

REFERENCES

- Hammermeister K, Sethi GK Henderson WG et al: Outcomes 15 years after valve replacement with a mechanical versus a bioprosthetic valve. J Am Coll Cardiol 2000;36:1152.
- Kang D-H, Park SW, Song JK et al: Long-term clinical and echocardiographic outcome of percutaneous mitral valvuloplasty. J Am Coll Cardiol 2000;35:169.

INFORMATION FOR PATIENTS

- www.drpen.com/394.0

WEB SITE

- www.priory.com/med/mitsten.htm

Mixed Aortic Valve Disease

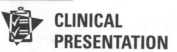 **KEY FEATURES**

ESSENTIALS OF DIAGNOSIS

- Moderate aortic regurgitation and stenosis (estimated aortic valve area 0.8–1.2 cm^2)

GENERAL CONSIDERATIONS

- In mixed aortic stenosis and regurgitation, one of the two lesions usually predominates and management is predicated on the dominant lesion
- When both lesions are moderate, the degree of hemodynamic disturbance is considerably more than one would expect from either lesion alone
- Moderate aortic regurgitation challenges the concentrically hypertrophied left ventricle from aortic stenosis by doing the following:
  - Adding diastolic volume, which moves the ventricle up its steep pressure-volume curve
  - Causing considerable diastolic pressure that is transmitted to the lungs, resulting in dyspnea and pulmonary congestion

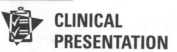 **CLINICAL PRESENTATION**

SYMPTOMS AND SIGNS

- Dyspnea
- Heart failure symptoms
- Effort syncope
- Angina pectoris

PHYSICAL EXAM FINDINGS

- Enlarged left ventricular impulse
- S_3 or S_4
- Ejection sound if bicuspid valve
- Diminished aortic S_2
- Typical harsh systolic ejection murmur and high-pitched diastolic decrescendo murmur in the aortic area
- Signs of heart failure may be present
- Peripheral signs of aortic regurgitation are usually absent because of the reduction in stroke volume from significant aortic stenosis

DIFFERENTIAL DIAGNOSIS

- Severe aortic regurgitation with mild aortic stenosis
- Severe aortic stenosis and mild regurgitation
- The murmur of patent ductus arteriosus may be mimicked by moderate aortic stenosis/aortic regurgitation

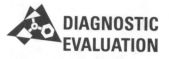 **DIAGNOSTIC EVALUATION**

LABORATORY TESTS

- Brain natriuretic peptide test: elevated in heart failure

ELECTROCARDIOGRAPHY

- ECG findings:
  - Left ventricular hypertrophy
  - Left atrial enlargement

IMAGING STUDIES

- Chest x-ray findings:
  - Enlarged left heart chambers
  - Aortic valve calcification
  - Pulmonary congestion
- Echocardiography:
  - Left ventricular hypertrophy
  - Left atrial enlargement
  - Thickened aortic valve
  - Dilated aorta
- Doppler echocardiography:
  - Continuous-wave Doppler measures the pressure gradient across the valve
  - The continuity equation accurately determines valve area
  - Color-flow Doppler assesses the severity of aortic regurgitation

DIAGNOSTIC PROCEDURES

- Transesophageal echocardiography can image the aortic valve orifice area in difficult cases
- Cardiac catheterization and angiography are frequently valuable:
  - To confirm the severity of aortic stenosis and regurgitation
  - To assess left ventricular performance

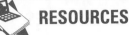

 TREATMENT

CARDIOLOGY REFERRAL

- Symptoms
- Suspected moderately severe disease

HOSPITALIZATION CRITERIA

- Evidence of heart failure
- Suspicion of endocarditis
- Significant arrhythmias

MEDICATIONS

- Use diuretics and digoxin for heart failure
- Vasodilator drugs are contraindicated because of the aortic stenosis

THERAPEUTIC PROCEDURES

- Aortic valvuloplasty contraindicated because of the aortic regurgitation

SURGERY

- Aortic valve replacement for symptoms or signs of left ventricular dysfunction
- Ross procedure should be considered in those < age 50 (pulmonary autograft to aortic valve and homograft to pulmonary valve)

MONITORING

- ECG in the hospital

DIET AND ACTIVITY

- Low-sodium diet
- Restricted activity if symptoms or signs of heart failure

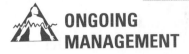 **ONGOING MANAGEMENT**

HOSPITAL DISCHARGE CRITERIA

- Resolution of heart failure
- Successful surgery

FOLLOW-UP

- After surgery: 3 months, 6 months, then yearly
- Baseline echo 3 months after surgery, then every 1–3 years, depending on the valve type
- Asymptomatic patients: yearly with an echo until evidence of left ventricular size increase or function decrease occurs, then every 3–6 months with echoes every 6 months until indications for surgery occur

COMPLICATIONS

- Infective endocarditis
- Heart failure
- Syncope
- Sudden death
- Arrhythmias

PROGNOSIS

- Moderate aortic stenosis and regurgitation progress to symptoms more rapidly than either lesion alone
- Preserving left ventricular performance is particularly critical in this double-loaded situation (systolic and diastolic loads increased)

RESOURCES

PRACTICE GUIDELINES

- Aortic valve replacement should be considered for symptoms or evidence of left ventricular dysfunction:
  – Ejection fraction 50–60 or left ventricular end-diastolic volume > 150 mL/m^2

REFERENCES

- Attenhofer Jost CH et al: Echocardiography in the evaluation of systolic murmurs of unknown cause. Am J Med 2000;108:614.
- Berglund H et al: Influence of ejection fraction and valvular regurgitation on the accuracy of a valve area determination. Echocardiography 2001;18:65.
- Oswalt JD e al: Highlights of a ten-year experience with the Ross procedure. Ann Thorac Surg 2001;71:S332.

INFORMATION FOR PATIENTS

- www.drpen.com/hd424.1

WEB SITE

- www.emedicine.com/med/ CARDIOLOGY.htm

Mixed Connective Tissue Disease and the Heart

 KEY FEATURES

ESSENTIALS OF DIAGNOSIS

- Raynaud's phenomenon, sclerodactyly
- Myopathy with high titers of ribonucleoprotein antibodies
- Pericarditis, pulmonary hypertension

GENERAL CONSIDERATIONS

- Patients with mixed connective tissue disease have clinical features that resemble other connective tissue diseases
- Characteristically, affected patients have high titers of antibodies to ribonucleoprotein and speckled antinuclear antibodies
- Rheumatoid agglutinins occur in about 50%
- Predominantly, females of all ages are affected
- Cardiac involvement is infrequent and usually related to pericarditis or pulmonary hypertension

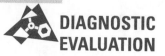 **CLINICAL PRESENTATION**

SYMPTOMS AND SIGNS

- Chest pain characteristic of pericarditis is common
- Symptoms of heart failure
  - Fatigue
  - Dyspnea
  - Edema

PHYSICAL EXAM FINDINGS

- Pulmonary hypertension
  - Right ventricular (RV) lift
  - Loud P_2
  - Edema
- Pericarditis
  - Friction rub
  - Elevated jugular venous pressure (JVP)

DIFFERENTIAL DIAGNOSIS

- Other connective tissue diseases
- Other causes of cardiac disease

DIAGNOSTIC EVALUATION

LABORATORY TESTS

- Antinuclear antibody titer, ribonucleoprotein level, rheumatoid factor
- Brain natriuretic peptide

ELECTROCARDIOGRAPHY

- RV and right atrial hypertrophy
- Diffuse ST elevation of pericarditis
- Supraventricular arrhythmias

IMAGING STUDIES

- Echocardiography:
  - Pericardial effusion
  - Right heart chamber enlargement
  - Verrucous mitral valve thickening
- Doppler echocardiography:
  - Elevated pulmonary pressure estimates
  - Mitral regurgitation
- Chest x-ray: enlarged cardiac silhouette

DIAGNOSTIC PROCEDURES

- Cardiac catheterization: may be required in some cases to evaluate possible coronary artery disease or cardiac tamponade

Mixed Connective Tissue Disease and the Heart

TREATMENT

CARDIOLOGY REFERRAL

- Suspected cardiac disease

HOSPITALIZATION CRITERIA

- Heart failure
- Pericarditis
- Rapid atrial fibrillation

MEDICATIONS

- Specific anti-inflammatory pharmacotherapy
- Appropriate therapy for pulmonary hypertension
- Steroids for pericarditis, eg, prednisone 5–50 mg PO daily

THERAPEUTIC PROCEDURES

- Pericardiocentesis if tamponade

MONITORING

- ECG in hospital as appropriate
- Blood pressure and JVP with pericarditis
- Pulmonary artery pressures during drug treatment of pulmonary hypertension

DIET AND ACTIVITY

- Low-sodium diet
- Restricted activity if heart failure

ONGOING MANAGEMENT

HOSPITAL DISCHARGE CRITERIA

- Resolution of problem

FOLLOW-UP

- Cardiology follow-up as appropriate to problem

COMPLICATIONS

- Atrial and ventricular arrhythmias
- Myocarditis
- Cardiac conduction disturbances

PROGNOSIS

- Mortality is 13% at 10 years

RESOURCES

PRACTICE GUIDELINES

- Although like other connective tissue diseases, any structure in the heart can become diseased, the usual clinical manifestations are pericarditis and pulmonary hypertension
- Rarely is cardiac disease the initial manifestation of mixed connective tissue

REFERENCE

- Rebollar-Gonzalez V et al: Cardiac conduction disturbances in mixed connective tissue disease. Rev Invest Clin 2001;53:330.

INFORMATION FOR PATIENTS

- www.aarda.org/patient_information.php

WEB SITE

- www.emedicine.com/MED/topic3417.htm

Mixed Mitral Valve Disease

KEY FEATURES
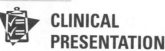

ESSENTIALS OF DIAGNOSIS

- Rheumatic mitral valve disease with moderate mitral regurgitation and a mean mitral diastolic gradient > 10 mm Hg and valve area of 1.1–1.5 cm^2 (moderate mitral stenosis)

GENERAL CONSIDERATIONS

- Mixed mitral valvular disease is frequently rheumatic in origin
- The clinical course is similar to that of mitral regurgitation alone
- The difference is that left atrial pressure rises proportionately more than left ventricular diastolic pressure, resulting in:
  - Earlier appearance of pulmonary congestion
  - More severe pulmonary hypertension
  - A higher incidence of atrial fibrillation
- Forward cardiac output is reduced more compared with pure mitral regurgitation owing to reduced left ventricular filling, resulting in earlier symptoms of fatigue and reduced exercise performance

CLINICAL PRESENTATION
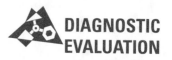

SYMPTOMS AND SIGNS

- Dyspnea on exertion, fatigue
- Edema, abdominal distention

PHYSICAL EXAM FINDINGS

- Jugular venous pressure may be elevated with a prominent *a* wave in sinus rhythm when pulmonary hypertension is present
- Evidence of edema, ascites, and pleural effusions
- Right ventricular lift
- Loud pulmonic component of S_2
- Opening snap followed by a low-pitched diastolic rumble at the apex
- Blowing pansystolic murmur at the apex

DIFFERENTIAL DIAGNOSIS

- Mild mitral regurgitation or mild mitral stenosis
- Severe mitral regurgitation or mitral stenosis; the severe lesion dominates management

DIAGNOSTIC EVALUATION

LABORATORY TESTS

- CBC: rarely, hemolytic anemia may be present from red cell trauma

ELECTROCARDIOGRAPHY

- ECG findings:
  - Right ventricular hypertrophy
  - Left ventricular voltage increased
  - Left atrial enlargement in sinus rhythm
  - Atrial fibrillation in some

IMAGING STUDIES

- Chest x-ray:
  - Enlargement of all four cardiac chambers
  - Dilated main pulmonary arteries
  - Pulmonary congestion
  - Pleural effusion
  - Relatively small aorta
- Echocardiography:
  - Enlargement of all four cardiac chambers
  - Thickened mitral valve with diastolic doming
  - Usually, normal left ventricular function
  - Doppler evidence of pulmonary hypertension
  - Doppler echocardiography of mitral stenosis
  - Color Doppler visualization of the mitral regurgitation

DIAGNOSTIC PROCEDURES

- Cardiac catheterization may be useful to quantify the degree of mitral stenosis and pulmonary hypertension

TREATMENT

CARDIOLOGY REFERRAL

- Symptoms
- Heart failure or other complications

HOSPITALIZATION CRITERIA

- Heart failure
- Rapid atrial fibrillation

MEDICATIONS

- Drugs to control heart rate in atrial fibrillation, such as beta blockers, selected calcium blockers, and anticoagulation agents
- Diuretics for congestion and edema
- Angiotension-converting enzyme inhibitors or receptor blockers for left ventricular dysfunction

THERAPEUTIC PROCEDURES

- Balloon valvuloplasty is contraindicated in mixed mitral disease because regurgitation often worsens

SURGERY

- Valve replacement is the treatment of choice for symptomatic patients and those with left ventricular dysfunction

MONITORING

- ECG monitoring in hospital

DIET AND ACTIVITY

- Low-sodium diet
- Restricted activity if heart failure is present

ONGOING MANAGEMENT

HOSPITAL DISCHARGE CRITERIA

- Resolution of heart failure
- Rate control of atrial fibrillation
- After successful surgery

FOLLOW-UP

- Asymptomatic patients: every 3–6 months with echocardiogram every 6–2 months
- After surgery: 3 months, 6 months then yearly

COMPLICATIONS

- Atrial fibrillation
- Heart failure
- Stroke from left atrial thrombi

PROGNOSIS

- Progression is more rapid than single-valve lesions
- After mitral valve replacement surgery: the 10-year survival rate is about 50%

PREVENTION

- Rheumatic fever prophylaxis
- Endocarditis prophylaxis

RESOURCES

PRACTICE GUIDELINES

- No specific guidelines are available and patients should be treated individually
- In general, mixed mitral valve disease should be treated like a more aggressive form of mitral regurgitation

REFERENCES

- Borrow RO et al: ACC/AHA guidelines for the management of patients with valvular heart disease. J Am Coll Cardol 1998;32:1486.
- Mavioglu I et al: Valve repair for rheumatic mitral disease. J Heart Valve Dis 2001;10:596.

INFORMATION FOR PATIENTS

- www.americanheart.org/presenter.jhtml?identifier=4709

WEB SITE

- www.emedicine.com/ped/topic2007.htm

Multifocal Atrial Tachycardia

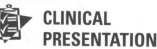 **KEY FEATURES**

ESSENTIALS OF DIAGNOSIS

- Heart rates up to 150 bpm
- Three or more distinct P waves in a single lead
- Variable P-P, P-R, and R-R intervals
- A majority (60–85%) of cases are associated with pulmonary disease

GENERAL CONSIDERATIONS

- Accounts for < 1% of all arrhythmias
- Chronic obstructive pulmonary disease exacerbation is the most common condition in which this arrhythmia is seen
- Respiratory failure, decompensated heart failure and infection may precipitate the condition
- Hypokalemia, hypomagnesemia, and hyponatremia may be associated with this arrhythmia
- Pulmonary embolism, valvular heart disease, and postoperative state may rarely be associated with this arrhythmia
- Abnormal automaticity is the most likely mechanism, although triggered activity is also proposed
- Multifocal atrial tachycardia is often misdiagnosed as atrial fibrillation

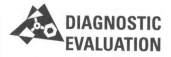 **CLINICAL PRESENTATION**

SYMPTOMS AND SIGNS

- Most of the symptoms are related to the underlying cause
- Most patients are short of breath secondary to underlying lung disease
- Palpitations
- Chest pain

PHYSICAL EXAM FINDINGS

- Variable S_1
- Other findings relate to underlying cause

DIFFERENTIAL DIAGNOSIS

- Atrial fibrillation

DIAGNOSTIC EVALUATION

LABORATORY TESTS

- CBC, basic metabolic panel
- Arterial blood gas analysis
- Cardiac biomarkers if there is a suspicion of myocardial infarction
- Chest x-ray and other investigation toward managing the underlying cause

ELECTROCARDIOGRAPHY

- ECG shows tachycardia with three or more distinct P waves in a single lead and variable P-P, P-R, and R-R intervals

IMAGING STUDIES

- Occasionally an echocardiogram may be used to assess right and left heart function

TREATMENT

CARDIOLOGY REFERRAL

- If patients are hemodynamically unstable
- If ventricular rate could not be controlled using conventional atrioventricular (AV) nodal blocking drugs

HOSPITALIZATION CRITERIA

- Most patients are hospitalized because of underlying respiratory failure

MEDICATIONS

- Treat the underlying cause (ie, respiratory failure)
- Verapamil is useful, 180–360 mg/day
- Cardiac selective beta blockers. such as metoprolol, may be used for ventricular rate control if tolerated
- Intravenous magnesium and potassium supplementation may convert a significant number to sinus rhythm
- Digoxin is usually not helpful and has the potential to initiate atrial tachycardia
- Theophylline and beta agonists should be titrated down to the least effective dose

THERAPEUTIC PROCEDURES

- In a rare patient, pacemaker implantation followed by AV nodal ablation may be required

MONITORING

- ECG monitoring in the hospital

DIET AND ACTIVITY

- As appropriate for the underlying cause

ONGOING MANAGEMENT

HOSPITAL DISCHARGE CRITERIA

- When ventricular rate is controlled and the precipitant cause is adequately treated

FOLLOW-UP

- As appropriate for the underlying disease

COMPLICATIONS

- Usually none

PROGNOSIS

- Prognosis depends on underlying cause

PREVENTION

- Prevention of exacerbations of underlying heart disease or lung disease

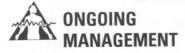

RESOURCES

PRACTICE GUIDELINES

- Therapy is directed toward pulmonary disease or electrolyte abnormality
- Chronic therapy may require calcium channel blocker
- No role for cardioversion, antiarrhythmic medication, or radiofrequency ablation of the arrhythmia

REFERENCES

- Engel TR, Radhagopalan S: Treatment of multifocal atrial tachycardia by treatment of pulmonary insufficiency: or is it vice versa? Chest 2000;117:7.
- Tucker KJ et al: Treatment of refractory recurrent multifocal atrial tachycardia with atrioventricular junction ablation and permanent pacing. J Invasive Cardiol 1995;7:207.

INFORMATION FOR PATIENTS

- www.nlm.nih.gov/medlineplus/arrhythmia.html

WEB SITE

- www.hrsonline.org

Myocardial Infarction, Acute Non–ST-Segment Elevation

 KEY FEATURES

ESSENTIALS OF DIAGNOSIS

- New or worsening angina pectoris or its equivalents
- ST-wave depression or T-wave inversion (less specific) on ECG in two or more contiguous leads
- Positive biologic markers for myocardial injury (ie, troponin or creatine kinase–MB)

GENERAL CONSIDERATIONS

- Acute myocardial infarctions (MI) make up 40–50% of all admissions to cardiac care units
- Usually caused by unstable plaque characterized by fissure or rupture of the fibrous cap
- Platelet aggregation leading to thrombus formation ensues
- Coagulation cascade gets activated, leading to thrombin formation
- Vasoconstriction occurs secondary to endothelial dysfunction
- Most episodes occur without antecedent increase in myocardial oxygen demand
- Worsening of stable coronary artery disease may be triggered by:
  - Severe anemia
  - Thyrotoxicosis
  - Acute tachyarrhythmias
  - Hypotension

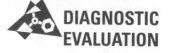 **CLINICAL PRESENTATION**

SYMPTOMS AND SIGNS

- Angina that lasts up to 20–30 minutes or longer
- Symptoms may occur at rest or during minimal accustomed exertion
- Associated symptoms occur such as sweating and fatigue
- Dyspnea with or without chest pain may be a primary manifestation
- Recurrence of ischemic symptoms within 4-6 weeks after an MI or coronary artery bypass graft

PHYSICAL EXAM FINDINGS

- No typical abnormal physical finding
- S_3 or S_4
- Transient ischemic mitral regurgitation
- Features of left ventricular dysfunction
- Hypotension may occur depending on the extent of myocardial involvement or secondary to an arrhythmia

DIFFERENTIAL DIAGNOSIS

- Stable angina pectoris
- Variant angina
- Unstable angina
- Aortic dissection
- Acute myopericarditis
- Acute pulmonary embolism
- Esophageal reflux
- Cholecystitis
- Peptic ulcer disease
- Cervical radiculopathy
- Costochondritis
- Pneumothorax

DIAGNOSTIC EVALUATION

LABORATORY TESTS

- CBC to exclude anemia
- Creatinine to assess renal function
- Cardiac biomarkers

ELECTROCARDIOGRAPHY

- 12-lead ECG (patients with resting ST-segment depression are considered high risk)

IMAGING STUDIES

- Echocardiogram to evaluate:
  - Regional wall motion analysis
  - Left ventricular function
  - Valvular heart disease
- In patients in whom medical management is chosen, stress perfusion study may be done 48 hours after the last episode of chest pain for further risk stratification

DIAGNOSTIC PROCEDURES

- Coronary angiogram

Myocardial Infarction, Acute Non–ST-Segment Elevation

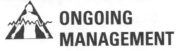

TREATMENT

CARDIOLOGY REFERRAL

- All patients with non–ST-segment MI should be seen by a cardiologist

HOSPITALIZATION CRITERIA

- All patients should be hospitalized

MEDICATIONS

- General:
  - Oxygen
  - Aspirin 165 mg
- Pain relief:
  - Sublingual nitroglycerin followed by IV morphine sulfate
- Specific pharmacologic therapy:
  - Beta blockers IV followed by oral unfractionated heparin or low-molecular-weight heparin
  - Clopidogrel for aspirin-sensitive patients or those likely to have percutaneous revascularization
  - Calcium channel blockers for refractory symptoms
  - Platelet glycoprotein IIb/IIIa inhibitors

THERAPEUTIC PROCEDURES

- Percutaneous coronary intervention (PCI) to the affected coronary artery when feasible
- Intra-aortic balloon counterpulsation to stabilize hemodynamically unstable patients for catheterization or surgery

SURGERY

- Coronary artery bypass graft (CABG) may be the best option in patients with left main artery disease, extensive disease, or disease not amenable to PCI

MONITORING

- In-hospital telemetry throughout hospitalization

DIET AND ACTIVITY

- Cardiac low-fat diet
- Bed rest initially

ONGOING MANAGEMENT

HOSPITAL DISCHARGE CRITERIA

- 24–48 hours after PCI or 5–7 days after CABG if no complications
- Patients chosen for medical management may be discharged if they have no symptoms for 72 hours on optimal medical therapy

FOLLOW-UP

- All patients must be followed up 2 weeks after discharge
- Consider a stress test 6 weeks to 3 months after revascularization

COMPLICATIONS

- ST-elevation MI
- Sudden cardiac death
- Heart failure

PROGNOSIS

- Difficult to predict because of the heterogeneous group of patients included
- TACTICS-TIMI 18 trial showed that 3.3% had 6 months mortality rate
- PRISM-PLUS trial showed refractory angina, MI, or death at 6 months of 10.6%, 8.3%, and 6.9%, respectively

PREVENTION

- Smoking cessation
- Low-fat diet
- Aerobic exercise
- Statin
- Control of diabetes and hypertension

RESOURCES

PRACTICE GUIDELINES

- Indications for coronary angiography:
  - Recurrent symptoms or ischemia despite adequate medical therapy
  - Congestive heart failure
  - Malignant ventricular arrhythmias or high-risk noninvasive test result (ejection fraction < 0.35, large anterior or multiple perfusion defects)
  - Previous PCI or CABG

REFERENCES

- Petersen JL, Mahaffey KW, Hasselblad V et al: Efficacy and bleeding complications among patients randomized to enoxaparin or unfractionated heparin for antithrombin therapy in non-ST-Segment elevation acute coronary syndromes: a systematic overview. JAMA 2004;292(1):89.
- Wallentin L et al: Outcome at 1 year after an invasive compared with a noninvasive strategy in unstable coronary-artery disease: The FRISC II invasive randomized trial. FRISC II Investigators. Fast Revascularization During Instability in Coronary Artery Disease. Lancet 2000;356:9.

INFORMATION FOR PATIENTS

- www.drpen.com/410.7

WEB SITES

- www.acc.org
- www.americanheart.org

Myocardial Infarction, Acute ST Elevation

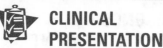 **KEY FEATURES**

ESSENTIALS OF DIAGNOSIS

- Evidence of myocardial injury:
  - Elevated marker protein such as troponin
- Evidence of acute myocardial ischemia:
  - Clinical symptoms and signs such as prolonged chest pain
  - Characteristic ECG changes:
  - ST-segment elevation of 1 mm in two chest leads or adjacent limb leads
- Cardiac imaging showing reduced regional perfusion or segmental wall motion abnormalities
- Diagnosis rests on:
  - Typical history
  - Abnormal ECG (ST elevation)
  - Cardiac biomarkers (troponin elevation)

GENERAL CONSIDERATIONS

- Injury to myocardial tissue caused by an imbalance between myocardial oxygen supply and demand, usually due to acute coronary artery occlusion by thrombosis in situ
- Each year, 1.1 million people experience myocardial infarction (MI)
- Six million patients are admitted for consideration of this diagnosis
- 460,000 succumb to coronary artery–related deaths
- Mortality rate has declined but still leads to death in one third of patients
- About 50% of deaths occur within 1 hour most frequently due to ventricular fibrillation

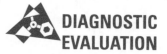 **CLINICAL PRESENTATION**

SYMPTOMS AND SIGNS

- Chest discomfort is usually in the center of the anterior chest radiating to the left arm or neck
- Individual patients may vary widely in the character, location, and radiation of chest discomfort
- The patient may place a hand over the sternum (Levine's sign)
- Women have more atypical symptoms
- Diabetics and the elderly may not complain of chest discomfort (silent infarct) but may have other features of an infarction such as heart failure
- Dyspnea, diaphoresis, nausea or vomiting may occur

PHYSICAL EXAM FINDINGS

- S_4 is heard frequently
- Signs of heart failure such as S_3, neck vein distention, and rales occur with larger infarcts
- Cold perspiration and skin pallor may be seen in those with left ventricular failure and sympathetic stimulation
- Sinus tachycardia is common (bradycardia not uncommon in inferior MI) and frequent premature ventricular beats
- Systolic blood pressure may be < 90 mm Hg in those with cardiogenic shock
- Murmurs or rubs may occur as complications of MI
  - Systolic murmur with mitral regurgitation
  - Pericardial rub in pericarditis

DIFFERENTIAL DIAGNOSIS

- Stable angina pectoris
- Variant angina
- Unstable angina
- Aortic dissection
- Acute myopericarditis
- Acute pulmonary embolism
- Esophageal reflux
- Cholecystitis
- Peptic ulcer disease
- Cervical radiculopathy
- Costochondritis
- Pneumothorax

DIAGNOSTIC EVALUATION

LABORATORY TESTS

- CBC, brain natriuretic peptide testing
- Cardiac biomarkers (creatine phosphokinase, MB, troponin T or I)
- Other tests depend on differential diagnosis, which may include amylase, lipase, liver function tests
- Arterial blood gas analysis if hypoxemia is found on pulse oximetry
- Urine analysis including drug screen for cocaine in young patients with MI or patients with history of drug use

ELECTROCARDIOGRAPHY

- ECG to identify the location and rhythm complications of acute MI

IMAGING STUDIES

- Echocardiogram:
  - To assess left ventricular function and extent of regional wall motion abnormalities
  - To evaluate complications such as papillary muscle dysfunction, ventricular septal defect, aneurysm, and pseudoaneurysm formation
- Resting nuclear perfusion studies are rarely done during acute MI but have been done to quantitate the size of the perfusion abnormality, size of the infarct, and left ventricular function, which helps in assessing the prognosis

DIAGNOSTIC PROCEDURES

- Coronary angiogram shows acute thrombotic obstruction in a large percentage of patients with acute ST-elevation MI
- In some patients, the atherosclerotic lesion may be the predominant problem with minimal thrombosis
- Rarely ST-elevation MI may be caused by vasospasm alone or in combination with a small atheromatous lesion

TREATMENT

CARDIOLOGY REFERRAL

- All patients should be managed by a cardiologist

HOSPITALIZATION CRITERIA

- All patients must be hospitalized

MEDICATIONS

- Aspirin 165 mg, or clopidogrel 75 mg if patient is aspirin sensitive
- Unfractionated heparin (60 units/kg bolus and 12 units/kg maintenance and adjust to partial thromboplastin time)
- Platelet IIb/IIIa glycoprotein inhibitor as part of percutaneous coronary intervention, preferably using abciximab
- Beta blockers: metoprolol 5 mg IV every 5 minutes so long as heart rate and blood pressure would permit and then orally 25–50 mg twice daily
- Morphine sulfate IV for pain: 2–4 mg initially; titrate as needed
- Sublingual followed by IV nitroglycerin for pain: start at 10 µg/min; titrate upward depending on blood pressure and heart rate
- Angiotensin-converting enzyme inhibitors (ACEIs) if blood pressure allows
- Oxygen if SaO_2 < 92%

THERAPEUTIC PROCEDURES

- Percutaneous coronary intervention (PCI) with stent placement
- Intra-aortic balloon counterpulsation to stabilize hemodynamically unstable patients for catheterization or surgery

PCI versus THROMBOLYTIC Therapy

- Symptom duration < 3 hours, PCI preferred if door-to-balloon time < 60 minutes; otherwise use thrombolytic therapy
- For symptom duration > 3 hours, PCI preferred for door-to-balloon time up to 90 minutes; otherwise use thrombolytic therapy
- PCI preferred: age > 75 years or left bundle branch block with cardiogenic shock that developed within 36 hours of MI, suitable for revascularization and within 18 hours of onset of shock

SURGERY

- Rarely CABG is needed; if so, preferable to operate after medical stabilization

MONITORING

- ECG monitor for arrhythmias

DIET AND ACTIVITY

- Cardiac low-fat diet
- Aerobic exercise as tolerated
- Cardiac phase II rehabilitation

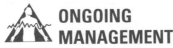

ONGOING MANAGEMENT

HOSPITAL DISCHARGE CRITERIA

- 3–5 days after uncomplicated MI
- Ability to ambulate (if ambulating before MI)
- Hemodynamic stability
- Absence of chest pain

FOLLOW-UP

- 2 weeks after discharge, 3 months after that; subsequently yearly with stress test

COMPLICATIONS

- Cardiogenic shock secondary to large size of infarct or complications
- Heart block
- Atrial fibrillation
- Ventricular tachycardia and fibrillation
- Mitral regurgitation
- Pseudoaneurysm
- Free wall rupture
- Aneurysm formation
- Pericarditis
- Dressler's syndrome

PROGNOSIS

- Depends on infarct size, presence of complications, and residual ischemia
- Uncomplicated inferior MI best prognosis

PREVENTION

- Smoking cessation
- Low-fat diet
- Aerobic exercise
- Statin drug therapy to LDL cholesterol < 80 mg/dL
- Control of diabetes and hypertension

RESOURCES

PRACTICE GUIDELINES

- Indication for thrombolytics: thrombolysis within first 12 hours if PCI cannot be performed within 90 minutes of presentation, provided there are no contraindications
- Indications for coronary angiography: primary PCI, if it can be accomplished within 60 minutes; rescue PCI after failed medical therapy; cardiogenic shock; presurgical evaluation of ventricular septal rupture or papillary muscle dysfunction; electrical or hemodynamic instability

REFERENCES

- Kloner RA, Rezkalla SH: Cardiac protection during acute myocardial infarction: where do we stand in 2004?J Am Coll Cardiol 2004 ;44:276.
- Zijlstra F et al: Clinical characteristics and outcome of patients with early (< 2 h), intermediate (2–4 h) and late (>4 h) presentation treated by primary coronary angioplasty or thrombolytic therapy for acute myocardial infarction. Eur Heart J 2002;23:550.

INFORMATION FOR PATIENTS

- www.drpen.com/410.9
- www.nhlbe.nih.gov/health/dci/Diseases/Cad/CAD_WhatIs.html

WEB SITES

- www.acc.org
- www.americanheart.org

KEY FEATURES

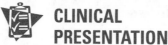 CLINICAL PRESENTATION

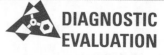 DIAGNOSTIC EVALUATION

ESSENTIALS OF DIAGNOSIS

- Acute myocardial infarction (MI) documented
- Normal or near-normal coronary angiography

GENERAL CONSIDERATIONS

- Ten percent of all patients and 25% of patients < 35 years do not have coronary atherosclerosis on angiography after an MI
- More common in Asian patients
- In the United States, coronary artery spasm occurs at sites of subcritical stenosis; in Japan, spasm occurs in completely normal arteries on angiogaphy
- In young patients, cocaine may induce vasospasm and MI
- Coronary embolism with subsequent recanalization occasionally may be a cause of acute MI
- Rarely, markedly elevated myocardial oxygen demand may precipitate an MI
- Rarely, pseudoephedrine and ephedra cause MI with normal coronary arteries
- Overall, smoking is a common risk factor in patients with MI and normal coronary arteries
- Coagulopathies or hyperviscosity syndromes can lead to in-situ coronary thrombosis

SYMPTOMS AND SIGNS

- Chest pain similar to that in MI that lasts > 30 minutes
- Dyspnea
- Palpitations
- Diaphoresis during chest pain

PHYSICAL EXAM FINDINGS

- S_3 and S_4 may occur depending on left ventricular function
- Bilateral pulmonary rales may occur if heart failure
- Elevated jugular venous distention may occur

DIFFERENTIAL DIAGNOSIS

- Rupture of a minimal (< 50% diameter narrowing) plaque with thrombus formation and subsequent dissolution
- Tako-Tsubo cardiomyopathy may mimic MI
- Myocarditis
- Arteritis
- Trauma

LABORATORY TESTS

- CBC, brain natriuretic peptide test
- Cardiac biomarkers such as creatine CPK-MB and troponin T or I

ELECTROCARDIOGRAPHY

- 12-lead ECG may show ST elevation or marked ST depression

IMAGING STUDIES

- Echocardiogram may show regional wall motion change
- Left ventricular function may be normal or abnormal

DIAGNOSTIC PROCEDURES

- Coronary angiogram
- Angiogram will be normal without evidence of atherosclerosis or show minimal change not enough to account for complete cessation of blood supply
- Ergonovine provocation test to provoke spasm no longer recommended
- Acetylcholine provocation test may be used to identify focal spasm
- Spontaneous focal spasm of coronary artery may occur
- Coronary vasodilator reserve may be assessed with adenosine and a Doppler flow wire

Myocardial Infarction with Normal Coronary Arteries, Acute

 ## TREATMENT

CARDIOLOGY REFERRAL

- All patients must be evaluated by a cardiologist

HOSPITALIZATION CRITERIA

- All patients must be hospitalized initially

MEDICATIONS

- Thrombolysis for suspected thrombosis or embolism
- Nitrates or calcium channel blockers to relieve spasm
- Specific therapy for or elimination of precipitating factors
- Secondary prevention measures as appropriate (eg, smoking cessation)
- Beta blockers generally avoided because of potential of unopposed alpha stimulation
- If coronary flow reserve is abnormal, a statin drug may be prescribed

THERAPEUTIC PROCEDURES

- Generally none required
- Rare patient with subcritical lesion and recurrent vasospasm of that site not adequately treated with vasodilators may benefit from percutaneous coronary intervention

SURGERY

- None required

MONITORING

- ECG monitoring in the hospital

DIET AND ACTIVITY

- Cardiac low-fat diet
- Aerobic exercise as tolerated

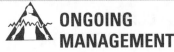 ## ONGOING MANAGEMENT

HOSPITAL DISCHARGE CRITERIA

- If no recurrent chest pain 48 to 72 hours after hospitalization

FOLLOW-UP

- Two weeks after discharge and 3 months after that
- Subsequently once a year

COMPLICATIONS

- Recurrent chest pain episodes not easily controllable with medication
- Rarely, sudden death

PROGNOSIS

- Generally better than coronary atherosclerosis
- Five-year survival rate 89–97%

PREVENTION

- Cessation of cigarette smoking
- Discontinuation of procoagulants such as birth control pills

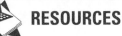 ## RESOURCES

PRACTICE GUIDELINES

- Recommended treatment:
  - Smoking must be discontinued
  - Calcium channel blockers and nitrates are mainstay of therapy

REFERENCES

- Chandrasekaran B, Kurbaan AS: Myocardial infarction with angiographically normal coronary arteries. J Roy Soc Med 2002;95:398.
- Sarda L et al: Myocarditis in patients with clinical presentation of myocardial infarction and normal coronary angiograms. J Am Coll Cardiol 2001;37:786.

INFORMATION FOR PATIENTS

- www.drpen.com/410.9

WEB SITES

- www.acc.org
- www.americanheart.org

Myocardial Infarction, Right Ventricular

 KEY FEATURES

ESSENTIALS OF DIAGNOSIS

- Symptoms consistent with acute myocardial infarction
- ECG changes of acute inferior or posterior ST-segment elevation myocardial infarction with ST elevation in V3R or V4R
- Elevated cardiac biomarkers
- Echocardiographic evidence of right ventricular wall motion abnormalities
- Hypotension and jugular venous distention with clear lung fields commonly observed
- In acute inferoposterior myocardial infarction, a mean right atrial to pulmonary wedge pressure ratio of ≥ 0.8

GENERAL CONSIDERATIONS

- Right ventricular (RV) involvement in acute inferior myocardial infarction (MI) is common
- Hemodynamically significant RV dysfunction is uncommon
- Of patients with acute inferoposterior MI, 20% may have hemodynamically significant RV involvement
- RV becomes noncontractile
- Cardiac output may be maintained in the initial phases by passive flow through the RV
- Right-sided heart pressures are elevated
- Left heart pressures are normal or minimally increased

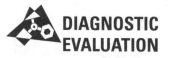 **CLINICAL PRESENTATION**

SYMPTOMS AND SIGNS

- Chest pain and symptoms of MI

PHYSICAL EXAM FINDINGS

- Elevated jugular venous distention
- Hypotension
- Cold and clammy extremities
- Cardiogenic shock
- Steep jugular venous y descent
- Kussmaul's sign

DIFFERENTIAL DIAGNOSIS

- Hypotension from other causes with inferoposterior myocardial infarction
- Pericarditis
- Pulmonary embolus
- Aortic dissection

DIAGNOSTIC EVALUATION

LABORATORY TESTS

- CBC
- Metabolic panel
- Arterial blood gases
- Chest x-ray: usually shows clear lung fields
- Cardiac enzymes including troponins

ELECTROCARDIOGRAPHY

- Evidence of acute inferior or posterior MI with ST elevation
- Shows ST elevation with right-sided chest leads V3R and V4R

IMAGING STUDIES

- Echocardiogram:
  - Shows RV regional wall motion abnormalities
  - May show depressed RV systolic function

DIAGNOSTIC PROCEDURES

- Right heart catheterization shows characteristic hemodynamic findings: steep y descent of right atrial pressure and ratio of mean right atrial to pulmonary capillary wedge pressure of > 0.8
- Coronary angiogram usually shows occlusion of the right or a dominant circumflex coronary artery

TREATMENT

CARDIOLOGY REFERRAL

- Patients with acute MI should be managed in consultation with a cardiologist
- Once hypotension occurs, the care should be transferred to a cardiologist

HOSPITALIZATION CRITERIA

- All acute MI patients have to be hospitalized
- Patients must be managed in a cardiac intensive care unit

MEDICATIONS

- Immediate coronary reperfusion
- IV fluids if left atrial pressure is low
- IV positive inotropic agents such as dobutamine to maintain blood pressure
- Avoid diuretics and vasodilators
- Other treatment similar to that for acute ST-elevation MI

THERAPEUTIC PROCEDURES

- Percutaneous coronary intervention
- Atrioventricular sequential pacing if a pacemaker required

SURGERY

- Coronary artery bypass graft if necessary

MONITORING

- Monitor for hypotension and cardiogenic shock

DIET AND ACTIVITY

- Low-fat diet
- Resume activity gradually as tolerated after hospital dismissal

ONGOING MANAGEMENT

HOSPITAL DISCHARGE CRITERIA

- Stable hemodynamic status
- No recurrence of chest pain
- Able to tolerate ambulation without difficulty in the hospital

FOLLOW-UP

- Two weeks after discharge and 3 months after that
- Subsequently yearly follow-up with a stress test
- Individual patients may have to be followed up more frequently

COMPLICATIONS

- Cardiogenic shock and death
- Life-threatening ventricular arrhythmia

PROGNOSIS

- Generally good, especially after reperfusion therapy
- RV function usually returns to normal after 3 months
- Long-term outcome depends on left ventricular function

PREVENTION

- Smoking cessation
- Low-fat diet
- Aerobic exercise
- Statin
- Control of diabetes mellitus and hypertension

RESOURCES

PRACTICE GUIDELINES

- Diagnosis:
  - Inferior MI and hemodynamic instability: right precordial lead (V4R) should be done to identify RV involvement
- Treatment:
  - Maintain preload (IV fluids)
  - Reduce afterload (reduce pulmonary pressure)
  - Inotropic support after 0.5–1 L of fluids and early percutaneous coronary intervention

REFERENCES

- Kosuge M et al: New electrocardiographic criteria for predicting the site of coronary artery occlusion in inferior wall acute myocardial infarction. Am J Cardiol 1998;82:1318.
- O'Rourke RA, Dell'Italia LJ: Diagnosis and management of right ventricular myocardial infarction. Curr Probl Cardiol 2004;29:6.

INFORMATION FOR PATIENTS

- www.drpen.com/410.9

WEB SITES

- www.acc.org
- www.americanheart.org

Myocardial Ischemia, Asymptomatic

KEY FEATURES

ESSENTIALS OF DIAGNOSIS

- Objective evidence of myocardial ischemia is the absence of angina pectoris or its equivalent
- Most patients have underlying coronary artery disease
- Ambulatory ECG monitoring shows ischemic ST transients during normal activities or a positive stress test documenting ischemia

GENERAL CONSIDERATIONS

- May occur in patients who have never developed symptoms or in patients who had prior symptomatic cardiac events
- Holter monitoring has increased the recognition of this condition
- Asymptomatic ST-segment deviation at night suggests two- or three-vessel disease
- Silent ischemia is a significant predictor of mortality
- Heart rate and blood pressure increase before silent ischemia
- Altered peripheral pain perception or cerebral cortical dysfunction have been proposed as mechanisms for silent ischemia
- Diabetics are more prone to silent ischemia

CLINICAL PRESENTATION

SYMPTOMS AND SIGNS

- Sudden death
- Patients may not experience chest pain even during acute myocardial infarction (MI)

PHYSICAL EXAM FINDINGS

- Generally noncontributory

DIFFERENTIAL DIAGNOSIS

- False-positive ECG or cardiac imaging studies
- Variant or vasospastic angina with atypical symptoms

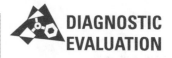 DIAGNOSTIC EVALUATION

LABORATORY TESTS

- CBC, metabolic panel
- Lipid panel
- hS-CRP (C-reactive protein)

ELECTROCARDIOGRAPHY

- ECG may show ischemic changes
- Ambulatory ECG monitoring showing ST transients is diagnostic
- Exercise stress test may be positive

IMAGING STUDIES

- Stress nuclear perfusion scan may be abnormal

DIAGNOSTIC PROCEDURES

- Coronary angiogram indicated if:
  - The perfusion scan shows high-risk changes (large area ischemia or left ventricular dilatation on stress)
  - There is asymptomatic nocturnal ST depression

TREATMENT

CARDIOLOGY REFERRAL

- High-risk patients require evaluation by a cardiologist

HOSPITALIZATION CRITERIA

- After coronary angiogram if percutaneous coronary intervention (PCI) or coronary artery bypass (CABG) planned

MEDICATIONS

- Beta-blockers are the mainstay of therapy because most episodes are associated with increased myocardial oxygen demand
- Nitrates and calcium channel blockers are less effective
- Revascularization is useful in selected patients
- Control any underlying atherosclerosis (ie, cholesterol lowering)

THERAPEUTIC PROCEDURES

- Percutaneous coronary intervention in selected patients

SURGERY

- CABG in selected patients

MONITORING

- ECG monitoring in hospital

DIET AND ACTIVITY

- Cardiac low-fat diet
- Aerobic exercise as tolerated

ONGOING MANAGEMENT

HOSPITAL DISCHARGE CRITERIA

- After adequate treatment

FOLLOW-UP

- Follow-up 3 months after initiation of treatment with follow-up ambulatory monitoring

COMPLICATIONS

- MI
- Sudden death

PROGNOSIS

- Silent ischemia is associated with adverse cardiac outcomes
- Size of perfusion defect predicts outcome

PREVENTION

- Smoking cessation
- Low-fat diet
- Aerobic exercise
- Statin
- Control of diabetes and hypertension

RESOURCES

PRACTICE GUIDELINES

- Holter monitoring is the usual way to detect this disorder
- Beta blockers are the mainstay of treatment

REFERENCES

- Almeda FQ, Kason TT, Nathan S, Kavinsky CJ: Silent myocardial ischemia: concepts and controversies. Am J Med 2004;116(2):112.

INFORMATION FOR PATIENTS

- www.nhlbi.nih.gov/health/dci/Diseases/Angina/Angina_WhatIs.html

WEB SITE

- www.americanheart.org

Myocarditis

KEY FEATURES

ESSENTIALS OF DIAGNOSIS

- New congestive heart failure with an antecedent viral syndrome
- Elevated erythrocyte sedimentation rate and/or cardiac biomarkers with acute myocarditis
- ECG shows sinus tachycardia, nonspecific ST-T changes, atrial or ventricular arrhythmias, or conduction abnormalities
- Echocardiogram demonstrates chamber enlargement, globally reduced left ventricular (LV) contractility, sometimes with regional variations
- Mural thrombi may be present

GENERAL CONSIDERATIONS

- Inflammatory disease of cardiac muscle
- Can be acute, subacute, or chronic
- Focal or diffuse myocardial inflammation that may also involve the endocardium, pericardium, or valvular structures
- Most commonly initiated by viral infection, although may occur as a result of other infectious organisms, drugs, toxins, collagen vascular diseases, or autoimmune or hypersensitivity reactions
- Most common virus associated with myocarditis is Coxsackie B; others include adenovirus, echovirus, influenza virus, hepatitis C, cytomegalovirus, and parvovirus B19
- Routine endomyocardial biopsy not recommended because inflammatory changes are often focal and nonspecific
- When positive, the inflammatory changes include inflammatory infiltrate with adjacent myocyte injury

CLINICAL PRESENTATION

SYMPTOMS AND SIGNS

- Clinical presentation is variable
- Most commonly asymptomatic
- Symptomatic patients may describe an antecedent viral syndrome, including fever, malaise, fatigue, arthralgias, myalgias, and skin rash
- Chest pain (pleuritic, ischemic, or atypical) is common
- Dyspnea, fatigue, decreased exercise tolerance
- Palpitations, dizziness or syncope
- Cardiogenic shock

PHYSICAL EXAM FINDINGS

- Exam findings vary widely
- Tachycardia (rarely, bradycardia)
- Hypotension
- Fever
- Signs of fluid overload
- Murmurs of mitral or tricuspid regurgitation (diastolic murmurs are rare)
- S_3 and occasionally S_4 gallops
- Pleural rubs and pericardial friction
- Circulatory collapse and shock (rare)

DIFFERENTIAL DIAGNOSIS

- Acute myocardial ischemia or infarction due to coronary artery disease
- Pneumonia
- Congestive heart failure due to other causes

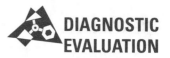 DIAGNOSTIC EVALUATION

LABORATORY TESTS

- Elevated erythrocyte sedimentation rate
- Elevated cardiac troponin T or I and CK-MB seen in some patients

ELECTROCARDIOGRAPHY

- May be normal but more commonly there are nonspecific changes
- Atrial or ventricular ectopic beats
- Atrial tachycardia or fibrillation
- Atrioventricular block or interventricular conduction block (eg, left bundle branch block)
- Regional ST elevations and Q waves that mimic acute myocardial infarction or diffuse ST elevations that simulate pericarditis

IMAGING STUDIES

- Chest x-ray: may be normal or demonstrate cardiomegaly with or without pulmonary edema
- Echocardiography: LV enlargement; globally reduced LV contractility, sometimes with regional variation mimicking myocardial infarction; increased LV wall thickness due to edematous inflammation occasionally in early disease; mural thrombi
- Gallium-67 imaging: highly sensitive for identifying active inflammation

DIAGNOSTIC PROCEDURES

- Cardiac catheterization: Not routinely performed but may be helpful when the presentation mimics myocardial infarction; hemodynamic findings include elevated LV end diastolic pressure and depressed cardiac output
- Endomyocardial biopsy: considered the gold standard for establishing the diagnosis; however, low sensitivity and specificity limit its diagnostic utility and the information it provides rarely determines specific therapy. It should be considered in patients with acute worsening rhythm disturbances (ventricular tachycardia); heart failure in the setting of peripheral eosinophilia, rash and fever; suspected giant cell myocarditis, infiltrative and storage diseases or neoplasms

TREATMENT

CARDIOLOGY REFERRAL

- Heart failure
- Suspected acute myocarditis
- Arrhythmias

HOSPITALIZATION CRITERIA

- Congestive heart failure
- Arrhythmias
- Syncope
- Hypotension/shock
- Thromboembolism

MEDICATIONS

- Narcotic analgesics for pain relief
- Specific antimicrobial treatment if an infectious agent is identified
- Immunosuppressive therapy is generally not helpful except in giant cell myocarditis and autoimmune diseases such as systemic lupus erythematosus
- Appropriate treatment of systolic dysfunction (angiotensin-converting enzyme inhibitors, beta blockers, digoxin, spironolactone, and diuretics)
- Avoid nonsteroidal anti-inflammatory drugs

THERAPEUTIC PROCEDURES

- Pericardiocentesis for pericardial effusion and signs of cardiac tamponade
- Pacemaker insertion for heart block

SURGERY

- Cardiac transplantation

MONITORING

- ECG monitoring in hospital
- Fluid balance

DIET AND ACTIVITY

- Low-sodium diet and fluid restriction in patients with congestive heart failure
- Strict bed rest (animal models show increased intensity of inflammation, morbidity, and mortality with exercise)

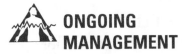 **ONGOING MANAGEMENT**

HOSPITAL DISCHARGE CRITERIA

- Compensated heart failure
- Stable cardiac rhythm

FOLLOW-UP

- See cardiologist within 2–4 weeks
- Serial echocardiograms every few months for the first year to assess progression or resolution of disease
- Holter monitoring for suspected arrhythmias

COMPLICATIONS

- Congestive heart failure
- Pulmonary edema
- Cardiogenic shock
- Recurrent myositis
- Dysrhythmias

PROGNOSIS

- Congestive heart failure:
  - Morbidity and mortality based on the degree of LV dysfunction
- New-onset congestive heart failure: 50% have improvement in cardiac function
  - 25% of patients have stabilization of reduced cardiac function
  - 25% continue to deteriorate
- Transplantation: patients have increased risk of recurrent myocarditis and transplant rejection

PREVENTION

- Avoidance of offending toxins and infectious organisms

RESOURCES

PRACTICE GUIDELINES

- Myocarditis may present subtly and should be considered in patients with chest pain and signs of heart failure
- Most patients respond to medical therapy alone
- Endomyocardial biopsy should be considered in patients with heart failure refractory to medical therapy, a rapidly deteriorating course or suspected secondary causes of dilated cardiomyopathy

REFERENCES

- Felker GM et al: Echocardiographic findings in acute and fulminant myocarditis. J Am Coll Cardiol 2000;36:227.
- Wu LA et al: Current role of endomyocardial biopsy in the management of patients with dilated cardiomyopathy and myocarditis. Mayo Clin Proc 2001;76:1030.

INFORMATION FOR PATIENTS

- http://www.medicinenet.com/myocarditis/article.htm
- http://patients.uptodate.com/topic.asp?file=myoperic/4988
- http://www.nlm.nih.gov/medlineplus/ency/article/000149.htm

WEB SITE

- http://www.emedicine.com/EMERG/topic326.htm

Neurocardiogenic Syncope

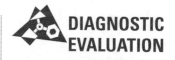

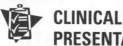

KEY FEATURES

ESSENTIALS OF DIAGNOSIS

- Most common mechanism of syncope in the young
- Bradycardia (vagal) and profound hypotension (vasodepressor) may occur either alone or in varying proportions
- Pain, fear, or emotion may precipitate syncope
- Many spells over several years are suggestive of this disorder
- Tilt testing is useful in the diagnosis

GENERAL CONSIDERATIONS

- Generally occurs with no structural heart disease
- Prolonged standing may precipitate this disorder
- Usually associated with prodrome such as nausea and diaphoresis
- Bezold-Jarisch reflex triggered by mechanoreceptors of the inferoposterior myocardium leads to sympathetic withdrawal and unopposed vagal input
- This reflex may be a contributor to syncope due to aortic stenosis and hypertrophic cardiomyopathy
- Fatigue, pallor, and diaphoresis after syncope is common

CLINICAL PRESENTATION

SYMPTOMS AND SIGNS

- Recurrent syncope with prodromal symptoms

PHYSICAL EXAM FINDINGS

- Generally normal in between syncopal episodes

DIFFERENTIAL DIAGNOSIS

- Sick sinus syndrome
- Orthostatic hypotension
- Iatrogenic syncope caused by antihypertensive medications

DIAGNOSTIC EVALUATION

LABORATORY TESTS

- CBC, basal metabolic panel

ELECTROCARDIOGRAPHY

- ECG to exclude heart disease

IMAGING STUDIES

- Echocardiogram to exclude structural heart disease

DIAGNOSTIC PROCEDURES

- Head-up tilt-table testing
- If regular tilt testing is negative, consider provocative tilt testing with isoproterenol or nitroglycerin
- Rare patient benefits from implantable loop recorder

TREATMENT

CARDIOLOGY REFERRAL

- Patient with frequent syncope should be referred to a cardiologist

HOSPITALIZATION CRITERIA

- Hospitalization seldom required
- Recurrent syncope especially with injuries

MEDICATIONS

- Salt and fluid loading; avoidance of dehydration
- Fludrocortisone 0.2 mg PO daily
- Beta blockers, such as metoprolol 50 mg/day
- Adrenergic agonist midodrine 10 mg 3 times daily
- Serotonin reuptake inhibitors, such as paroxetine 20 mg/day
- Disopyramide 600 mg/day in divided doses

THERAPEUTIC PROCEDURES

- Dual-chamber pacemaker with rate-drop feature in a rare patient

SURGERY

- None required

MONITORING

- After initiation of therapy, tilt test may be repeated to document efficacy

DIET AND ACTIVITY

- Additional salt intake
- Avoid dehydration

ONGOING MANAGEMENT

HOSPITAL DISCHARGE CRITERIA

- After therapy is started

FOLLOW-UP

- Three months after initial assessment
- If symptoms are frequent, earlier follow-up may be required
- Stable patient may be returned to primary care physician

COMPLICATIONS

- Trauma associated with syncope
- Accidents at work or during driving

PROGNOSIS

- Benign outcome

PREVENTION

- Avoid precipitating factors such as prolonged standing, dehydration

RESOURCES

PRACTICE GUIDELINES

- Indications for tilt testing:
  - No history of organic cardiovascular disease
  - History suggestive of vasovagal episodes
  - Organic cardiovascular disease, but history suggestive of vasovagal episodes and other causes of syncope not identified
  - Unexplained syncope

REFERENCES

- Goldschlager N et al: Etiologic considerations in the patient with syncope and an apparently normal heart. Arch Intern Med 2003;163:151.
- Sutton R: Has cardiac pacing a role in vasovagal syncope? J Interv Card Electrophysiol 2003; 9:145.

INFORMATION FOR PATIENTS

- www.drpen.com/780.2
- www.hlm.nih.gov/medlineplus/arrhythmia.html

WEB SITES

- www.hrsonline.org
- www.acc.org

Nonparoxysmal Junctional Tachycardia

 KEY FEATURES

ESSENTIALS OF DIAGNOSIS

- Heart rate 60–120 bpm
- Atrioventricular (AV) dissociation
- Gradual onset and termination
- When rhythm is caused by digoxin, AV dissociation is common
- Usually seen with organic heart disease

GENERAL CONSIDERATIONS

- Causes include:
  - Digoxin toxicity
  - Inferior myocardial infarction
  - Open-heart surgery
  - Myocarditis
  - Rarely congenital heart disease
- This arrhythmia is not episodic
- P waves may be before or after or buried in the QRS complex
- Antegrade AV block and intermittent atrial capture may give the appearance of irregular rhythm
- Enhanced vagal tone may slow the arrhythmia but not terminate it
- Digoxin toxicity is the cause of 60% of cases
- Regular ventricular rhythm in atrial fibrillation treated with digoxin should raise suspicion of this arrhythmia
- Twenty percent of cases are secondary to inferior infarction and usually disappear within days
- Valve surgery and myocarditis are other causes of this arrhythmia

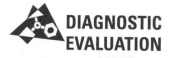 **CLINICAL PRESENTATION**

SYMPTOMS AND SIGNS

- Depends on precipitating cause
- Symptoms of digoxin toxicity may be present
- Myocardial infarction or valve surgery history will be self-evident

PHYSICAL EXAM FINDINGS

- Cannon *a* waves if there is AV dissociation
- Variable S_1 may be present
- Other features depend on underlying cause

DIFFERENTIAL DIAGNOSIS

- Atrial tachycardia
- Atrioventricular nodal reentry tachycardia (AVNRT) (slower heart rate, gradual onset and termination, lack of termination with vagal maneuvers differentiate the rhythm from AVNRT)

DIAGNOSTIC EVALUATION

LABORATORY TESTS

- CBC, metabolic panel

ELECTROCARDIOGRAPHY

- ECG to detect and document the rhythm
- Continuous telemetry until the rhythm resolves

IMAGING STUDIES

- Echocardiogram to evaluate left ventricular function

DIAGNOSTIC PROCEDURES

- Overdrive pacing transiently suppresses the rhythm

TREATMENT

CARDIOLOGY REFERRAL

- All patients should be evaluated by a cardiologist

HOSPITALIZATION CRITERIA

- Most patients are hospitalized at the time of the arrhythmia
- If patients present to the emergency room, they require hospitalization until the rhythm resolves

MEDICATIONS

- No treatment is usually indicated
- Rhythm spontaneously resolves as the inciting event subsides
- If the rhythm is hemodynamically disturbing, AV sequential pacing at a rate faster than the tachycardia may suppress the rhythm and restore the atrial contribution to cardiac output

THERAPEUTIC PROCEDURES

- None required

MONITORING

- No need for monitoring after the rhythm resolves

ONGOING MANAGEMENT

HOSPITAL DISCHARGE CRITERIA

- Once the rhythm resolves, provided that the patient is stable otherwise

FOLLOW-UP

- Two weeks after discharge
- Underlying cardiac conditions may need follow-up
- Avoid digoxin or use lowest possible dose

COMPLICATIONS

- Usually no long-term complications

PROGNOSIS

- Most patients recover from this arrhythmia without adverse outcome

PREVENTION

- Use the smallest therapeutic doses of digoxin necessary

RESOURCES

PRACTICE GUIDELINES

- Management guidelines:
  - Withhold digoxin or use digibind if ventricular tachycardia or high-grade heart block occurs
  - For persistent tachycardia, use beta blockers, calcium channel blockers, and if necessary, overdrive atrial pacemaker

REFERENCE

- Hamdan MH, Badhwar N, Scheinman MM: Role of invasive electrophysiologic testing in the evaluation and management of adult patients with focal junctional tachycardia. Card Electrophysiol Rev 2002;6:431.

INFORMATION FOR PATIENTS

- www.nlm.nih.gov/medlineplus/ arrhythmia.html

WEB SITES

- www.acc.org
- www.hrsonline.org

Obesity and Heart Disease

KEY FEATURES

ESSENTIALS OF DIAGNOSIS

- Body mass index > 30 kg/m^2
- Increased left ventricular mass by imaging in the absence of hypertension or diabetes
- Heart failure and cardiac arrhythmias common

GENERAL CONSIDERATIONS

- Obesity is not only a risk factor for coronary artery disease, but can cause left ventricular hypertrophy, heart failure, and arrhythmias independent of hypertension
- Fatty infiltration of the conduction system and sleep apnea have been found in obese individuals; both can lead to arrhythmias
- Eccentric left ventricular hypertrophy may be related to increased plasma volume and metabolic demands
- Obesity is also part of the metabolic syndrome, which predisposes to atherosclerosis

CLINICAL PRESENTATION

SYMPTOMS AND SIGNS

- Dyspnea, fatigue are common
- Chest pain and palpitations can occur

PHYSICAL EXAM FINDINGS

- Increased body mass index:
  - Normal 18.8–25 kg/m^2
  - Overweight 25–30 kg/m^2
  - Obese >30 kg/m^2
- Central (truncal or android) obesity (waist circumference > 102 cm men, > 88 cm women) is a risk factor for atherosclerosis
- Lower body (gynecoid) obesity is *not* a risk factor for coronary disease
- Systemic hypertension
- Left ventricular lift or heave
- Signs of heart failure may be present
- S$_3$ or S$_3$ may be present

DIFFERENTIAL DIAGNOSIS

- Coronary artery disease
- Dilated cardiomyopathy
- Hypertrophic cardiomyopathy
- Diabetic cardiomyopathy

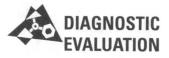 DIAGNOSTIC EVALUATION

LABORATORY TESTS

- Elevated lipids
- Abnormal liver function tests from fatty accumulation

ELECTROCARDIOGRAPHY

- Prolonged QTc

IMAGING STUDIES

- CT and MRI: useful to confirm excess internal fat accumulation
- Echocardiography:
  - Shows left ventricular hypertrophy, usually eccentric but sometimes concentric
  - Evidence of systolic or diastolic dysfunction may be present

DIAGNOSTIC PROCEDURES

- Underwater weighing for determination of lean body mass
- Skinfold thickness measures with calipers

TREATMENT

CARDIOLOGY REFERRAL

- Suspected cardiac disease
- Difficult to control hypertension

HOSPITALIZATION CRITERIA

- Heart failure
- Respiratory failure
- Planned procedure or surgery

MEDICATIONS

- Weight loss through diet, exercise, and approved drugs
- Assessment and treatment of comorbid conditions, such as hyperlipidemia and hypertension
- Indicated treatment for heart failure or arrhythmias

SURGERY

- Bariatric surgery in selected cases

MONITORING

- ECG in hospital as appropriate
- Daily weight

DIET AND ACTIVITY

- Diet of 500–1000 kcal/day: 30% total fat, 7% saturated fat
- Aerobic exercise for at least 30 minutes a day

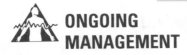

ONGOING MANAGEMENT

HOSPITAL DISCHARGE CRITERIA

- Resolution of problem
- After successful surgery

FOLLOW-UP

- Close follow-up involving behavior modification interventions for at least 6 months

COMPLICATIONS

- Sudden death
- Heart failure
- Acute coronary syndromes

PROGNOSIS

- A body mass index of $> 30 \text{ kg/m}^2$ increases mortality rate 50–100%

PREVENTION

- A prudent diet and daily physical activity can prevent obesity in most people

RESOURCES

PRACTICE GUIDELINES

- The initial goal of weight loss therapy is a 10% decrease from baseline
  - This is best achieved by diet, exercise, and behavioral modification strategies
  - If this goal is achieved, further weight loss can be considered to ultimately get body mass index to $< 25 \text{ kg/m}^2$

REFERENCE

- Vega GL: Obesity, the metabolic syndrome and cardiovascular disease. Am Heart J 2001;142:1108.

INFORMATION FOR PATIENTS

- www.drpen.com/278.01

WEB SITE

- www.emedicine.com/med/topic1653.htm

Orthostatic Hypotension

KEY FEATURES

ESSENTIALS OF DIAGNOSIS

- Symptoms of reduced cerebral perfusion upon assuming an upright position—dizziness to frank syncope
- Marked fall in blood pressure within 3 minutes of standing (> 20 mm Hg systolic or > 10 mm Hg diastolic)

GENERAL CONSIDERATIONS

- This disorder may be symptomatic or asymptomatic
- Symptoms are worse in the morning, after meals, and after exercise
- Usual causes include volume depletion (usually secondary to diuretics), vasodilators, and neurogenic causes such as primary and secondary causes of autonomic failure
- Elderly population is most commonly affected owing to reduced baroreceptor sensitivity, impaired thirst mechanism, and reduced cerebral blood flow
- Parkinson's disease and multiple-system atrophy (Shy-Drager syndrome) may cause orthostatic hypotension

CLINICAL PRESENTATION

SYMPTOMS AND SIGNS

- Lightheadedness
- Dizziness
- Blurred vision
- Weakness
- Palpitation
- Tremulousness
- Syncope

PHYSICAL EXAM FINDINGS

- Postural drop in blood pressure of > 20 mm Hg systolic or > 10 mm Hg diastolic
- Features of neurologic disease if present

DIFFERENTIAL DIAGNOSIS/CAUSES

- Fluid loss, anemia, dehydration
- Primary autonomic dysfunction: Shy-Drager syndrome
- Secondary dysautonomia:
  - Parkinson's disease
  - Diabetes mellitus
  - Amyloidosis
  - Human immunodeficiency virus infection
  - Multiple sclerosis
- Vasoactive medications:
  - Antihypertensive agents
  - Ethanol
  - Psychoactive drugs
- Advanced age: akinetic falling spells of the aged

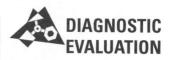 DIAGNOSTIC EVALUATION

LABORATORY TESTS

- CBC,; metabolic panel

ELECTROCARDIOGRAPHY

- ECG to screen for cardiac disease

IMAGING STUDIES

- None required for diagnosis

DIAGNOSTIC PROCEDURES

- Autonomic nervous system studies may be indicated

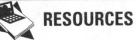

 TREATMENT

CARDIOLOGY REFERRAL

- Seldom required unless initial management is not successful or diagnosis is in question

HOSPITALIZATION CRITERIA

- Syncope secondary to profound volume depletion
- Recurrent syncope
- Trauma secondary to syncope

MEDICATIONS

- Treat underlying cause if possible
- Wear elastic stockings
- Maintain adequate salt and water intake
- Administer fludrocortisone 0.1-1.0 mg PO daily
- Give alpha-1-adrenergic agonists, eg, midodrine 10 mg 3 times PO daily

THERAPEUTIC PROCEDURES

- None required

MONITORING

- Orthostatic blood pressure monitoring after initiation of treatment

DIET AND ACTIVITY

- Liberal salt intake to maintain euvolemia

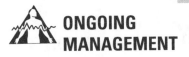 **ONGOING MANAGEMENT**

HOSPITAL DISCHARGE CRITERIA

- After initiation of therapy

FOLLOW-UP

- Initially 2 weeks; after that 3 months, depending on response

COMPLICATIONS

- Trauma secondary to syncope

PROGNOSIS

- Prognosis depends on precipitating cause
- Multisystem atrophy carries the worst prognosis
- Medication-related condition usually responds to withdrawal of offending medication

PREVENTION

- Check orthostatic blood pressure whenever vasodilators are added or dose adjusted

RESOURCES

PRACTICE GUIDELINES

- Elderly patients who complain of dizziness must have their orthostatic blood pressure measured

REFERENCES

- Pavri BB, Ho RT: Syncope. Identifying cardiac causes in older patients. Geriatrics 2003;58:26.
- Weimer LH: Syncope and orthostatic intolerance for the primary care physician. Prim Care 2004;31:175.

INFORMATION FOR PATIENTS

- www.ninds.nih.gov/health_and_medical/disorders/orthosta_doc.html

WEB SITES

- www.hrsonline.org
- www.acc.org

Pacemaker Malfunction

 KEY FEATURES

ESSENTIALS OF DIAGNOSIS

- Failure to capture:
  - Pacing spike is not followed by a depolarization
- Oversensing:
  - Typically, the T wave or skeletal muscle potentials are sensed as depolarization, and a pacing spike is not initiated
- Pacemaker-mediated tachycardia:
  - Pacing at or near the programmed upper rate limit secondary to retrograde conduction of the ventricular complex to the atrium, which is sensed as a P wave
- Lead fracture is suspected when there is high impedance
- Lead insulation failure leads to low lead impedance
- Electromagnetic interference (eg, by antitheft devices) may interfere with pacemaker function

GENERAL CONSIDERATIONS

- Component failure can be intermittent, and a complete evaluation may not identify the problem initially
- Activity before the clinical event is useful and should be sought
- Pacemaker interrogation is critical in the evaluation
- A complete evaluation includes history, examination, indication for pacemaker insertion, and review of imaging studies
- Medications influence the pacing thresholds and should be examined
- Lead dislodgement usually occurs soon after implantation
- Exit block is a chronic problem, presumably related to fibrosis disturbing the electrode-myocardium interface (reduced by steroid eluting leads)
- Perforation and metabolic alteration (including medication) may raise pacing thresholds
- Air in the pocket may result in pacing failure of unipolar pacemaker
- Loose set screw manifests as failure to pace or capture
- Overall, pacemakers are extraordinarily reliable; component failure is rare
- Diaphragmatic stimulation is rare but may occur

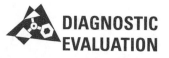 **CLINICAL PRESENTATION**

SYMPTOMS AND SIGNS

- Dizziness
- Syncope
- Fatigue
- Palpitations secondary to excessive response from a sensor-driven pacemaker

PHYSICAL EXAM FINDINGS

- Usually no change in findings
- Myopotential oversensing can be brought on by isometric maneuver
- Diaphragmatic pacing may be observed

DIFFERENTIAL DIAGNOSIS

- Lead dislodgement
- Loose connection between the lead and the pulse generator
- Metabolic abnormalities such as hyperkalemia
- Antiarrhythmic medication adverse effects

DIAGNOSTIC EVALUATION

LABORATORY TESTS

- Cardiac biomarker if undersensing is an issue and is not explained by other conditions
- Metabolic panel to evaluate the causes of undersensing or failure to capture

ELECTROCARDIOGRAPHY

- ECG with rhythm strip to identify the problem

IMAGING STUDIES

- Echocardiogram may be useful when there is an intervening event like myocardial infarction
- Chest x-ray may help in evaluating lead fracture and definitely macrodislodgement
- CT scan and echocardiogram may be helpful in cardiac perforation

DIAGNOSTIC PROCEDURES

- Device interrogation

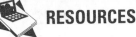

 TREATMENT

CARDIOLOGY REFERRAL

• Electrophysiologic evaluation is recommended for all patients

HOSPITALIZATION CRITERIA

• Depends on underlying problem
• If patient is pacemaker dependent, hospitalization is recommended

MEDICATIONS

• Antiarrhythmic drug adjustment as necessary

THERAPEUTIC PROCEDURES

• Treatment depends on the cause of malfunction
• Pacemaker-mediated tachycardia can be treated by prolongation of the postventricular atrial refractory period
• Diaphragmatic stimulation may be reduced or eliminated by reducing the output within the safety margin; if not, repositioning may be needed
• Lead repositioning
• New lead placement
• Revision or implantation of a new pacemaker

SURGERY

• Epicardial pacing is rarely required

MONITORING

• ECG monitoring in the hospital

DIET AND ACTIVITY

• General healthy life style
• No specific change required

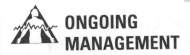 **ONGOING MANAGEMENT**

HOSPITAL DISCHARGE CRITERIA

• Once the problem is eliminated

FOLLOW-UP

• One week after hospital discharge
• On symptom recurrence
• Routine follow-up every 3 months

COMPLICATIONS

• Depends on the cause

PROGNOSIS

• Generally very good prognosis because most problems can be resolved

PREVENTION

• Good implantation technique
• Proper monitoring

RESOURCES

PRACTICE GUIDELINES

• Goals of transtelephonic monitoring:
  – Determine the intrinsic rhythm or continuous pacing at programmed parameters
  – Identify atrial rhythm sinus versus atrial fibrillation and assess sensing function in both chambers
  – Assess magnet mode functions

REFERENCE

• Scher DL: Troubleshooting pacemakers and implantable cardioverter-defibrillators. Curr Opin Cardiol 2004;19:36.

INFORMATION FOR PATIENTS

• www.nlm.nih.gov/medlineplus/arrhythmia.html

WEB SITE

• www.hrsonline.org

Pacemaker Syndrome

KEY FEATURES

ESSENTIALS OF DIAGNOSIS

- Weakness, orthopnea, dizziness, breathlessness, presyncope, syncope, pulmonary congestion, and altered mental status
- Atrial rhythm and rate are dyssynchronous with the ventricular rhythm and rate
- Appropriately timed atrial contraction does not precede the paced ventricular event

GENERAL CONSIDERATIONS

- Prevalence is 10–50% and more common in the elderly
- Common with VVI pacing and reduced with dual-chamber pacing
- Diagnosis established by the objective findings of ventricular-atrial conduction, cannon waves, and transient mitral regurgitation
- Atrial contraction and resultant atrial stretch activate the baroreceptors to produce vagally mediated vasodilatation and decrease in heart rate
- May occur in any pacing mode when AV synchrony is uncoupled
- Incidence has a wide range depending on whether patients were switched from an AV synchronous mode to VVI mode or were studied in VVI mode
- In VVI mode, incidence is 7–10%
- When switched from DDD to VVI mode, symptoms are experienced by 80% of patients

CLINICAL PRESENTATION

SYMPTOMS AND SIGNS

- Pulsations in the neck
- Palpitations
- Fatigue, weakness, apprehension
- Chest pain
- Dyspnea
- Dizziness
- Presyncope, syncope

PHYSICAL EXAM FINDINGS

- Arterial blood pressure in supine and standing position with ventricular pacing and sinus rhythm (drop of 20 mm Hg suggests pacemaker syndrome)
- Cannon *a* waves
- Pulsatile liver
- S_3 gallop, pulmonary rales

DIFFERENTIAL DIAGNOSIS

- Newer forms of pacemaker syndromes such as prolonged AV conduction (intrinsic AV node problem or drug induced) in AAI or AAIR mode
- AV dyssynchrony caused by mode switching

DIAGNOSTIC EVALUATION

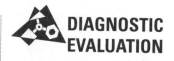

LABORATORY TESTS

- CBC, basal metabolic panel

ELECTROCARDIOGRAPHY

- ECG may be used to document VA conduction during symptoms
- Ambulatory ECG monitoring may be useful in confirming the diagnosis

IMAGING STUDIES

- Doppler echocardiogram may be used to document hemodynamic changes secondary to VVI pacemaker

DIAGNOSTIC PROCEDURES

- Hemodynamic measurements with and without pacemaker rhythm (20 mm Hg drop)
- Relief of patient's symptoms with SR or AV synchrony

TREATMENT

CARDIOLOGY REFERRAL

- Patients should be evaluated by an electrophysiolgist

HOSPITALIZATION CRITERIA

- Usually can be managed as outpatient
- If syncope or serious symptoms occur, patient has to be hospitalized

MEDICATIONS

- Trial of antiarrhythmic drugs to eliminate retrograde ventriculoatrial conduction

THERAPEUTIC PROCEDURES

- Atrial pacing and sensing unless contraindicated
- In VVI pacing, upgrading to DDD mode with physiologic AV pace intervals
- Reducing the lower rate of VVI pacing to reduce the number of paced events

SURGERY

- Rarely may need epicardial pacemaker upgrade secondary to lack of venous access

MONITORING

- Monitor for symptoms after VVI pacemaker insertion

DIET AND ACTIVITY

- Symptomatic patients may have to restrict activity until treated

ONGOING MANAGEMENT

HOSPITAL DISCHARGE CRITERIA

- Twenty-four hours after an upgrade to DDD pacemaker

FOLLOW-UP

- Every 3 months after pacemaker insertion

COMPLICATIONS

- Patients may sustain injuries secondary to syncope

PROGNOSIS

- Once treated, symptoms resolve

PREVENTION

- Insertion of AV synchronous pacemaker except in patients with atrial fibrillation

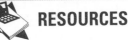

RESOURCES

PRACTICE GUIDELINES

- This condition is rare
- Consider upgrading single-chamber ventricular pacemaker if the patient is not in atrial fibrillation

REFERENCES

- Mitrani RD et al: Cardiac pacemakers: Current and future status. Curr Probl Cardiol 1999;24:341.
- Ross RA, Kenny RA. Pacemaker syndrome in older people. Age Ageing 2000;29:13.

INFORMATION FOR PATIENTS

- www.nlm.nih.gov/medlineplus/ arrhythmia.html

WEB SITE

- www.hrsonline.org

Paroxysmal Atrial Tachycardia With Block

KEY FEATURES

ESSENTIALS OF DIAGNOSIS

- Atrial rate of 150–250 bpm
- Atrioventricular (AV) block of 2:1
- Often associated with digitalis toxicity

GENERAL CONSIDERATIONS

- Increasingly seen in advanced organic heart disease and severe pulmonary disease
- When seen, digoxin toxicity must be suspected
- A ventriculophasic response is often seen (P-P intervals containing QRS complexes are shorter than those that do not)
- May be secondary to auotmaticity or triggered activity
- Exacerbated by hypokalemia, particularly when associated with digoxin excess

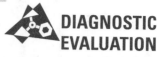 CLINICAL PRESENTATION

SYMPTOMS AND SIGNS

- Related underlying cardiac disease and ventricular rate
- Shortness of breath
- Rarely chest pain
- Palpitations
- Gastrointestinal symptoms secondary to digitalis toxicity

PHYSICAL EXAM FINDINGS

- Varying S_1
- Disproportionate jugular *a* waves compared with pulse (2:1)
- Carotid sinus massage may slow pulse rate (not advised in digitalis toxicity owing to induction of serious ventricular arrhythmia)

DIFFERENTIAL DIAGNOSIS

- Other forms of atrial tachycardia
- Atypical AV nodal reentrant tachycardia
- Atrial flutter

DIAGNOSTIC EVALUATION

LABORATORY TESTS

- CBC, metabolic panel
- Serum digoxin level (may not correlate with toxicity, which is a clinical diagnosis)
- Arterial blood gas analysis if there is evidence of advanced lung disease

ELECTROCARDIOGRAPHY

- Shows atrial tachycardia usually with 2:1 AV block
- The ventricular rate is often within the normal range
- Varying block may also be noted

IMAGING STUDIES

- Echocardiogram to assess underlying heart disease

DIAGNOSTIC PROCEDURES

- None required

TREATMENT

CARDIOLOGY REFERRAL

- When secondary to digitalis toxicity usually can be managed by a generalist
- When tachycardia is persistent with advanced heart disease, cardiology referral is required

HOSPITALIZATION CRITERIA

- Almost all patients require hospitalization secondary to advanced nature of underlying disease

MEDICATIONS

- Withdraw digoxin when appropriate
- In life-threatening conditions, consider digoxin (Digibind) 228 mg (6 vials); life-threatening ingestions may require more
- Correct electrolyte abnormalities
- Therapies targeted at abolishing the arrhythmia are unrewarding
- In persistent cases, AV block with medication may be achieved to control ventricular rate

THERAPEUTIC PROCEDURES

- If the tachycardia is secondary to advanced heart disease and not related to digitalis toxicity, then radiofrequency ablation may be attempted with a mapping (contact or noncontact) system

SURGERY

- Usually not required

MONITORING

- ECG monitoring in hospital
- Digoxin level monitoring during Digibind therapy

DIET AND ACTIVITY

- Related to underlying heart disease

ONGOING MANAGEMENT

HOSPITAL DISCHARGE CRITERIA

- Resolution of arrhythmia
- Symptomatic stability

FOLLOW-UP

- Two weeks after hospital discharge
- Subsequent follow-up depends on underlying heart disease

COMPLICATIONS

- Depends on underlying heart disease
- May precipitate heart failure

PROGNOSIS

- Depends on underlying heart disease

PREVENTION

- Monitoring patients on digoxin, giving the lowest therapeutic dose and early recognition of toxicity

RESOURCES

PRACTICE GUIDELINES

- Discontinue digoxin
- Persistent advanced AV block: consider using Digibind

REFERENCES

- Ma G, Brady WJ, Pollack M, Chan TC: Electrocardiographic manifestations: digitalis toxicity. J Emerg Med 2001;20:145.
- Spodick DH: Electrocardiology teacher analysis and review: atrial flutter vs. (paroxysmal) atrial tachycardia with block. Am J Geriatr Cardiol 1999;8:143.

INFORMATION FOR PATIENTS

- www.nlm.nih.gov/medlineplus/ arrhythmia.html

WEB SITE

- www.hrsonline.org

Partial Anomalous Pulmonary Venous Connection

 KEY FEATURES

ESSENTIALS OF DIAGNOSIS

- Young adult with dyspnea, recurrent respiratory infections, hemoptysis, and palpitations
- Physical findings of atrial septal defect (ASD):
  - Right ventricular heave
  - Systolic ejection murmur at the left sternal border
  - Wide fixed split S_2 and a diastolic flow rumble over the tricuspid area
- Incomplete right bundle branch block on ECG
- Pulmonary vascular congestion, enlarged right heart, and occasionally evidence of the anomalous vein on chest radiograph
- Cardiac imaging evidence of anomalous pulmonary venous connection and ASD in many patients

GENERAL CONSIDERATIONS

- This condition is present in approximately 10% of patients with ASD (usually of the sinus venous type)
- Excessive pulmonary venous return to the right heart over years causes right atrial and ventricular dilation
- Atrial arrhythmias, right heart failure and rarely pulmonary hypertension may develop
- Symptomatic patients or those with a large shunt (Qp/Qs ratio > 2.0) should have surgical repair, including repair of any associated congenital heart defects
- Surgical repair is contraindicated in patients with an associated ASD who have developed pulmonary vascular disease

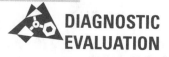 **CLINICAL PRESENTATION**

SYMPTOMS AND SIGNS

- Dyspnea
- Signs of right heart failure
- Recurrent respiratory infections
- Hemoptysis
- Palpitations

PHYSICAL EXAM FINDINGS

- Right ventricular heave
- Systolic ejection murmur at the left sternal border
- Wide fixed split S_2 consistent with an associated ASD
- Diastolic flow rumble over the tricuspid valve

DIFFERENTIAL DIAGNOSIS

- ASD alone
- Right-heart failure from other causes
- Pulmonary hypertension from other causes

DIAGNOSTIC EVALUATION

LABORATORY TESTS

- No specific tests

ELECTROCARDIOGRAPHY

- Incomplete right bundle branch block
- Right axis deviation
- Right ventricular hypertrophy
- Right atrial enlargement

IMAGING STUDIES

- Chest x-ray:
  - Enlarged right atrium and right ventricle
  - Pulmonary vascular congestion, rarely enlarged pulmonary vein
- Echocardiography:
  - Enlarged right atrium and right ventricle, sometimes color-flow Doppler evidence of an ASD
  - Transesophageal echocardiography can usually demonstrate anomalous drainage of one or more pulmonary veins into the right atrium (usually the right upper pulmonary vein)
  - A sinus venous type ASD may be present at the junction of the superior vena cava and right atrium

DIAGNOSTIC PROCEDURES

- Cardiac catheterization:
  - Oxygen saturation step-up in the right atrium (usually the high right atrium). Qp/Qs ratio may be calculated
  - Pulmonary artery pressures are often elevated owing to increased flow
  - Pulmonary vascular resistance may be elevated rarely

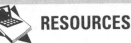

TREATMENT

CARDIOLOGY REFERRAL

- Signs and symptoms of right heart failure
- Suspected ASD

HOSPITALIZATION CRITERIA

- Heart failure
- Tachyarrhythmias

MEDICATIONS

- Supportive care in nonsurgical cases for heart failure, arrhythmias, and pulmonary vascular disease

THERAPEUTIC PROCEDURES

- No specific procedures

SURGERY

- Surgical correction for patients with Qp/Qs shunt ratio > 2:1

MONITORING

- ECG monitoring in the hospital

DIET AND ACTIVITY

- Low-sodium diet for patients with heart failure

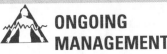

ONGOING MANAGEMENT

HOSPITAL DISCHARGE CRITERIA

- Resolution of heart failure
- Stabilization of cardiac arrhythmias
- After successful surgery

FOLLOW-UP

- Exam within 3 months after surgery, then every 1–2 years
- For patients with uncorrected anomalous pulmonary veins, every 6–12 months depending on the shunt magnitude and comorbid conditions
- Echocardiography if symptoms arise or worsen

COMPLICATIONS

- Superior vena cava obstruction after surgery
- Arrhythmias or right heart failure may develop in patients with uncorrected lesions and/or when the shunt ratio is underestimated

PROGNOSIS

- Few data are available on mortality rates
- Major morbidity is due to arrhythmias, right heart failure, and rarely pulmonary hypertension

PREVENTION

- Prevention of progressive right-sided cardiac enlargement and failure, arrhythmias, and pulmonary hypertension by early surgery when the condition is diagnosed in patients with a significant shunt ratio

RESOURCES

PRACTICE GUIDELINES

- Definitive surgical repair should be performed in patients with significant shunts and no significant pulmonary vascular disease

REFERENCES

- Okumura L et al: Intraatrial rerouting by atrial flaps for partial anomalous pulmonary venous return. Ann Thorac Surg 2003;76:1726.
- Vanderheyden G et al: Partial anomalous pulmonary venous connection or scimitar syndrome. Heart 2003;89:761.

INFORMATION FOR PATIENTS

- http://www.healthsystem.virginia.edu/ internet/childrens-heart/pted/ pcdt024.cfm

WEB SITES

- www.emedicine.com/ped/ topic2522.htm
- www.pubmedcentral.nih.gov/ articlerender.fcgi?artid=341862
- http://www.emedicine.com/ped/ topic2816.htm

Patent Ductus Arteriosus

 KEY FEATURES

ESSENTIALS OF DIAGNOSIS

- Continuous machinery-like murmur, loudest below the left clavicle
- Left ventricular hypertrophy
- Pulmonary plethora, left atrial and ventricular enlargement
- In older adults, calcification of the ductus on chest radiograph
- Left atrial and ventricular dilatation with normal right heart chambers on echocardiography
- Continuous high-velocity color Doppler jet with retrograde flow along lateral wall of main pulmonary artery near left branch

GENERAL CONSIDERATIONS

- Remnant of the normal fetal circulation with a connection between the left pulmonary artery and descending aorta distal to the left subclavian artery
- A nonrestrictive patent ductus arteriosus (large left-to-right shunt) usually causes congestive heart failure within first year of life
- Causes volume overload and enlargement of the left heart chambers due to recirculation of blood from the aorta to pulmonary circulation and back to the left atrium
- Usually associated with other defects, such as pulmonary or tricuspid atresia
- In a minority of patients, pulmonary vascular disease may develop with reversal of the shunt
- Differential cyanosis may develop when the shunt reverses and results in desaturated blood flowing into the descending aorta distal to the left subclavian artery

 CLINICAL PRESENTATION

SYMPTOMS AND SIGNS

- Usually presents in childhood
- Rarely presents in a young adult
- Congestive heart failure
- Adults may present with exertional dyspnea, chest pain, palpitations

PHYSICAL EXAM FINDINGS

- Acyanotic upper extremities
- Sometimes clubbing and cyanosis of the lower extremities and occasionally the left hand
- Widened pulse pressure
- Hyperdynamic, laterally displaced apical impulse
- Continuous, machinery-like murmur, loudest below the left clavicle
- Murmur decreases and may disappear as pulmonary vascular resistance increases and shunt reverses
- S_3 gallop
- Diastolic murmur across the mitral valve

DIFFERENTIAL DIAGNOSIS

- Other causes of exertional dyspnea, chest pain, and palpitations
- Other causes of left-heart dilatation and failure
- The characteristic continuous murmur can be mimicked by aortic stenosis with regurgitation, mitral stenosis with regurgitation, and ventricular septal defect with aortic regurgitation

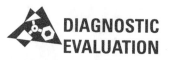 **DIAGNOSTIC EVALUATION**

LABORATORY TESTS

- No specific tests

ELECTROCARDIOGRAPHY

- Normal when the shunt is small
- Left atrial enlargement
- Left ventricular hypertrophy
- P-pulmonale, right axis deviation, right ventricular hypertrophy if pulmonary hypertension develops and the shunt reverses

IMAGING STUDIES

- Chest x-ray:
  - Normal if the shunt is small
  - Left ventricular enlargement, pulmonary vascular plethora
  - Enlarged pulmonary artery and peripheral pulmonary artery pruning in the presence of pulmonary hypertension
  - Patent ductus arteriosus may be calcified in the adult
- Echocardiography:
  - Left atrial and left ventricular enlargement
  - Continuous high-velocity Doppler flow in the main pulmonary artery near the left branch
  - Right ventricular hypertrophy and high-velocity Doppler tricuspid regurgitant jet may be present if pulmonary hypertension develops

DIAGNOSTIC PROCEDURES

- Cardiac catheterization:
  - Oxygen saturation step-up occurs at the level of the pulmonary artery
  - Contrast dye injection may reveal the ductus
  - Pulmonary artery pressure, pulmonary vascular resistance, and flow ratio (Qp/Qs ratio) may be determined

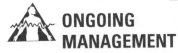

TREATMENT

CARDIOLOGY REFERRAL

- Continuous murmur
- Congestive heart failure
- Signs or symptoms of pulmonary hypertension
- Differential cyanosis

HOSPITALIZATION CRITERIA

- Heart failure
- Suspected endocarditis
- Tachyarrhythmias

MEDICATIONS

- Antibiotic prophylaxis is needed for infective endocarditis

THERAPEUTIC PROCEDURES

- Percutaneous occlusion of the duct with a coil, Amplatzer duct occluder, or Rashkind umbrella device is often feasible and reduces the risk of endocarditis

SURGERY

- Surgical closure should be done for left-to-right shunts > 2:1
- Surgical risk is elevated with pulmonary vascular resistance > 10 U/m^2 and older age

MONITORING

- ECG monitoring during hospitalization

DIET AND ACTIVITY

- Low-sodium diet in patients with heart failure

ONGOING MANAGEMENT

HOSPITAL DISCHARGE CRITERIA

- After successful closure of the patent ductus arteriosus

FOLLOW-UP

- Within 3 months

COMPLICATIONS

- Endocarditis
- Pulmonary hypertension
- Heart failure

PROGNOSIS

- Large, uncorrected shunts generally lead to congestive heart failure or pulmonary hypertension by age 30 years
- Most adults with a patent ductus arteriosus and a pulmonary vascular resistance < 4 Wood units have good results with surgical ligation or percutaneous closure
- Survival is poor for patients with large shunts and severe pulmonary vascular disease (pulmonary vascular resistance > 10 Wood units)
- Approximately 15% of patients > 40 years have calcification or aneurysmal dilation of the ductus

PREVENTION

- Endocarditis prophylaxis for the first 6 months after shunt closure
- Continued endocarditis prophylaxis for persistent shunts

RESOURCES

PRACTICE GUIDELINES

- Surgical ductal ligation remains the standard of practice for treatment of infants
- Percutaneous coil occlusion is widely accepted as the treatment of choice for most children and adults with small- to medium-sized patent ductus arteriosus

REFERENCE

- Jaeggi ET et al: Transcatheter occlusion of the patent ductus arteriosus with a single device technique: comparison of the Cook detachable coil and the Rashkind umbrella device. Int J Cardiol 2001;79:71.

INFORMATION FOR PATIENTS

- http://www.heartcenteronline.com/myheartdr/common/articles.cfm?ARTID=291
- http://www.nhlbi.nih.gov/health/dci/Diseases/pda/pda_what.html

WEB SITES

- http://www.emedicine.com/ped/topic1747.htm
- http://tchin.org/resource_room/c_art_16.htm
- http://www.emedicine.com/ped/topic2834.htm

Patent Foramen Ovale/Atrial Septal Aneurysm

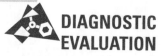 KEY FEATURES

ESSENTIALS OF DIAGNOSIS

- Cryptogenic stroke due to paradoxical embolus
- Echocardiographic evidence of patent foramen ovale and/or atrial septal aneurysm

GENERAL CONSIDERATIONS

- A patent foramen ovale (PFO) is a flap-like opening between the atrial septal primum and secundum at the level of the fossa ovalis that persists after age 1 year
- An atrial septal aneurysm (ASA) is a congenital outpouching in the region of the fossa ovalis that is frequently associated with a PFO
- PFO is detected in 10–15% of the population by contrast echocardiography, and 25% have a probe-patent foramen ovale at autopsy
- Potential cause of transient ischemic attack (TIA) or cryptogenic stroke due to paradoxical emboli
- Combination of PFO and ASA the highest risk of recurrent stroke
- Any condition that increases right atrial pressure more than left atrial pressure (including the Valsalva maneuver) can cause paradoxical right-to-left shunting across the PFO and lead to embolic events
- At present, no consensus guidelines exist for the treatment of PFO

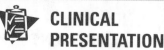 CLINICAL PRESENTATION

SYMPTOMS AND SIGNS

- Most patients are asymptomatic
- Cryptogenic stroke or TIA

PHYSICAL EXAM FINDINGS

- Physical exam is usually normal except for neurologic deficits in patients with stroke

DIFFERENTIAL DIAGNOSIS

- Atrial septal defect
- Bowed, hypermobile, but intact atrial septum without aneurysm
- Other causes of cryptogenic stroke, such as mitral valve prolapse, left atrial myxoma, and infective endocarditis

DIAGNOSTIC EVALUATION

LABORATORY TESTS

- No specific lab tests

ELECTROCARDIOGRAPHY

- No specific findings

IMAGING STUDIES

- Transthoracic echocardiography with saline contrast:
  - The appearance of "microbubbles" in the left atrium within three cardiac cycles of their appearance in the right atrium after agitated saline contrast injection suggests a PFO
  - A PFO may also be detected with color flow Doppler in the middle region of the atrial septum
  - When clinically indicated, a transesophageal echocardiogram is recommended for patients with "negative" transthoracic echocardiogram results because of the higher sensitivity

DIAGNOSTIC PROCEDURES

- Transesophageal echocardiography:
  - Provides superior visualization of the atrial septum and is therefore preferred over contrast transthoracic echocardiography
  - Distinguishes a PFO from a small atrial septal defect and diagnosis ASAs

TREATMENT

CARDIOLOGY REFERRAL

- Patients with an embolic event and findings of a PFO and/or ASA by echocardiographic imaging

HOSPITALIZATION CRITERIA

- Stroke or other embolic event

MEDICATIONS

- Asymptomatic patients:
  - No specific treatment is warranted, although antiplatelet therapy (aspirin) may be considered
- Patients with first neurologic event and PFO alone:
  - Aspirin or warfarin 81 mg/day PO
- Patients with first neurologic event and PFO and/or ASA:
  - Antiplatelet agent
- Patients with recurrent neurologic events:
  - Should have the PFO closed

THERAPEUTIC PROCEDURES

- Percutaneous PFO device closure is FDA-approved for patients with recurrent neurologic events due to presumed paradoxical embolism that occurred despite medical therapy
- Percutaneous PFO closure probably should not be done in patients with an ASA because device closure does not prevent platelet/fibrin deposition
- The procedure requires 6 months of antiplatelet therapy (aspirin or clopidogrel) after the procedure

SURGERY

- Surgical closure of the interatrial communication should be considered in patients with cerebral events that are prolonged or recurrent or are followed by residual neurologic deficits
- Surgical resection of an ASA with closure of the defect is preferred over catheter-based PFO closure in patients with PFO and ASA who have recurrent neurologic events despite medical therapy

MONITORING

- Neurologic examination every 1 hour in patients with acute stroke

DIET AND ACTIVITY

- All patients with a PFO should avoid maneuvers that provoke transient right-to-left shunting, such as occurs with the Valsalva maneuver, including straining to defecate, lifting, or vigorous, repetitive coughing

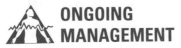

ONGOING MANAGEMENT

HOSPITAL DISCHARGE CRITERIA

- Stabilization after stroke
- After successful percutaneous or surgical closure of the atrial septal abnormality

FOLLOW-UP

- Cardiologist visit within 2–4 weeks
- Transthoracic echocardiography with saline contrast after percutaneous device or surgical closure of the PFO

COMPLICATIONS

- Catheter-based closure may be complicated by: device embolism (rare), entrapment within the right atrial Chiari network, frame fracture, vessel damage, atrial wall perforation, air embolism during device delivery, thrombus formation around the device with possible embolic event, and infective endocarditis
- Surgical closure is associated with all the potential complications of cardiac surgery, including those associated with general anesthesia and sternal wound complications

PROGNOSIS

- Risk of first or recurrent neurologic event in patients with isolated PFO is unknown
- It is unclear whether patients with isolated ASA have an increased risk of recurrent stroke
- Patients with both PFO and ASA have the highest risk (about 15%) of recurrent stroke

PREVENTION

- Endocarditis prophylaxis not indicated

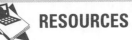

RESOURCES

PRACTICE GUIDELINES

- PFO and/or ASA should be considered in the differential of a TIA or cryptogenic stroke
- Transesophageal echocardiography with agitated saline contrast is the preferred diagnostic modality because of its superior visualization of the atrial septum compared with transthoracic echocardiography
- No consensus guidelines regarding management of PFO and ASA exist; no specific therapy is required for asymptomatic patients with PFO. Patients with isolated PFO after their first neurologic event may be treated with aspirin or warfarin, although surgical or device closure should be considered for patients with prolonged or residual neurologic deficits

REFERENCE

- Mas JL et al: Recurrent cerebrovascular events associated with patent foramen ovale, atrial septal aneurysm or both. N Engl J Med 2001;345:1740.

INFORMATION FOR PATIENTS

- http://www.clevelandclinic.org/health/ health-info/docs/3400/3454.asp? index=11626

WEB SITE

- http://www.emedicine.com/med/ topic1766.htm

Pericardial Effusion

KEY FEATURES

ESSENTIALS OF DIAGNOSIS

- Echocardiographic demonstration of pericardial fluid

GENERAL CONSIDERATIONS

- Normal pericardial space contains 15–25 mL of plasma ultrafiltrate
- Symptoms are largely related to the rate of fluid accumulation
- Causes of pericardial effusion:
  - Idiopathic
  - Congestive heart failure
  - Valvular heart disease
  - Neoplastic
  - Infection (bacterial, viral, fungal, parasitic, tuberculosis, HIV)
  - Autoimmune or connective tissue diseases
  - Trauma
  - Uremia
  - Drugs
  - Postpericardiotomy syndrome
  - Heart transplantation
  - Chylopericardium
  - Myxedema
  - Radiation
- Most common malignant effusions are lung, breast, and leukemia/lymphoma

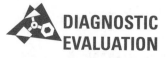

CLINICAL PRESENTATION

SYMPTOMS AND SIGNS

- Small pericardial effusions are usually asymptomatic
- Patients with pericarditis may complain of chest pain, pressure, discomfort, palpitations
- Patients with large pericardial effusions may experience a cough, hiccups, dyspnea, or hoarseness
- Patients with cardiac tamponade may present with lightheadedness, syncope, anxiety, and confusion

PHYSICAL EXAM FINDINGS

- Muffled heart sounds in patients with large effusions
- Pericardial friction rub in patients with pericarditis
- Tachycardia
- Signs of cardiac tamponade:
  - Beck's triad (hypotension, muffled heart sounds, jugular venous distention)
  - Pulsus paradoxus (exaggerated fall in systemic blood pressure > 10 mm Hg with inspiration)
- Decreased pulse pressure
- Ewart's sign (dullness to percussion beneath the angle of the left scapula from compression of the left lung by pericardial fluid)
- Hepatosplenomegaly
- Edema
- Cyanosis

DIFFERENTIAL DIAGNOSIS

- Pericardial fat is indistinguishable on echocardiogram
- Chylous pericardial fluid may be present from thoracic duct obstruction

DIAGNOSTIC EVALUATION

LABORATORY TESTS

- CBC with differential
- Cardiac enzymes, such as troponin
- Thyroid-stimulating hormone
- Rheumatoid factor, antinuclear antibodies, immunoglobulin complexes, and complement levels in some cases of suspected rheumatologic illness

ELECTROCARDIOGRAPHY

- Low voltage
- Sinus tachycardia
- Electrical alternans
- PR-segment depression and diffuse ST elevation in the presence of pericarditis

IMAGING STUDIES

- Chest x-ray: enlarged cardiac silhouette ("water bottle heart")
- Echocardiography:
  - The effusion appears as an "echo-free" space between the visceral and parietal pericardium
- Chest CT scan

DIAGNOSTIC PROCEDURES

- Transesophageal echocardiography: useful in characterizing loculated effusions

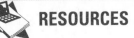

TREATMENT

CARDIOLOGY REFERRAL

- A newly diagnosed patient should probably be seen at least once by a cardiologist
- Symptomatic patient with a known pericardial effusion
- Enlarging pericardial effusion by serial echocardiography

HOSPITALIZATION CRITERIA

- Large pericardial effusion
- Suspected cardiac tamponade
- Patients who undergo elective percutaneous or surgical pericardial drainage

MEDICATIONS

- Small effusion: treat underlying cause (eg, hypothyroidism)
- Moderate effusion: monitor carefully during specific causal therapy
- Corticosteroids and nonsteroidal anti-inflammatory drugs for patients with autoimmune conditions
- Antineoplastic therapy (eg, systemic chemotherapy, radiation) for patients with malignant effusions

THERAPEUTIC PROCEDURES

- – Pericardiocentesis
- – A catheter may be left within the pericardial space for 24–48 hours for continued drainage
- Balloon pericardiotomy may be useful for recurrent effusions but is rarely performed
- Pericardial sclerosis may be performed for recurrent effusions

SURGERY

- Surgical creation of a pericardial window (usually via a subxyphoid approach) to the pleura

MONITORING

- ECG monitoring during hospitalization
- Frequent vital signs for patients with rapidly enlarging effusions

DIET AND ACTIVITY

- No specific diet or activity restrictions for patients who have no impending cardiac tamponade

ONGOING MANAGEMENT

HOSPITAL DISCHARGE CRITERIA

- Asymptomatic patients with small to moderate effusions (with appropriate follow-up)
- After successful percutaneous or surgical pericardial drainage and/or symptoms have resolved

FOLLOW-UP

- Clinical evaluation every few weeks to months for signs or symptoms of increasing pericardial effusion or constrictive pericarditis for at least 1 year
- Serial cardiac imaging studies every few weeks to months in asymptomatic patients with persistent moderate- to large-sized effusions to detect early signs of cardiac tamponade

COMPLICATIONS

- Pericardial tamponade
- Chronic pericardial effusion, effusive-constrictive pericarditis, or constrictive paricarditis may develop after months or years
- Complications of pericardiocentesis: myocardial and/or coronary artery lacerations, ventricular rupture, pneumothorax, dysrhythmias, and infections
- Complications of pericardial sclerosis: intense pain, fevers, infections, and atrial dysrhythmias

PROGNOSIS

- Depends on the underlying cause
- Idiopathic effusions are associated with a good prognosis
- Symptomatic patients with pericardial effusions related to HIV/AIDS or cancer have poor survival rates

PREVENTION

- Preventing conditions that are associated with the development of pericardial effusions may help prevent their formation, enlargement, or recurrence

RESOURCES

PRACTICE GUIDELINES

- In hemodynamically stable patients, the subxyphoid pericardial window procedure may be preferred over pericardiocentesis as the initial treatment because evidence suggests that it is safe and more effective at reducing recurrence

REFERENCE

- Tsang TS et al: Outcomes of clinically significant idiopathic pericardial effusion requiring intervention. Am J Cardiol 2002;91:704.

INFORMATION FOR PATIENTS

- http://www.mayoclinic.com/invoke.cfm?id=HQ01198
- http://www.nlm.nih.gov/medlineplus/ency/article/000182.htm
- http://patients.uptodate.com/topic.asp?file=myoperic/5426

WEB SITE

- http://www.emedicine.com/med/topic1786.htm

Pericarditis, Acute

KEY FEATURES

ESSENTIALS OF DIAGNOSIS

- Central chest pain aggravated by coughing, inspiration, or recumbency
- Pericardial friction rub on auscultation
- Characteristic ECG changes

GENERAL CONSIDERATIONS

- Acute pericarditis is an inflammatory condition of the pericardium
- Causes include viral, tuberculosis, other bacterial, immune-mediated, uremia, neoplastic, post-myocardial infarction, post-cardiac surgery, trauma, and idiopathic
- Pericarditis should also be considered in the setting of persistent fevers with a pericardial effusion or unexplained new cardiomegaly on chest x-ray

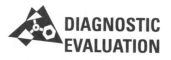 CLINICAL PRESENTATION

SYMPTOMS AND SIGNS

- Chest pain (sharp, anteriorly located and pleuritic in nature)
  - Pain intensity may decrease by sitting upright and forward, and it may radiate to one or both trapezius ridges
  - Sometimes the chest pain is dull in nature with variable location and intensity
- Many have prodromal symptoms suggestive of a viral infection

PHYSICAL EXAM FINDINGS

- Fever and tachycardia
- Pericardial friction rub:
  - Typically scratchy
  - Consisting of one to three components (corresponding to ventricular systole, early diastole, and atrial contraction)
  - Localized or widespread, but most commonly at the left sternal border
  - May be postural and better detected in the seated upright position or during suspended respiration

DIFFERENTIAL DIAGNOSIS

- Acute myocardial infarction
- Aortic dissection
- Pulmonary embolus
- Pneumothorax
- Pneumonia

DIAGNOSTIC EVALUATION

LABORATORY TESTS

- CBC: mild leukocytosis
- Erythrocyte sedimentation rate: modestly elevated
- Elevated C-reactive protein
- Cardiac biomarkers (troponin I, creatine kinase MB fraction) are often modestly elevated
- Antinuclear antibody titer
- Tuberculin skin test
- Additional diagnostic lab tests tailored to the clinical presentation

ELECTROCARDIOGRAPHY

- Four stages of ECG changes:
  - Stage I: Widespread, concave upward ST-segment elevation with reciprocal ST depressions in AVR and V1; PR depression in leads other than AVR; PR elevation in AVR
  - Stage II: Normalization of the ST and PR segments several days later
  - Stage III: Isoelectric or depressed ST segments with inverted T waves—these changes may never occur or may persist indefinitely
  - Stage IV: Normalization of the T waves, which may occur weeks or months later
- Sustained arrhythmias are uncommon and may suggest concomitant myocarditis or other cardiac disease

IMAGING STUDIES

- Chest x-ray:
  - Often normal unless associated with a pericardial effusion of at least 200 mL, in which case the cardiac silhouette may be enlarged
- Echocardiography:
  - Often normal unless associated with a pericardial effusion

DIAGNOSTIC PROCEDURES

- Pericardial biopsy in selected cases

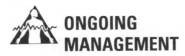

Pericarditis, Acute

TREATMENT

CARDIOLOGY REFERRAL

- Suspected myocarditis
- If pericardiocentesis is being considered
- Recurrent or chronic pericarditis
- Arrhythmias

HOSPITALIZATION CRITERIA

- High fever (> 100.4° F or 38° C) and leukocytosis
- Immunosuppressed state
- Suspected myocarditis or cardiac tamponade
- Hemodynamic instability
- Failure to respond within a few days to nonsteroidal anti-inflammatory (NSAID) therapy
- Large pericardial effusion
- Acute trauma

MEDICATIONS

- Treat underlying cause (eg, uremia)
- NSAID, eg, ibuprofen 200–400 mg PO every 6 hours
- Steroids if unresponsive to NSAIDs
- Colchicine 0.6–1.2 mg PO daily for recurrent pericarditis

THERAPEUTIC PROCEDURES

- Pericardiocentesis for:
  - Cardiac tamponade
  - Suspected purulent, tuberculosis or neoplastic pericarditis
  - Persistent large pericardial effusion

SURGERY

- Pericardiectomy in rare cases

MONITORING

- ECG monitoring in the hospital

DIET AND ACTIVITY

- No dietary restrictions
- Encourage adequate fluid intake
- Activity as tolerated

ONGOING MANAGEMENT

HOSPITAL DISCHARGE CRITERIA

- Stable vital signs
- Stable cardiac rhythm
- Absence of evidence of an enlarging pericardial effusion or impending cardiac tamponade

FOLLOW-UP

- Clinic visit within 2 weeks or earlier as symptoms dictate
- Echocardiography 1–2 weeks and thereafter, depending on the clinical situation

COMPLICATIONS

- Recurrent acute pericarditis
- Chronic pericarditis
- Effusive-constrictive pericarditis
- Cardiac tamponade
- Constrictive pericarditis

PROGNOSIS

- Approximately 15–30% of patients with idiopathic acute pericarditis have recurrent pericarditis or develop chronic pericardial disease

PREVENTION

- No therapy has been proven to prevent sequelae such as cardiac tamponade, pericardial constriction, and recurrent pericarditis

RESOURCES

PRACTICE GUIDELINES

- A patient with simple uncomplicated acute pericarditis can usually be managed in the outpatient setting
- Patients with high-risk features should be admitted to the hospital:
  - Evidence suggesting cardiac tamponade
  - Failure to respond within a few days to NSAID therapy
  - High fever
  - Immunosuppressed state
- The goal of therapy is the relief of pain
- The use of corticosteroids is reserved for the patient who is clearly refractory to NSAIDs

REFERENCE

- Maisch B et al: Guidelines on the diagnosis and management of pericardial diseases executive summary: the Task Force on the Diagnosis and Management of Pericardial Diseases of the European Society of Cardiology. Eur Heart J 2004;25:587.

INFORMATION FOR PATIENTS

- http://patients.uptodate.com/topic.asp?file=myoperic/5163
- www.patient.co.uk/showdoc/40000589

WEB SITE

- http://www.emedicine.com/med/topic1781.htm

Pericarditis, Constrictive

 ## KEY FEATURES

ESSENTIALS OF DIAGNOSIS

- Markedly elevated (JVP) venous pressure with accentuated *x* and *y* descents and Kussmaul's sign
- Pericardial knock on auscultation
- MRI, CT, or echocardiographic imaging showing a thickened pericardium

GENERAL CONSIDERATIONS

- Results from scarring as the aftermath of almost any pericardial injury or inflammation
- Most common cause in the United States is cardiac surgery
- Other common causes:
  - Radiation therapy
  - Idiopathic and connective tissue disease; tuberculous constriction is the most common cause in underdeveloped countries
- Pericardium becomes thickened, fibrotic, and sometimes calcified (especially with tuberculosis)
- The noncompliant pericardium encases the heart and results in a fixed cardiac volume
- Diastolic filling is abruptly halted in early diastole when the volume limit of the noncompliant pericardium is attained
- It is sometimes difficult to distinguish from restrictive cardiomyopathy but is important to do so because constriction may be cured with pericardiectomy
- Some patients have normal pericardial thickness
- Some patients undergo spontaneous resolution or respond to medical therapy
- Although most patients have relief of symptoms after pericardiectomy, some do not

CLINICAL PRESENTATION

SYMPTOMS AND SIGNS

- Fatigue
- Dyspnea
- Increased abdominal girth
- Edema
- Malabsorptive diarrhea
- Chest pain
- Dizziness

PHYSICAL EXAM FINDINGS

- Markedly elevated JVP with *x* and *y* troughs more prominent than the *a* and *v* peaks
- Pulsus paradoxus in some
- Kussmaul's sign (lack of inspiratory decline in JVP)
- Pericardial knock (early diastolic sound) on auscultation
- Abdominal distention with fluid wave from ascites
- Pulsatile hepatomegaly
- Profound cachexia
- Edema or anasarca

DIFFERENTIAL DIAGNOSIS

- Cardiac tamponade
- Restrictive cardiomyopathy
- Right heart failure
- Cirrhosis with ascites
- Malabsorption syndrome

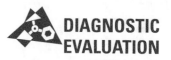 ## DIAGNOSTIC EVALUATION

LABORATORY TESTS

- Antinuclear antibody titer
- Rheumatoid factor
- Tuberculin skin test

ELECTROCARDIOGRAPHY

- No specific ECG findings with constriction
- Nonspecific ST- and T-wave changes common
- Low voltage sometimes present
- Atrial fibrillation common in advanced cases
- P mitrale common in less severe and less chronic cases

IMAGING STUDIES

- Chest x-ray: pericardial calcification is specific but uncommon
- MRI is the procedure of choice to image pericardial thickness
- CT is also extremely useful
- Echocardiography is an essential adjunctive test
  - Abrupt posterior septal motion during inspiration "septal bounce," and moderate biatrial enlargement
  - Doppler mitral E velocity is typically increased, and exaggerated respirophasic variation in mitral inflow (mitral E velocity decreases by at least 25% with inspiration) is characteristic. The inferior vena cava is dilated and does not collapse with inspiration. Hepatic vein flow does not increase with inspiration

DIAGNOSTIC PROCEDURES

- Right and left heart catheterization:
  - Sometimes needed for diagnosis in suspected cases and often used for confirmation of pericardial constriction
  - Findings include elevated and equalized diastolic pressures; prominent *x* and *y* descents (M or W sign) in venous and atrial pressure tracings; "square root" sign (diastolic dip and plateau in the left ventricle and right ventricle pressure tracings); discordant right ventricular and left ventricular peak systolic pressures during inspiration; Kussmaul's sign in the central venous pressure tracing

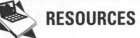

 TREATMENT

CARDIOLOGY REFERRAL

- Heart failure signs or symptoms
- Suspected pericardial constriction

HOSPITALIZATION CRITERIA

- Decompensated heart failure
- Tachyarrhythmias

MEDICATIONS

- Unless there is evidence of chronic constriction (cachexia, atrial fibrillation, hepatic dysfunction, or pericardial calcification), a trial of nonsteroidal anti-inflammatory drugs (or steroids, antibiotics, or chemotherapy, depending on the clinical situation) and diuretics or simple observation is recommended

SURGERY

- Surgical pericardiectomy

MONITORING

- ECG monitoring in the hospital

DIET AND ACTIVITY

- Low-sodium diet
- Fluid restriction
- Activity as tolerated

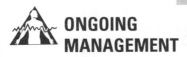 **ONGOING MANAGEMENT**

HOSPITAL DISCHARGE CRITERIA

- After medical stablization
- After successful pericardial stripping

FOLLOW-UP

- Clinic visit within 2 weeks of hospital discharge
- Echocardiography 3 months after surgery and annually thereafter, depending on symptoms

COMPLICATIONS

- Surgical pericardiectomy has a significant (6–12%) operative mortality
- Postoperative heart failure requiring inotropic support due to myocardial fibrosis and atrophy
- Atrial arrhythmias

PROGNOSIS

- Diastolic function returns to normal in only 41% of patients during the first 3 months after surgery
- Approximately 24% of patients have persistently abnormal diastolic filling patterns by echo and remain symptomatic
- The poorest outcome is seen in patients with radiation-induced disease
- Long-term survival is inferior to that of an age- and sex-matched population, with a 5- and 10-year survival rate of approximately 78% and 57%, respectively
- Recurrent constriction may occur

PREVENTION

- Medical treatment of inflammatory pericarditis, as clinically indicated
- Minimize exposure of the heart during radiation therapy for malignancy

RESOURCES

PRACTICE GUIDELINES

- Because the primary form of therapy for constriction is surgical, the diagnosis must be correct
- With the combined use of Doppler echocardiography, MRI, and CT to image the pericardium, careful hemodynamic studies, and endomyocardial biopsy (in some cases), it should be possible to distinguish pericardial constriction from restrictive cardiomyopathy in most cases
- A trial of conservative management is recommended because some patients have transient pericardial constriction and resolution of symptoms with medical therapy or observation
- For persistent or recurrent symptoms after surgery, consider three possibilities:
  - Myocardial dysfunction from severe, prolonged compression
  - Incomplete or inadequate pericardiectomy
  - Recurrence of constriction
- Surgery should be considered cautiously in patients with mild or very advanced pericardial disease and in those with radiation-induced constriction, myocardial dysfunction, or significant renal dysfunction, because the operative risk is very high and these patients show little or no benefit

REFERENCES

- Maisch B et al: Guidelines on the diagnosis and management of pericardial diseases executive summary: The Task Force on the Diagnosis and Management of Pericardial Diseases of the European Society of Cardiology. Eur Heart J 2004;25:587.

INFORMATION FOR PATIENTS

- http://patients.uptodate.com/topic.asp?file=myoperic/4613
- http://patients.uptodate.com/topic.asp?file=myoperic/4613&title=Constrictive+pericarditis

WEB SITE

- www.emedicine.com/med/topic1783.htm

Pericarditis, Effusive-Constrictive

KEY FEATURES

ESSENTIALS OF DIAGNOSIS

- Echocardiographic demonstration of pericardial fluid with fibrinous strands and constrictive physiology
- Persistence of elevated intracardiac filling pressures after pericardiocentesis with constrictive features
- The most identifiable cause is uremia, although any cause of pericarditis can produce this condition

GENERAL CONSIDERATIONS

- Effusive-constrictive pericarditis combines features of pericardial effusion and constrictive pericarditis
- The syndrome is dynamic and may represent an intermediate stage of constrictive pericarditis
- It appears to be relatively uncommon
- Most cases are idiopathic
- Common causes are uremia, malignancy, radiation, and tuberculosis
- Although pericardiocentesis may be associated with symptomatic improvement, some patients require pericardiectomy

CLINICAL PRESENTATION

SYMPTOMS AND SIGNS

- Fatigue
- Dyspnea
- Increased abdominal girth
- Edema
- Malabsorptive diarrhea
- Chest pain
- Dizziness

PHYSICAL EXAM FINDINGS

- Markedly elevated jugular venous pressure with x and y troughs that are more prominent than the a and v peaks
- Pulsus paradoxus
- Kussmaul's sign (lack of inspiratory decline in jugular venous pressure) in some
- Abdominal distention with fluid wave from ascites
- Pulsatile hepatomegaly
- Cachexia
- Edema/anasarca

DIFFERENTIAL DIAGNOSIS

- Cardiac tamponade
- Constrictive pericarditis
- Restrictive cardiomyopathy with incidental pericardial effusion

DIAGNOSTIC EVALUATION

LABORATORY TESTS

- Antinuclear antibody titer
- Rheumatoid factor
- Tuberculin skin test

ELECTROCARDIOGRAPHY

- Nonspecific ST- and T-wave changes
- Low-voltage QRS
- Atrial fibrillation

IMAGING STUDIES

- Chest x-ray:
  - The cardiac silhouette may be small, normal, or enlarged
  - Pericardial calcification is uncommon
- Echocardiography:
  - Usually shows a small-to-moderate–sized effusion with strands of solid material between the visceral and parietal pericardium
  - Pericardial thickening and/or adhesions may be apparent
  - Doppler evidence of exaggerated respirophasic variation in mitral E velocity may be present
  - The inferior vena cava may be dilated

DIAGNOSTIC PROCEDURES

- Right heart catheterization during or after pericardiocentesis establishes the diagnosis
- After the effusion is drained, elevation of intracardiac filling pressures persists and the recorded waveforms may exhibit the classic appearance of constriction

TREATMENT

CARDIOLOGY REFERRAL

- Heart failure
- Chronic pericardial disease
- Persistent symptoms or evidence of right heart failure after pericardial fluid drainage

HOSPITALIZATION CRITERIA

- Decompensated heart failure
- Evidence of cardiac tamponade

MEDICATIONS

- Treat underlying cause if known

THERAPEUTIC PROCEDURES

- Pericardiocentesis alone may produce at least temporary relief of symptoms in most patients

SURGERY

- Pericardial resection of the visceral pericardium is often required

MONITORING

- ECG monitoring
- Vital signs

DIET AND ACTIVITY

- Low-sodium diet
- Activity as tolerated unless evidence of cardiac tamponade or impending tamponade exists

ONGOING MANAGEMENT

HOSPITAL DISCHARGE CRITERIA

- Stable hemodynamics and cardiac rhythm
- Absence of enlarging pericardial effusion
- After successful pericardiocentesis or pericardiectomy

FOLLOW-UP

- Clinic visit within 2 weeks
- Echo within 2 weeks and serially thereafter, based on the clinical situation

COMPLICATIONS

- Progressive pericardial constriction or effusion after pericardiocentesis
- Incomplete relief of symptoms due to incomplete or inadequate pericardiectomy
- The visceral component of the pericardiectomy is difficult and stripping may damage the coronary arteries, resulting in myocardial ischemia or infarction

PROGNOSIS

- Clinical course after pericardiectomy depends on the underlying cause of pericardial disease and the patient's general condition

PREVENTION

- Treatment of the underlying condition; otherwise no specific therapy has been shown to prevent effusive-constrictive pericarditis

RESOURCES

PRACTICE GUIDELINES

- Right heart pressures and systemic arterial pressures should ideally be measured during elective pericardiocentesis
- Persistence of elevated right atrial pressure suggests effusive-constrictive pericarditis
- Pericardiectomy should be considered in patients with persistent or recurrent symptoms after pericardiocentesis

REFERENCES

- Hoit BD: Management of effusive and constrictive pericardial heart disease. Circulation 2002;105:2939.
- Maisch B et al: Guidelines on the diagnosis and management of pericardial diseases executive summary: the Task Force on the Diagnosis and Management of Pericardial Diseases of the European Society of Cardiology. Eur Heart J 2004;25:587.

INFORMATION FOR PATIENTS

- http://patients.uptodate.com/topic.asp?file=myoperic/4613&title=Constrictive+pericarditis

WEB SITE

- http://www.emedicine.com/med/topic1783.htm

Peripheral Arterial Atherosclerosis Obliterans

 KEY FEATURES

ESSENTIALS OF DIAGNOSIS

- Intermittent claudication
- Resting leg pain, ulceration, or gangrene
- Reduced amplitude or absence of peripheral pulses
- Iliofemoral bruits
- Ankle–brachial artery pressure ratio < 0.9
- Cool feet when supine that blanch on elevation and become rubrous and warm when dependent

GENERAL CONSIDERATIONS

- The major cause of peripheral arterial disease in developed countries is atherosclerosis
- Asymptomatic peripheral atherosclerosis is 3 or 4 times more common than symptomatic disease
- Men and women have the same prevalence of this disease

CLINICAL PRESENTATION

SYMPTOMS AND SIGNS

- Intermittent claudication is the hallmark of peripheral arterial disease
  - Pelvic artery disease results in thigh or buttock claudication
  - Femoral or popliteal disease results in calf claudication
- Chronic leg ischemia can cause persistent rest pain, ulcerations, or gangrene of the foot

PHYSICAL EXAM FINDINGS

- Femoral or iliac bruits
- Weak distal pulses
- Distal extremity ulcerations, especially at pressure points
- Leg elevation results in a pale color
- Sitting after leg raising results in a slow return of color (1 or more minutes), which develops into a red-blue hue
- Decreased nail growth and hair loss in the extremity
- Extremity cool to the touch

DIFFERENTIAL DIAGNOSIS

- Sciatica from lower back disease
- Arterial embolism
- Erythromelalgia
- Vascular compartment compression syndromes

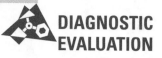 **DIAGNOSTIC EVALUATION**

LABORATORY TESTS

- CBC, erythrocyte sedimentation rate, prothrombin time, fibrinogen
- Plasma viscosity

IMAGING STUDIES

- Duplex ultrasound images the vessel and the flow inside it
- Vital capillaroscopy can assess the capillaries in the skin

DIAGNOSTIC PROCEDURES

- Angiography can delineate stenoses
- Intravascular ultrasound can clarify lesion characteristics

TREATMENT

CARDIOLOGY REFERRAL

- Suspected coronary artery disease

HOSPITALIZATION CRITERIA

- Threatened limb loss
- Gangrene
- Planned surgery

MEDICATIONS

- Stop smoking
- Exercise training
- Antiplatelet drugs—aspirin 81 mg/day, clopidogrel 75 mg/day PO
- Vasodilators: pentoxifylline 400 mg PO tid
- Prostacyclin analogues are under study
- Anticoagulants in selected cases
- Vascular endothelial growth factor is experimental

THERAPEUTIC PROCEDURES

- Hyperbaric oxygen may help wound healing in chronic limb ischemia
- Angioplasty in selected cases
- Thrombectomy in selected cases

SURGERY

- Revascularization
- Amputation

MONITORING

- Monitor blood pressure; low pressure may retard healing

DIET AND ACTIVITY

- Exercise as tolerated
- Low saturated fat diet

ONGOING MANAGEMENT

HOSPITAL DISCHARGE CRITERIA

- Resolution of problem
- After successful surgery

FOLLOW-UP

- Depends on nature and severity of the problem

COMPLICATIONS

- Gangrene and limb loss
- Infection

PROGNOSIS

- In patients with claudication
  - Annual mortality rate is about 5%;
  - Fifty percent have developed critical limb ischemia or are dead at 5 years
- Amputation carries a 50% mortality rate at 2–3 years

PREVENTION

- Same as for prevention of atherosclerosis in general:
  - Reduce cholesterol, blood pressure, and blood sugar
  - Stop smoking
  - Exercise and lose weight

RESOURCES

PRACTICE GUIDELINES

- Amputation is a last resort, so attempts at revascularization are justifiable if there is a 25% or greater chance of success

REFERENCES

- Feiring AJ et al: Primary stent-supported angioplasty for treatment of below-knee critical limb ischemia and severe claudication: early and one-year outcomes. J Am Coll Cardiol 2004;44:2307.
- Gardner AW et al: Natural history of physical function in older men with intermittent claudication. J Vasc Surg 2004;40:73.
- McDermott MM et al: Functional decline in peripheral arterial disease: associations with the ankle brachial index and leg symptoms. JAMA 2004;292:453.
- Mernard JR et al: Long-term results of peripheral arterial disease rehabilitation. J Vasc Surg 2004;39:1186.

INFORMATION FOR PATIENTS

- www.drpen.com/443.9

WEB SITE

- www.emedicine.com/med/topic391.htm

Periprosthetic Valve Leaks

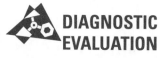

KEY FEATURES

ESSENTIALS OF DIAGNOSIS

- New murmur in a patient with a prosthetic valve or a regurgitant murmur ascribed to the prosthetic valve
- Echocardiographic evidence of perivalvular leak
- Clinical deterioration, embolism, or hemolysis

GENERAL CONSIDERATIONS

- A periprosthetic valve leak is regurgitation between the native valve ring and the prosthesis sewing ring
- Small periprosthetic leaks often occur immediately after surgery and are detected by transesophageal echocardiography in the operating room
  - Resolve in days to weeks as the prosthetic ring becomes endothelialized
- Persistent periprosthetic leaks can enlarge rapidly, requiring reoperation, but they usually remain stable for years
- The incidence of persistent perivalvular leak is high with calcified mitral annulus and preoperative endocarditis
- A new periprosthetic leak suggests infective endocarditis
- Rarely, a periprosthetic leak causes enough sheer stress on red cells to produce clinically significant hemolysis

CLINICAL PRESENTATION

SYMPTOMS AND SIGNS

- Usually asymptomatic
- Fatigue and dyspnea on exertion if anemic due to hemolysis
- Fever, sweats, malaise if endocarditis is present
- Heart failure symptoms if leak is hemodynamically significant

PHYSICAL EXAM FINDINGS

- New systolic murmur (mitral and tricuspid)
- New diastolic murmur (aortic and pulmonic)
- Pallor
- Enlarged ventricular impulses
- Thrill
- Peripheral signs of endocarditis
- Signs of heart failure

DIFFERENTIAL DIAGNOSIS

- Prosthetic valve malfunction: thrombus vegetation, or pannus
- Infective endocarditis without periprosthetic leak
- Hemolysis due to prosthesis malfunction or other causes
- Embolism from thrombus formation
- Clinical deterioration for other reasons (eg, prosthesis too small)

DIAGNOSTIC EVALUATION

LABORATORY TESTS

- Low hematocrit, elevated lactic dehydrogenase, elevated bilirubin, hemoglobinuria and a positive blood smear for fragmented cells if hemolysis is present
- Positive blood cultures if endocarditis is present

ELECTROCARDIOGRAPHY

- ECG findings:
  - Tachycardia
  - Chamber enlargement

IMAGING STUDIES

- Chest x-ray finding: cardiac chamber enlargement
- Fluoroscopy can detect:
  - Abnormal mechanical prosthetic valve function
  - The rocking motion of partial valve dehiscence
- Echocardiography findings:
  - Chamber enlargement is seen with hemodynamically significant lesions
  - Prosthetic valve rocking may be seen with partial dehiscence
  - Evidence of vegetations may be present
  - Prosthetic valve abnormalities may be detected, suggesting a valvular rather than perivalvular etiology
- Doppler echocardiography:
  - Color-flow Doppler usually is critical in identifying the site and cause of regurgitation and defining its severity

DIAGNOSTIC PROCEDURES

- Transesophageal echocardiography may be necessary to define the exact site and cause of regurgitation and diagnose prosthetic valve dysfunction or endocarditis
- Cardiac catheterization is rarely needed to make the diagnosis but may be necessary to define coronary anatomy or confirm the hemodynamic consequences of valve malfunction before repeat surgery

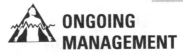

 ## TREATMENT

CARDIOLOGY REFERRAL

- New murmur in a patient with a prosthetic valve
- Hemodynamically significant regurgitation
- Hemolytic anemia discovered

HOSPITALIZATION CRITERIA

- Suspected endocarditis
- Heart failure
- Severe anemia

MEDICATIONS

- Beta blockers may reduce sheer forces, eg, metoprolol 25 mg bid
- Transfusion can arrest hemolytic anemia because a higher hematocrit increases the viscosity of blood and reduces sheer forces
- Vasodilators are helpful for hemodynamically significant aortic periprosthetic regurgitation, eg, amlodipine 5 mg/day PO

THERAPEUTIC PROCEDURES

- Transcatheter occlusion devices are being perfected

SURGERY

- Replacement of the prosthetic valve is often required with endocarditis, severe leaks, and refractory hemolytic anemia

MONITORING

- ECG monitoring in the hospital
- Outpatient: monitoring of hematocrit and physical exam

DIET AND ACTIVITY

- Low-sodium diet
- Restrict exercise with hemodynamically significant lesions or severe anemia

ONGOING MANAGEMENT

HOSPITAL DISCHARGE CRITERIA

- Resolution of hemolysis
- Resolution of heart failure
- After successful surgery

FOLLOW-UP

- Every 3–6 months, depending on the severity of the leak and the propensity to hemolysis
- Echocardiograms if change is suspected
- Echocardiogram 3 months after surgery, then every 1 or 3 years, depending on whether the valve is tissue or mechanical, respectively
- After reoperation: at 3 months, 6 months, then every 6–12 months

COMPLICATIONS

- Infective endocarditis
- Hemolysis
- Heart failure
- Valve dehiscence

PROGNOSIS

- Most periprosthetic leaks are well tolerated and require no specific interaction
- Endocarditis as a cause is associated with a 20–30% mortality rate
- Repeat surgery carries increased risks, and if the condition that contributed to the leak is still present (eg, annular calcium), there is no guarantee that it will not happen again

PREVENTION

- Meticulous surgical technique in at-risk patients, such as those with annular calcium or endocarditis
- Maintaining hematocrit > 30 will decrease hemolysis

RESOURCES

PRACTICE GUIDELINES

- Patients with severe leaks or endocarditis causing the leak usually require repeat surgery, as do those with a moderate leak and symptoms or signs of hemodynamic compromise
- Mild leaks can usually be managed medically unless refractory hemolytic anemia occurs

REFERENCES

- Ansingkar K et al: Transesophageal three-dimensional color Doppler echocardiographic assessment of valvular and paravalvular mitral prosthetic regurgitation. Echocardiography 2000;17:579.
- Okumiya T et al: Evaluation of intravascular hemolysis with erythrocyte creatine in patients with cardiac valve prostheses. Chest 2004;125:2115.

INFORMATION FOR PATIENTS

- www.yoursurgery.com/Procedure Details.cfm?BR=3&Proc=24

WEB SITE

- www.nlm.nih.gov/medlineplus/ tutorials/heartvalvereplacement.html

Permanent Junctional Reciprocating Tachycardia

KEY FEATURES

ESSENTIALS OF DIAGNOSIS

- Commonly observed in children
- Heart rate may vary from 120 to 250 bpm
- Tachycardia cardiomyopathy may occur because the tachycardia tends to be incessant
- This is a reentrant tachycardia and quite sensitive to autonomic manipulation
- Tachycardia tends to slow down with age because retrograde conduction through the accessory pathway tends to slow down

GENERAL CONSIDERATIONS

- This is reentrant arrhythmia induced by a retrogradely conducting (concealed) decremental accessory pathway
- It may occur in the perioperative period in infants and children
- The perioperative form is self-limiting; however heart rates > 200 bpm may cause marked hypotension
- The idiopathic form can persist for years, leading to tachycardia cardiomyopathy
- P waves precede the QRS complexes (long RP tachycardia)
- The P waves are inverted in inferior leads
- The pathway causing this type of orthodromic reciprocating tachycardia is commonly located at or near the os of the coronary sinus
- Drug therapy does not control this arrhythmia secondary to prolonged conduction property of the accessory pathway, although rate control can be achieved

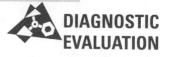 CLINICAL PRESENTATION

SYMPTOMS AND SIGNS

- Palpitations
- Shortness of breath
- Features of congestive heart failure

PHYSICAL EXAM FINDINGS

- Elevated jugular venous distention
- S_3 may be heard during sinus rhythm
- Bilateral pulmonary rales

DIFFERENTIAL DIAGNOSIS

- Automatic atrial tachycardia
- Atypical atrioventricular nodal reentrant tachycardia

DIAGNOSTIC EVALUATION

LABORATORY TESTS

- CBC, metabolic panel

ELECTROCARDIOGRAPHY

- ECG shows a narrow QRS with inverted P waves in the inferior leads
- Holter monitor is used to detect and document rhythm disturbance

IMAGING STUDIES

- Echocardiogram to evaluate left ventricular function

DIAGNOSTIC PROCEDURES

- Electrophysiologic study to define mechanism of rhythm disturbance and determine suitability for ablation

TREATMENT

CARDIOLOGY REFERRAL

• Patients suspected to have this disorder should be referred to an electrophysiologist

HOSPITALIZATION CRITERIA

• Patients in active heart failure
• Post-ablation for 24 hours

MEDICATIONS

• Drug therapy is frequently *not* helpful
• Type 1C drug or amiodarone may achieve rate control
• Digoxin has no effect, and verapamil may accelerate the tachycardia
• Beta blockers may control heart rate in adults

THERAPEUTIC PROCEDURES

• Radiofrequency ablation is successful in 95% of patients

SURGERY

• Not required

MONITORING

• ECG monitoring in the hospital

DIET AND ACTIVITY

• General healthy life style

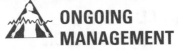 ## ONGOING MANAGEMENT

HOSPITAL DISCHARGE CRITERIA

• Adequate treatment of heart failure
• After ablation

FOLLOW-UP

• Two weeks after ablation
• Three months' follow-up to reevaluate left ventricular function

COMPLICATIONS

• Cardiomyopathy

PROGNOSIS

• Once ablation is done, prognosis is very good

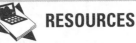 ## RESOURCES

PRACTICE GUIDELINES

• Consider this in the differential diagnosis of a young patient with supraventricular tachycardia and heart failure

REFERENCES

• Critelli G: Recognizing and managing permanent junctional reciprocating tachycardia in the catheter ablation era. J Cardiovasc Electrophysiol 1997;8:226.
• Gaita F, Antonio M, Riccardi R et al: Cryoenergy catheter ablation: a new technique for treatment of permanent junctional reciprocating tachycardia in children. J Cardiovasc Electrophysiol 2004;15:263.

INFORMATION FOR PATIENTS

• www.nlm.nih.gov/medlineplus/ arrhythmia.html

WEB SITES

• www.hrsonline.org
• www.acc.org

Pheochromocytoma

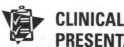

KEY FEATURES

ESSENTIALS OF DIAGNOSIS

- Headache, palpitations, and sweating in conjunction with either hypertension (may be paroxysmal) or orthostatic hypotension
- Pressor response to anesthesia induction or to antihypertensive or sympathomimetic drugs
- Biochemical evidence of excess catecholamines
- Adrenal tumor or tumor along the sympathetic chain (paraganglioma)

GENERAL CONSIDERATIONS

- Pheochromocytoma is a catecholamine-producing tumor of the sympathoadrenal system
- Hypertension is the major manifestation of these tumors, which is sustained in the majority
- Episodic hypertension due to catecholamine release is the classic manifestation but occurs in about one-third of patients

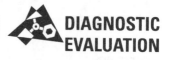

CLINICAL PRESENTATION

SYMPTOMS AND SIGNS

- Episodic palpitation
- Headache
- Sweating
- Tremor
- Pallor

PHYSICAL EXAM FINDINGS

- Sustained or episodic hypertension
- Orthostatic hypotension
- Café au lait spots

DIFFERENTIAL DIAGNOSIS

- Other causes of hypertension, headaches, palpitations, and orthostatic hypotension

DIAGNOSTIC EVALUATION

LABORATORY TESTS

- A plasma epinephrine and noreprinephrine > 2000 pg/mL is diagnostic
- Twenty-four-hour urine for metanephrine and normetanephrine
- If plasma catecholamine 1000–2000 pg/mL, repeat 3 hours after clonidine 0.3 mg PO; > 500 pg/mL suggests pheochromocytoma

IMAGING STUDIES

- CT or MRI of the abdomen to localize the tumor after a positive serum catecholamine study
- I^{131} MIBG scan to find tumors not seen by CT or MRI

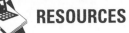

TREATMENT

CARDIOLOGY REFERRAL

• Suspected pheochromocytoma

HOSPITALIZATION CRITERIA

• Blood pressure > 220/120 mm Hg
• Planned surgery

MEDICATIONS

• Preoperative alpha and beta blockade

SURGERY

• Surgical removal of the catecholamine-producing tumor(s)

MONITORING

• ECG and blood pressure in hospital and during clonidine suppression test

DIET AND ACTIVITY

• Low-sodium diet
• Restriction of vigorous exercise until tumor is removed

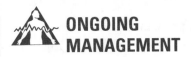

ONGOING MANAGEMENT

HOSPITAL DISCHARGE CRITERIA

• After successful surgery

FOLLOW-UP

• Routine postsurgical follow-up

COMPLICATIONS

• Stroke
• Heart failure
• Aortic dissection
• Myocardial infarction
• Renal failure

PROGNOSIS

• Excellent with successful removal of the tumor

RESOURCES

PRACTICE GUIDELINES

• Beta blockers or alpha blockers should never be used alone in patients with suspected or proven pheochromocytoma
• Both systems need to be blocked (eg, beta blockade alone would leave the patient susceptible to unopposed alpha stimulation by the tumor and severe hypertension)

REFERENCE

• Plouin P et al: Factors associated with perioperative morbidity and mortality in patients with pheochromocytoma: analysis of 165 operations at a single center. J Clin Endocrinol Metab 2001;86:1480.

INFORMATION FOR PATIENTS

• www.drpen.com/227.0

WEB SITE

• www.emedicine.com/medtopic1816.htm

Polymyositis/Dermatomyositis and the Heart

 ## KEY FEATURES

ESSENTIALS OF DIAGNOSIS

- Muscle weakness, characteristic skin lesions
- Arrhythmias or conduction disturbances and myocarditis
- Pericarditis, coronary arteritis, and valve disease, especially mitral valve prolapse

GENERAL CONSIDERATIONS

- Polymyositis/dermatomyositis is a chronic inflammatory myopathy that presents as symmetric proximal muscle weakness and a rash, usually over the extensor surfaces of the hands
- The incidence is about 1–5 per million per year in the United States
- It strikes adults in their fourth to sixth decades
- African American women are more often affected
- Occasionally the condition is associated with other connective tissue diseases
- Cardiovascular disease is a common cause of mortality

CLINICAL PRESENTATION

SYMPTOMS AND SIGNS

- Palpitation due to ectopic beats
- Congestive heart failure findings, such as dyspnea on exertion and edema
- Chest pain due to pericarditis

PHYSICAL EXAM FINDINGS

- Pericardial rub, elevated jugular venous pressure
- Pulmonary rales, S_3, enlarged apical impulse
- Right ventricular lift, loud P_2

DIFFERENTIAL DIAGNOSIS

- Other connective tissue diseases
- Other causes of cardiac disease

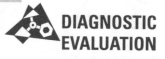 ## DIAGNOSTIC EVALUATION

LABORATORY TESTS

- Elevated creatine kinase and the MB fraction

ELECTROCARDIOGRAPHY

- ST-T–wave abnormalities in about 50%
- Fascicular and bundle branch blocks
- Atrioventricular blocks
- Premature atrial and ventricular beats

IMAGING STUDIES

- Chest x-ray:
  - Cardiomegaly
  - Pulmonary congestion
- Echocardiography:
  - Pericardial effusion
  - Left ventricular wall motion abnormalities and reduced ejection fraction
  - Enlarged right heart and Doppler evidence of increased pulmonary pressure
  - Mitral valve prolapse in about 50%
  - Hyperkinetic heart syndrome in some
- Myocardial perfusion imaging with technetium-99m pyrophosphate shows myocardial uptake

DIAGNOSTIC PROCEDURES

- Cardiac catheterization may be required if coronary vasculitis is suspected

TREATMENT

CARDIOLOGY REFERRAL

• Suspected heart disease

HOSPITALIZATION CRITERIA

• Pericarditis
• Heart failure
• Significant arrhythmias or heart block

MEDICATIONS

• Specific anti-inflammatory pharmacotherapy
• Specific cardiac therapy as indicated

THERAPEUTIC PROCEDURES

• Percutaneous coronary intervention may be required

SURGERY

• Valve, coronary, or pericardial surgery is rare

MONITORING

• ECG monitoring in hospital as appropriate

DIET AND ACTIVITY

• Low-sodium diet if heart failure
• Restricted activity if heart failure or myocarditis

ONGOING MANAGEMENT

HOSPITAL DISCHARGE CRITERIA

• Resolution of cardiac problem

FOLLOW-UP

• As appropriate for cardiac problem

COMPLICATIONS

• Sudden death
• Heart failure
• Cardiac tamponade
• Myocardial infarction
• Pulmonary hypertension

PROGNOSIS

• Overall survival rate is 50–60% at 10 years
• Cardiopulmonary disease reduces survival

RESOURCES

PRACTICE GUIDELINES

• Cardiac manifestations of polymyositis/dermatomyositis are managed as appropriate for the problem

REFERENCE

• Spiera R, Kagen L: Extramuscular manifestations in idiopathic inflammatory myopathies. Curr Opin Rheumatol 1998;10:556.

INFORMATION FOR PATIENTS

• www.drpen.com/710.3

WEB SITES

• www.emedicine.com/med/topic3441.htm
• www.emedicine.com/med/topic2608.htm

Postural Tachycardia Syndrome

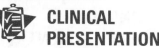 KEY FEATURES

ESSENTIALS OF DIAGNOSIS

- Chronic orthostatic symptoms with a dramatic rise in heart rate (> 28 bpm) on standing (within 5 minutes) with no orthostatic hypotension (frank syncope is rare)
- Evidence of dysautonomia on functional testing

GENERAL CONSIDERATIONS

- May be primary or secondary to another disorder
- Many patients have a dramatic increase in heart rates up to 120–170 bpm within 2–5 minutes of upright tilt
- Many patients may have been previously labeled as suffering from panic attacks or chronic anxiety
- May be familial
- Norepinephrine reuptake transporter protein gene mutation leading to excessive serum epinephrine is identified in familial form
- Autonomic neuropathies and acetylcholine receptor antibodies in the peripheral autonomic ganglia have been seen in postfebrile illness (postviral) postural tachycardia syndrome (POTS)
- Possible link between Ehlers-Danlos syndrome III and POTS
- May occur in diabetes mellitus, amyloidosis, sarcoidosis, alcoholism, chemotherapy (particularly with the vinca alkaloids), heavy metal poisoning, Sjögren's syndrome, and lupus erythematosus
- May occur after pregnancy
- May be a paraneoplastic manifestation

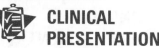 CLINICAL PRESENTATION

SYMPTOMS AND SIGNS

- Exercise intolerance
- Extreme fatigue
- Lightheadedness
- Diminished concentration
- Tremulousness
- Nausea, headache
- Near syncope
- Occasionally syncope

PHYSICAL EXAM FINDINGS

- Generally normal other than orthostatic tachycardia

DIFFERENTIAL DIAGNOSIS

- Prolonged immobilization
- Significant rapid weight loss
- Orthostatic hypotension
- Neurocardiogenic syndrome
- Chronic fatigue syndrome
- Other neuropathies (eg, syringomyelia)
- Supraventricular tachyarrhythmias

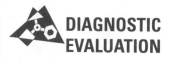 DIAGNOSTIC EVALUATION

LABORATORY TESTS

- CBC, basal metabolic panel
- Fasting glucose
- In appropriate situations: serum protein electrophoresis, paraneoplastic panel
- Antinuclear antibody test

ELECTROCARDIOGRAPHY

- Usually normal in supine resting position

IMAGING STUDIES

- Echocardiogram to exclude structural heart disease

DIAGNOSTIC PROCEDURES

- Tilt-table testing shows an excessive increase in heart rate without any or minimal drop in blood pressure

TREATMENT

CARDIOLOGY REFERRAL

- Patients not responding to conservative measures may benefit from cardiac electrophysiology consultation

HOSPITALIZATION CRITERIA

- If there is syncope, brief hospitalization may be required
- POTS generally can be managed as outpatient

MEDICATIONS

- Avoid dehydration, extreme heat, and alcohol consumption
- Elevate head end of the bed to help condition orthostatic stress
- Aerobic exercise and strength training (if deconditioned consider water exercise)
- Patients response to individual drugs vary substantially
- Combination therapy may be better
- Salt and fluid replacement
- Fludrocortisone 0.2 mg/day PO
- Autonomic agents: alpha-1-adrenergic agonists (midodrine 10 mg 3 times/day), cardioselective beta blockers (metoprolol 50 mg/day)
- Selective serotonin reuptake inhibitor (SSRI) such as paroxetine 20 mg/day
- Epoetin alpha 50–100 U subcutaneously or IV, 3 times/week until desired hematocrit is attained
- Patient and family education

MONITORING

- Frequent monitoring of symptoms

DIET AND ACTIVITY

- Liberal salt intake
- Aerobic exercise
- Strength training

ONGOING MANAGEMENT

HOSPITAL DISCHARGE CRITERIA

- Most patient can be managed as an outpatient

FOLLOW-UP

- Depends on symptomatology and the response to treatment
- May require follow-up every 2 weeks to 3–6 months until symptoms abate or are tolerable

COMPLICATIONS

- Persistent symptoms leading to disability

PROGNOSIS

- Postviral POTS tends to improve over 2–5 years
- Prognosis is guarded in primary form

PREVENTION

- None known

RESOURCES

PRACTICE GUIDELINES

- Diagnosis:
  - Tilt testing heart rate (HR) increase of 30 bpm (HR >120 bpm) in 5–10 minutes
  - Absence of orthostatic hypotension
  - Absence of autonomic neuropathy and development of orthostatic symptoms
- Management:
  - Fluids
  - Resistance training
  - High-salt diet (10–15 g/day)
  - Fludrocortisone, midodrine, clonidine, SSRI, and rarely octreotide and erythropoietin
- No single agent is appropriate for all patients

REFERENCES

- Jacob G et al: The neuropathic postural tachycardia syndrome. N Engl J Med 2000;343:1008.
- Kanjwal MY, Kosinski DJ, Grubb BP. Treatment of postural orthostatic tachycardia syndrome and inappropriate sinus tachycardia. Curr Cardiol Rep 2003;5:402.

INFORMATION FOR PATIENTS

- www.hlm.nih.gov/medlineplus/ arrhythmia.html

WEB SITE

- www.hrsonline.org

Pulmonary Atresia with Intact Ventricular Septum

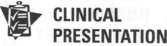 KEY FEATURES

ESSENTIALS OF DIAGNOSIS

- History of cyanosis at birth, which worsens at the time of ductal closure
- Single S_2; continuous murmur is rare
- Oligemic lung fields, enlarged cardiac silhouette on chest x-ray
- Atrial septal defect, small right ventricle, absent pulmonary valve

GENERAL CONSIDERATIONS

- Rarely encountered in adults with congenital heart disease
- Pulmonary valve is absent or imperforate
- Pulmonary blood flow is retrograde through patent ductus arteriosus in the newborn in most cases
- Left atrium receives all the systemic and pulmonary venous return through an atrial septal defect
- Cyanosis may worsen acutely when the ductus closes shortly after birth
- A palliative shunt may be placed to increase pulmonary blood flow
- The right ventricle may be diminutive, normal, or enlarged depending on the size of the tricuspid valve orifice and the degree of tricuspid regurgitation, if any
- Many have ventriculocoronary connections with coronary perfusion dependent on right ventricular systolic events

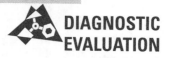 CLINICAL PRESENTATION

SYMPTOMS AND SIGNS

- History of cyanosis that worsens shortly after birth when the ductus closes

PHYSICAL EXAM FINDINGS

- Infant with cyanosis
- Physical exam variable and depends on the size of the right ventricle and the presence of tricuspid regurgitation
- Single S_2
- Continuous murmur rare

DIFFERENTIAL DIAGNOSIS

- Tricuspid atresia
- Other causes of cyanosis

DIAGNOSTIC EVALUATION

LABORATORY TESTS

- CBC may show polycythemia

ELECTROCARDIOGRAPHY

- Prominent left ventricular forces

IMAGING STUDIES

- Chest x-ray:
  - Oligemic lung fields and an enlarged cardiac silhouette caused by an enlarged left ventricle
- Echocardiogram:
  - Atrial septal defect
  - Small, hypertrophied right ventricle
  - Patent, small tricuspid valve
  - Thickened, immobile, atretic pulmonary valve with no Doppler evidence of flow through it
  - The ductus possibly running from the aortic arch to pulmonary artery

DIAGNOSTIC PROCEDURES

- Cardiac catheterization:
  - Systemic or suprasystemic right ventricular pressures
  - Catheter cannot be passed from the right ventricle to the pulmonary artery
  - Angiography of the right ventricle fails to opacify the pulmonary arteries
  - Contrast may fill the sinusoid vessels that often communicate with the coronary arteries

TREATMENT

CARDIOLOGY REFERRAL

- Regular cardiology follow-up throughout childhood and adulthood is recommended
- Worsened cyanosis
- Heart failure

HOSPITALIZATION CRITERIA

- Heart failure
- Sudden death
- Angina
- Arrhythmias

MEDICATIONS

- Diuretics for heart failure

SURGERY

- In the older child with an adequate-sized right ventricle, a right ventricle to main pulmonary artery conduit is placed (Rastelli procedure)
- In those with a rudimentary right ventricle, a Fontan procedure is done (cavocaval baffle to pulmonary artery connection)

MONITORING

- ECG monitoring during hospitalization
- Fluid intake and output

DIET AND ACTIVITY

- Low-sodium diet for patients with heart failure
- Activity as tolerated

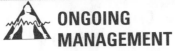

ONGOING MANAGEMENT

HOSPITAL DISCHARGE CRITERIA

- After successful surgery

FOLLOW-UP

- Within 2 weeks of hospital discharge
- Every 3–6 months thereafter, depending on the clinical situation

COMPLICATIONS

- Decompression of the right ventricle by connection with the pulmonary artery may cause myocardial ischemia by reversal of coronary blood flow in some patients with right ventricular dependent coronary artery blood flow with resultant sudden death, angina, or arrhythmias
- Congestive heart failure
- Valvular or conduit obstruction
- Progressive cyanosis with resultant polycythemia and hyperviscosity syndrome

PROGNOSIS

- Overall prognosis is limited:
  - 65–80% survival at age 1 year
  - 75% survival at age 5 years
- Prognosis depends on systemic-to-pulmonary blood flow ratio, presence of right ventricular dependent coronary blood flow, degree of tricuspid or pulmonary valvular (in those with a conduit) regurgitation, or other congenital defects

PREVENTION

- Antibiotic prophylaxis for endocarditis

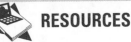

RESOURCES

PRACTICE GUIDELINES

- Definitive surgical repair in neonates with pulmonary atresia and intact ventricular septum are generally dictated by morphologic characteristics of the right ventricle
- These patients require careful follow-up for evidence of postoperative complications
- Cardiac transplantation should be considered for patients who develop inoperable complications after prior palliative surgeries

REFERENCES

- Ashburn DA: Determinates of mortality and type of repair in neonates with pulmonary atresia and intact ventricular septum. J Thorac Cardiovasc Surg 2004;127:1000.
- Gatzoulis MA et al: Definitive palliation with cavopulmonary or aortopulmonary shunts for adults with single ventricle physiology. Heart 2000;83:51.

INFORMATION FOR PATIENTS

- http://www.americanheart.org/presenter.jhtml?identifier=1303
- http://www.heartcenteronline.com/myheartdr/Common/articles.cfm?ARTID=522

WEB SITE

- http://www.emedicine.com/ped/topic2526.htm

Pulmonary Atresia with Ventricular Septal Defect

KEY FEATURES

ESSENTIALS OF DIAGNOSIS

- Often associated with velocardiofacial syndrome or DiGeorge syndrome
- Neonate or infant with cyanosis and hypoxia (or congestive heart failure in 25%) and single accentuated S_2, pansystolic murmur along the left lower sternal border
  - Continuous murmurs in the presence of patent ductus arteriosus and/or systemic to pulmonary collateral arteries
- Cardiac imaging:
  - Large aortic valve overriding a malaligned large membranous or infundibular ventricular septal defect (VSD) and a blind hypoplastic right ventricular infundibulum
  - Atrial septal defects (ASDs) and muscular VSDs may by present
  - Patent ductus arteriosus (PDA) may be identified; right aortic arch in 50%

GENERAL CONSIDERATIONS

- Sometimes pulmonary atresia with VSD is considered the most severe in the spectrum of tetralogy of Fallot
- Clinical presentation and surgical options depend on the amount of pulmonary blood flow
- Pulmonary circulation is supplied by a PDA, systemic to pulmonary collateral arteries, or plexuses of bronchial and pleural arteries
- Other associated congenital conditions: tricuspid atresia or stenosis, complete atrioventricular canal defects, complete or corrected transposition of the great arteries, left superior vena cava, anomalies of the coronary sinus, dextrocardia, and asplenia or polysplenia syndromes
- Surgical options depend on the anatomy of the individual

CLINICAL PRESENTATION

SYMPTOMS AND SIGNS

- Most patients present with cyanosis and hypoxia, which becomes severe when the ductus arteriosus closes
- Rarely patients present around ages 4–6 weeks with heart failure, increased blood flow, and minimal cyanosis in the setting of a large PDA or well-developed systemic to pulmonary collateral arteries
- Hemoptosis may occur owing to rupture of collateral arteries
- Infections may occur, especially with DiGeorge syndrome

PHYSICAL EXAM FINDINGS

- Cyanosis
- Normal S_1; single, often accentuated S_2 (aortic valve closure)
- Pansystolic murmur along the left lower sternal border; some with severe cyanosis do not have a detectable murmur
- Continuous murmurs in the presence of a PDA or systemic to pulmonary collateral arteries
- An early diastolic murmur of aortic regurgitation may be present

DIFFERENTIAL DIAGNOSIS

- Tetralogy of Fallot
- PDA
- Truncus arteriosus
- Other causes of cyanosis and heart failure

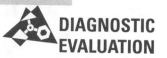 DIAGNOSTIC EVALUATION

LABORATORY TESTS

- Arterial blood gases: show hypoxemia and hypocarbia
- CBC: reactive polycythemia

ELECTROCARDIOGRAPHY

- Right ventricular hypertrophy and right axis deviation
- Right atrial enlargement
- Sometimes left ventricular hypertrophy and left atrial enlargement

IMAGING STUDIES

- Chest x-ray: normal or mildly enlarged, boot-shaped heart; absent main pulmonary arterial shadow; heterogeneous reticular pattern in lung fields from systemic to pulmonary artery collateral vessels; enlarged, right-sided aortic arch in 50% of cases; variable pulmonary vascular markings
- Echocardiography: large aortic valve overriding a large membranous or infundibular VSD and a hypoplastic right ventricular infundibulum with an absent pulmonary valve; an ASD may be present; muscular VSDs may be detected; a right-sided aortic arch may be present in 50% of cases
- MRI: helpful for defining the larger, surgically relevant pulmonary artery anatomy, but inadequate for defining peripheral pulmonary circulation

DIAGNOSTIC PROCEDURES

- Cardiac catheterization and angiography: typical hemodynamic findings include normal right atrial pressure; systemic-level right ventricular pressures due to the VSD; normal arterial pulmonary resistance; normal or wide aortic pulse pressure depending on presence of significant systemic to pulmonary shunting; the pulmonary artery cannot be accessed through the right side; angiography helps to delineate the size and distribution of the true pulmonary arteries and collateral vessels

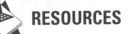
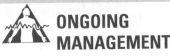

TREATMENT

CARDIOLOGY REFERRAL

- Neonates or infants with hypoxemia and cyanosis or congestive heart failure should be seen immediately by a pediatric cardiologist and cardiac surgeon
- Patients with previous surgery for this condition and dyspnea, congestive heart failure, arrhythmias, cyanosis syncope or new murmurs

HOSPITALIZATION CRITERIA

- Most patients diagnosed in the hospital shortly after birth
- Infants who develop new or worsened cyanosis shortly after closure of the ductus arteriosus around ages 2–4 weeks
- Infants with congestive heart failure or hemoptosis

MEDICATIONS

- Initial management of infants with ductal-dependent pulmonary circulation is prostaglandin E_1 administration

THERAPEUTIC PROCEDURES

- Phlebotomy for severe polycythemia
- Percutaneous needle perforation and balloon dilatation in some patients with isolated pulmonary atresia
- Percutaneous stenting of stenosed aortopulmonary collateral arteries in some

SURGERY

- Palliative surgeries: aortopulmonary shunts; bidirectional Glenn (superior cavopulmonary shunt); repair of interatrial, subpulmonic, or subaortic obstruction
- Corrective surgery involves the Fontan operation or one of its modifications (bicaval to pulmonary artery connection) after age 1 or 2 years
- Heart-lung transplantation is a viable option for patients with completely atretic pulmonary arteries

MONITORING

- Pulse oximetry
- ECG monitoring in the hospital
- Fluid balance

DIET AND ACTIVITY

- Low-sodium, fluid-restricted diet for infants with congestive heart failure
- Restricted activity if hypoxic, cyanotic patients

ONGOING MANAGEMENT

HOSPITAL DISCHARGE CRITERIA

- After successful palliative or corrective surgical repair or heart-lung transplantation
- After treatment for infective endocarditis or other complications

FOLLOW-UP

- Visit with pediatric or adult cardiologist within 2–4 weeks of hospital discharge
- Bi-annual visits with the cardiologist after surgery in stable patients or more frequently for patients with complications

COMPLICATIONS

- Congestive heart failure
- Erythrocytosis
- Infective endocarditis, brain abscess, or other infections
- Delayed growth
- Arrhythmias and sudden death
- Systemic venous hypertension with protein-losing enteropathy
- Aortic root dilatation and/or aortic regurgitation
- Shunt or neo-pulmonary artery restenoses

PROGNOSIS

- Patients often require repeated surgeries for complete repair and/or postoperative complications

PREVENTION

- Antibiotics are recommended for endocarditis prophylaxis

RESOURCES

PRACTICE GUIDELINES

- Upon diagnosis, a pediatric cardiologist, pediatric cardiothoracic surgeon, and geneticist should be consulted
- Patients with ductal-dependent circulation should receive prostaglandin E_1 to maintain ductal patency until surgery can be performed
- Surgical options depend on the anatomy of the patient and may involve several procedures to complete the repair
- Patients should be carefully monitored for adequacy of repair and postoperative complications
- Heart-lung transplantation remains a viable option in patients with completely atretic left pulmonary arteries
- Parents should have genetic counseling for future pregnancies

REFERENCES

- De Giovanni JV: Timing, frequency, and results of catheter intervention following recruitment of major aortopulmonary collaterals in patients with pulmonary artresia and ventricular septal defect. J Interv Cardiol 2004;17:47.
- Gupta A: Staged repair of pulmonary artresia with ventricular septal defect and major aortopulmonary collateral arteries. J Thorac Cardiovasc Surg 2003;126:1746.
- Lim JS: Dil-catheter balloon occlusion aortography in pulmonary artresia with ventricular septal defect and major aorto-pulmonary collaterals. Pediatr Cardiol 2004;25:500.
- Lofland GK: Pulmonary artresia, ventricular septal defect, and multiple aorta pulmonary collateral arteries. Semin Thorac Cardiovasc Surg Pediatr Card Surg Annu 2004;7:85.

INFORMATION FOR PATIENTS

- http://www.americanheart.org/ presenter.jhtml?identifier=1303

WEB SITE

- http://www.emedicine.com/ped/ topic2898.htm

Pulmonary Edema, Acute

 KEY FEATURES

ESSENTIALS OF DIAGNOSIS

- Acute onset of profound dyspnea and orthopnea
- Jugular venous distention, diffuse pulmonary rales, and tachycardia
- Left ventricular (LV) systolic or diastolic dysfunction

GENERAL CONSIDERATIONS

- Clinical syndrome characterized by sudden development of respiratory distress and interstitial pulmonary edema
- Primary pathogenic mechanism is an elevation in pulmonary capillary pressure due to LV systolic or diastolic dysfunction
- Compensatory mechanisms result in neurohumoral activation, tachycardia and elevated systemic vascular resistance that further increase LV filling pressures and worsen pulmonary edema
- Can occur in the absence of heart disease with fluid overload due to blood transfusion or severe renal disease
- Results in reduced diffusion capacity and lung compliance, hypoxia, and dyspnea
- Rate of increase in pulmonary edema related to pulmonary venous pressure and capacity of the lymphatic vessels to remove excess fluid
- Causes of acute pulmonary edema:
  - Myocardial ischemia
  - Acute aortic insufficiency
  - Acute mitral regurgitation
  - Mitral stenosis
  - Renal vascular hypertension
  - Other conditions in the presence of preexisting diastolic dysfunction (eg, fever, sepsis, anemia, thyroid disease, cardiac dysrhythmia)

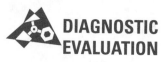 **CLINICAL PRESENTATION**

SYMPTOMS AND SIGNS

- Acute onset or worsening of cough and dyspnea
- Chest discomfort
- Diaphoresis

PHYSICAL EXAM FINDINGS

- Tachypnea and use of accessory respiratory muscles
- Tachycardia
- Jugular venous pressure may be elevated
- Diffuse pulmonary rales
- Hypertension or hypotension
- New or changed murmur
- S_3 or S_4
- Peripheral edema may be present

DIFFERENTIAL DIAGNOSIS

- Pulmonary emboli
- Bilateral pneumonia
- Acute respiratory distress syndrome

DIAGNOSTIC EVALUATION

LABORATORY TESTS

- Arterial blood gases: can quantify the level of hypoxia
- CBC: may suggest infection or identify anemia as precipitating events
- Electrolyte, blood urea nitrogen and creatinine: may identify renal dysfunction
- Cardiac enzymes (eg, troponin): may be elevated in the presence of myocardial ischemia
- Thyroid function tests

ELECTROCARDIOGRAPHY

- Sinus tachycardia
- Left atrial enlargement
- Atrial fibrillation or flutter with a rapid ventricular response
- ST- and T-wave changes suggestive of myocardial ischemia
- LV hypertrophy

IMAGING STUDIES

- Chest x-ray:
  - Variable pulmonary vascular redistribution and interstitial edema
  - Perihilar alveolar edema ("butterfly" appearance)
  - Cardiac silhouette may be normal or enlarged
  - Pleural effusions may or may not be present
- Transthoracic echocardiography:
  - To assess the degree of LV systolic and/or diastolic dysfunction
  - To identify the presence of valvular disease
  - To estimate the pulmonary artery systolic pressure and right atrial pressure
  - New wall motion abnormalities may suggest myocardial ischemia or injury

DIAGNOSTIC PROCEDURES

- Right heart catheterization: often not necessary but typically reveals the following:
  - Marked elevations in pulmonary capillary wedge pressure
  - Pulmonary artery pressure and sometimes right atrial pressure
  - Cardiac output may be reduced or normal

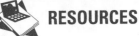

TREATMENT

CARDIOLOGY REFERRAL

- Any patient with suspected cardiogenic pulmonary edema

HOSPITALIZATION CRITERIA

- Hypoxia
- Respiratory distress
- Suspected myocardial ischemia or infarction

MEDICATIONS

- Oxygen, morphine sulfate
- IV diuretics
- IV catecholamines
- IV phosphodiesterase inhibitors
- IV vasodilators (eg, nitrates, nitroprusside, enalaprilat, hydralazine)
- IV b-type natriuretic peptide (nesiritide)

THERAPEUTIC PROCEDURES

- Mechanical ventilation
- Intra-aortic balloon pump counter-pulsation
- Ultrafiltration in some cases
- Hemodialysis for patients with end-stage renal disease
- Cardiac catheterization considered in suspected acute coronary syndrome

MONITORING

- Pulse oximetry
- Telemetry
- Blood pressure
- Fluid balance
- Blood gas analysis

DIET AND ACTIVITY

- Nothing by mouth until stabilized
- Fluid and sodium restriction
- Bed rest until stabilized

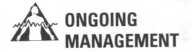

ONGOING MANAGEMENT

HOSPITAL DISCHARGE CRITERIA

- Adequate oxygenation
- Compensated heart failure
- Stable cardiac rhythm and blood pressure

FOLLOW-UP

- Cardiologist within 2 weeks
- Serial cardiac imaging and laboratory studies depending on the clinical situation

COMPLICATIONS

- Recurrent acute pulmonary edema
- Acute myocardial infarction (MI)
- Cardiogenic shock
- Atrial or ventricular arrhythmias
- Electrolyte disturbances

PROGNOSIS

- Variable morbidity and mortality rates; up to 15–20% in-hospital mortality
- Mortality rate up to 40% in patients with acute MI and acute pulmonary edema

PREVENTION

- Primary and secondary MI prevention
- Blood pressure control
- Medical compliance
- Adequate diuresis
- Treatment of cardiorenal disease
- Percutaneous treatment of renal artery stenosis

RESOURCES

PRACTICE GUIDELINES

- Aggressive medical therapy to decrease LV preload (diuretics) and afterload (vasodilators) are the mainstays of initial therapy
- Hypotensive patients with severe LV systolic dysfunction and/or acute valvular disorders may benefit from inotropic support
- Patients with severe LV dysfunction and signs of ischemia or severe mitral regurgitation may benefit from intra-aortic balloon pump insertion
- Ventilatory support is indicated for patients with inadequate oxygenation despite supplemental oxygen
- Adequate treatment of the underlying precipitating cardiovascular disorder is important to prevent recurrences

REFERENCES

- Crane SD, Elliott MW, Gilligan P et al: Randomised controlled comparison of continuous positive airways pressure, bilevel non-invasive ventilation, and standard treatment in emergency department patients with acute cardiogenic pulmonary edema. Emerg Med J 2004;21:155.
- Poole-Wilson PA, Xue SR: New therapies for the management of acute heart failure. Curr Cardiol Rep 2003;5:229

INFORMATION FOR PATIENTS

- http://www.mayoclinic.com/ invoke.cfm?id=DS00412

WEB SITE

- http://www.emedicine.com/med/ topic1955.htm

Pulmonary Edema, Noncardiogenic

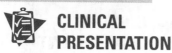 KEY FEATURES

ESSENTIALS OF DIAGNOSIS

- Bilateral diffuse alveolar infiltrates are present with severe hypoxemia
- Pulmonary capillary wedge pressure (PCWP) is < 18 mm Hg
- Arterial PO_2/ inspired oxygen concentration (PaO_2/FiO_2) of ≤ 200 mm Hg

GENERAL CONSIDERATIONS

- Acute respiratory distress syndrome (ARDS) is the most severe form of acute lung injury
- ARDS may be a manifestation of several conditions, such as sepsis, aspiration, hypertransfusion, toxic inhalation, severe nonthoracic trauma, and cardiopulmonary bypass
- Other incompletely understood causes include high-altitude pulmonary edema, neurogenic pulmonary edema, narcotic overdose, eclampsia, and cardioversion
- Clinically one third of ARDS patients have sepsis
- The mechanism of lung injury varies, but the common result is pulmonary endothelial damage with increased capillary permeability

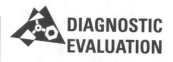 CLINICAL PRESENTATION

SYMPTOMS AND SIGNS

- Tachydyspnea, labored breathing

PHYSICAL EXAM FINDINGS

- Pulmonary rales

DIFFERENTIAL DIAGNOSIS

- Cardiogenic pulmonary edema (PCWP is typically > 18 mm Hg)
- Lymphangitic carcinomatosis (PCWP is < 18 mm Hg)
- Unilateral pulmonary edema after evacuation of large pleural effusion (PCWP is normal)

DIAGNOSTIC EVALUATION

LABORATORY TESTS

- Blood cultures may be positive in sepsis

IMAGING STUDIES

- Chest x-ray:
  - Shows diffuse patchy bilateral infiltrates initially; then confluence with air bronchograms
  - The costophrenic angles are spared and effusions are unusual
  - Heart size is normal
- Echocardiography: shows normal left ventricular function

DIAGNOSTIC PROCEDURES

- Right heart catheterization may be necessary to exclude cardiogenic shock

TREATMENT

CARDIOLOGY REFERRAL

- Suspected cardiogenic shock

HOSPITALIZATION CRITERIA

- All patients with ARDS are hospitalized

MEDICATIONS

- Treat the underlying cause if possible
- Give supplemental oxygen and noninvasive ventilatory support in early stages of acute lung injury
- Give mechanical ventilatory support with positive end-expiratory pressure and low tidal volumes (6–10 mL/kg) in established ARDS

THERAPEUTIC PROCEDURES

- Endotracheal intubation is almost always required

MONITORING

- ECG monitoring in hospital as appropriate
- Routine right-heart catheter monitoring is not recommended

DIET AND ACTIVITY

- ICU protocol for parenteral nutrition in the critically ill

ONGOING MANAGEMENT

HOSPITAL DISCHARGE CRITERIA

- Resolution of ARDS
- Correction of the underlying problem

FOLLOW-UP

- Depends on the cause

COMPLICATIONS

- Multiorgan failure

PROGNOSIS

- Mortality rate 30–40%, can be higher if due to sepsis

PREVENTION

- No known measures

RESOURCES

PRACTICE GUIDELINES

- The treatment of ARDS involves two aspects:
  - Identification and treatment of the underlying cause
  - Meticulous respiratory support

REFERENCES

- Vincent JL et al: Epidemiology and outcome of acute respiratory failure in intensive care unit patients. Crit Care Med 2003;31:S296.
- Ware LB et al: The acute respiratory distress syndrome. N Engl J Med 2000;342:1334.

INFORMATION FOR PATIENTS

- www.drpen.com/428

WEB SITE

- www.emedicine.com/med/topic70.htm

Pulmonary Embolism

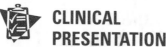

KEY FEATURES

ESSENTIALS OF DIAGNOSIS

- Otherwise unexplained dyspnea, tachypnea, or chest pain
- Clinical, ECG, or echocardiographic evidence of acute cor pulmonale
- Elevated plasma D-dimer enzyme-linked immunosorbent assay
- Positive spiral chest CT scan with contrast
- High-probability ventilation-perfusion lung scan or high-probability perfusion lung scan with a normal chest radiograph
- Positive venous ultrasound for thrombus in the legs, with a convincing clinical history and a suggestive lung scan
- Diagnostic pulmonary angiogram

GENERAL CONSIDERATIONS

- Pulmonary embolism is seen in:
  - Immobilized patients, such as after surgery
  - Patients with congestive heart failure, malignancies, pelvic trauma, and deep venous thrombosis
- In the absence of surgery or trauma, pulmonary embolism often is due to a hypercoagulable state, which may be genetic or secondary to cancer or hormone therapy
- The most common genetic causes of venous thromboembolism are factor V Leiden and the prothrombin gene
- Venous thromboembolism is a major problem for women because it is associated with oral contraceptives, hormone replacement therapy, and pregnancy

CLINICAL PRESENTATION

SYMPTOMS AND SIGNS

- Dyspnea
- Chest pain
- Syncope
- Hemoptysis

PHYSICAL EXAM FINDINGS

- Tachycardia
- Hypotension
- Cyanosis
- Elevated jugular venous pressure
- Right ventricular lift
- S_3
- Tachypnea
- Evidence of deep venous thrombosis

DIFFERENTIAL DIAGNOSIS

- Pneumonia
- Myocardial infarction
- Pulmonary disorder with pleurisy
- Respiratory distress secondary to pulmonary edema, asthma, or pleural effusion
- Early sepsis
- Psychogenic hyperventilation

DIAGNOSTIC EVALUATION

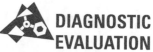

LABORATORY TESTS

- Arterial blood gases: may be abnormal
- Plasma D-dimer: elevated
- Troponin: may be elevated
- Brain natriuretic peptide: may be elevated

ELECTROCARDIOGRAPHY

- Acute cor pulmonale: S1, Q3, T3 pattern
- New right bundle branch block
- Evidence of right ventricular hypertrophy with strain
- P pulmonale

IMAGING STUDIES

- Chest x-ray: a peripheral pie-shaped infiltrate is unusual but diagnostic
- Lung scan for ventilation-perfusion defect
- CT of chest with contrast: can show arterial filling defects that are diagnostic
- CT of the legs: can also demonstrate deep venous thrombosis and can be combined with CT of the chest
- Venous ultrasonography: can demonstrate deep venous thrombosis
- Echocardiography may show:
  - Thrombi in the main pulmonary arteries
  - Dilated hypokinetic right ventricle with normal left ventricle
  - Elevated pulmonary pressures detected by Doppler

DIAGNOSTIC PROCEDURES

- Transesophageal echocardiography can be used in critically ill patients to directly visualize thrombi in the main pulmonary arteries (especially useful in patients with pulseless electrical activity)
- Pulmonary angiography is usually reserved for therapeutic purposes, such as suction catheter embolectomy
- Pulmonary angioscopy is reserved for diagnosing chronic pulmonary emboli before surgical removal

TREATMENT

CARDIOLOGY REFERRAL

- Evidence of right heart strain, failure, or pressure overload
- Elevated troponin

HOSPITALIZATION CRITERIA

- Hemodynamic compromise or instability
- Hypoxia
- Deep venous thrombosis
- Hypotension
- Heart failure
- Evidence of right ventricular dysfunction
- Elevated pulmonary pressure
- Elevated troponin

MEDICATIONS

- Acute anticoagulation with heparin for several days, with warfarin instituted concurrently and continuing for 6 months
- Thrombolytic therapy in patients with hemodynamic compromise (no proven effect on mortality)

THERAPEUTIC PROCEDURES

- IV filter placement in the inferior vena cava for patients who are not candidates for anticoagulation (because of bleeding) or are unresponsive to anticoagulation
- Catheter embolectomy in selected cases

SURGERY

- Acute embolectomy in selected cases
- Embolectomy for chronic emboli in selected cases

MONITORING

- ECG monitoring in hospital
- Oxygen saturation monitoring in hospital

DIET AND ACTIVITY

- Adequate physical exercise encouraged

ONGOING MANAGEMENT

HOSPITAL DISCHARGE CRITERIA

- Resolution of acute problems with adequate anticoagulation established
- After successful procedure with adequate anticoagulation established

FOLLOW-UP

- INR should be kept at 2–3 for 6 months, longer for patients with persistent predisposing factors

COMPLICATIONS

- Sudden death
- Right heart failure
- Shock
- Chronic pulmonary emboli
- Chronic pulmonary hypertension

PROGNOSIS

- Depends on associated and predisposing conditions, extent of lung injury, and resultant pulmonary hypertension severity

PREVENTION

- All hospitalized patients should undergo the following prophylaxis for pulmonary embolism based on their level of risk:
  - Compression stockings
  - Pneumatic compression devices
  - Ambulation as indicated
  - Low-dose heparin for patients at highest risk, such as those with hip replacement surgery

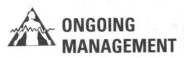

RESOURCES

PRACTICE GUIDELINES

- An integrated algorithm for diagnosing pulmonary embolism begins with clinical suspicion:
  - If suspicion is low and D-dimer is normal, then the diagnosis is excluded and no further testing is required
  - If D-dimer is elevated or clinical suspicion is high, imaging tests are indicated, preferably a CT scan

REFERENCES

- Aklog L et al: Acute pulmonary embolectomy: a contemporary approach. Circulation 2002; 105:1416.
- Dalen JE: Pulmonary embolism: what have we learned since Virchow? Natural history, pathophysiology, and diagnosis. Chest 2002;122:1440.
- Wicki J et al: Predicting adverse outcome in patients with acute pulmonary embolism: a risk score. Thromb Haemost 2000; 84:548.

INFORMATION FOR PATIENTS

- www.nhlbi.nih.gov/health/dci/diseases/pe/pe_what.html

WEB SITE

- www.emedicine.com/med/topic/958.htm

Pulmonary Hypertension, Primary

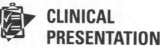 KEY FEATURES

ESSENTIALS OF DIAGNOSIS

- No evidence of either lung or heart disease
- Dyspnea, malaise, chest pain, or exertional syncope
- Right ventricular (RV) lift
- Increased intensity of the pulmonic component of S_2
- ECG evidence of RV hypertrophy
- Elevated pulmonary artery pressures by Doppler echocardiography or cardiac catheterization

GENERAL CONSIDERATIONS

- Rare disorder (1–3 cases/million/year) mostly seen in young women
- Characterized by elevated pulmonary artery pressure (PAP) and pulmonary vascular resistance (PVR) without an apparent cause, progressive right heart failure, and very poor survival
- Bone morphogenetic protein receptor type II (BMPR2) gene mutations identified in 50% of familial cases and approximately 10% of sporadic cases
- Pathophysiology is pulmonary vasoconstriction, vascular remodeling, and in situ thrombosis
- Options for treatment are increasing but data are limited and overall prognosis remains poor
- Pregnancy should be strongly discouraged because of high maternal and fetal mortality
- Noncardiac surgery is associated with high peri-operative morbidity and mortality

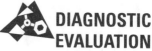 CLINICAL PRESENTATION

SYMPTOMS AND SIGNS

- Symptoms may be vague and subtle
- Dyspnea
- Exercise intolerance
- Exertional chest pain (angina)
- Dizziness and pre-syncope
- Syncope
- Palpitations
- Increased abdominal girth (ascites)
- Extremity swelling

PHYSICAL EXAM FINDINGS

- Tachycardia
- Hypotension
- Hypoxia may or may not be present
- Normal or elevated jugular venous pressure with prominent *a* waves
- Left parasternal lift (enlarged RV)
- Increased intensity of P_2
- Holosystolic murmur of tricuspid regurgitation at the lower sternal border
- Diastolic murmur of pulmonic insufficiency at the left sternal border
- Hepatomegaly; pulsatile liver with severe tricuspid regurgitation
- Peripheral edema

DIFFERENTIAL DIAGNOSIS

- Mitral stenosis
- Sleep apnea
- Chronic pulmonary embolism
- Autoimmune diseases such as scleroderma
- Left ventricular failure
- Congenital heart disease
- Cirrhosis of the liver with portopulmonary hypertension
- Pulmonary veno-occlusive disease

DIAGNOSTIC EVALUATION

LABORATORY TESTS

- CBC (polycythemia suggests respiratory disease or congenital heart disease)
- Electrolytes, blood urea nitrogen, creatinine (prerenal azotemia suggests poor forward cardiac output or overdiuresis)
- Liver function tests (may be elevated with passive liver congestion from right heart failure)
- Serum brain type natriuretic peptide and uric acid levels have prognostic value
- Tests to exclude secondary causes: antinuclear antibody, rheumatoid factor, HIV serology, thyroid function tests, urine toxicology for amphetamines/cocaine

ELECTROCARDIOGRAPHY

- Sinus tachycardia
- Atrial flutter or fibrillation
- Right atrial enlargement
- RV hypertrophy
- Right bundle branch block

IMAGING STUDIES

- Chest x-ray: RV enlargement
- Transthoracic echocardiography:
  - Findings associated with poor survival are right atrial enlargement and a pericardial effusion
  - Typical findings are variable RV enlargement, hypertrophy, and systolic dysfunction; D-shaped left ventricle due intraventricular septal flattening during systole; the left ventricle and atrium appear small and underfilled; the pulmonary artery systolic pressure can be estimated by the peak tricuspid regurgitant jet velocity; variable degrees of functional tricuspid and pulmonary regurgitation are present
- Ventilation-perfusion lung scan, contrast CT chest, or pulmonary angiography: must be obtained to exclude thromboembolic pulmonary hypertension
- High-resolution chest CT: to exclude interstitial lung disease

DIAGNOSTIC PROCEDURES

- Right heart catheterization (required to establish the diagnosis): defined by a mean pulmonary arterial pressure > 25 mm Hg at rest or > 30 mm Hg during exercise and a pulmonary wedge pressure ≤ 15 mm Hg; typical findings:

– Increased pulmonary vascular resistance

– Normal or low cardiac output and normal or elevated right atrial pressure

– Vasodilators (eg, nitric oxide, epoprostenol, adenosine, sildenafil) are administered to determine acute vasoreactivity ("responders" have a drop in the mean PAP of at least 10 mm Hg to a level of ≤ 40 mm Hg)

• Screening pulse oximetry or formal sleep study: to exclude obstructive sleep apnea

• Complete pulmonary function tests:

– Excludes or characterizes the contribution of obstructive or restrictive respiratory disorder

– The diffusion capacity for carbon monoxide is often reduced in patients with primary pulmonary hypertension

TREATMENT

CARDIOLOGY REFERRAL

• Referral to a designated center for pulmonary arterial hypertension care

HOSPITALIZATION CRITERIA

• Syncope
• Hypoxia
• Symptomatic hypotension
• Decompensated right heart failure
• Many patients are hospitalized to initiate intravenous pulmonary vasal dilator therapies

MEDICATIONS

• Oxygen supplementation for hypoxia (some patients may have exercise-related hypoxia)
• Empiric anticoagulation may confer survival benefit
• Digoxin may be used cautiously in patients with right heart failure
• Diuretics for right heart failure
• Pulmonary vasodilator therapies: prostacyclin analogs (eg, epoprostenol) require intravenous administration, oral endothelin antagonists (eg, Tracleer); oral phosphodiesterase type V inhibitors (eg, sildenafil and cialis) are being studied but are not yet approved for treatment of PAH
• Calcium channel blockers typically used in patients with a significant response to acute vasodilator testing, although the efficacy is uncertain
• Two methods of birth control for women of childbearing age

THERAPEUTIC PROCEDURES

• Palliative atrial septostomy may be considered in patients with severe right heart failure and low forward cardiac output

SURGERY

• Bilateral lung with or without combined heart transplantation is a last resort for eligible patients with severe disease and poor quality of life

MONITORING

• Pulse oximetry
• Telemetry
• Systemic blood pressure
• Critical patients may benefit by hemodynamic monitoring with a pulmonary arterial catheter to tailor therapy

DIET AND ACTIVITY

• Fluid and sodium restriction for patients with right heart failure
• Activity as tolerated

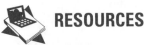

ONGOING MANAGEMENT

HOSPITAL DISCHARGE CRITERIA

• Stable vital signs
• Adequate oxygenization
• Evidence of adequate organ perfusion

FOLLOW-UP

• Pulmonary hypertension specialist within 2 weeks
• Serial echocardiography is recommended approximately every 3–6 months to monitor treatment response or disease progression
• Six-minute walk test every 3–4 months for prognosis and to monitor response to treatment
• Some centers perform right heart catheterization annually or semiannually to monitor response to therapy or progression of disease

COMPLICATIONS

• Syncope
• Arrhythmias
• Progressive right heart failure
• Sudden death
• Increasing oxygen requirements

• Line infections in patients receiving intravenous pulmonary vasodilators

PROGNOSIS

• Median survival for *untreated* patients is 2.8 years; 1-year, 3-year, and 5-year survival rates are approximately 68%, 48%, and 34%, respectively
• Survival is improved in *treated* patients but remains poor: 1, 3, and 5-year survival rates of 87%, 63%, and 54% respectively, with intravenous epoprostenol
• Survival after bilateral lung transplantation is 70%, 45%, and 20% at 1, 5, and 10 years, respectively
• Pregnancy is poorly tolerated and associated with a very high maternal and fetal mortality rate

PREVENTION

• Avoidance of risk factors associated with pulmonary arterial hypertension, including amphetamines and anorexogens

RESOURCES

PRACTICE GUIDELINES

• Right heart catheterization is required to confirm the diagnosis
• Secondary causes should be excluded
• Once identified, patients should be referred to a designated center with expertise in the diagnosis and treatment of pulmonary hypertension

REFERENCES

• Rubin LJ: Executive summary: diagnosis and management of pulmonary arterial hypertension: ACCP evidence-based clinical practice guidelines. Chest 2004;126:4S.
• Simonneau G et al: Clinical classification of pulmonary arterial hypertension. J Am Coll Cardiol 2004;43:5S.

INFORMATION FOR PATIENTS

• http://www.americanheart.org/presenter.jhtml?identifier=4752
• http://www.phassociation.org/

WEB SITES

• http://www.emedicine.com/med/topic1962.htm
• http://www.phassociation.org/Medical/

Pulmonic Regurgitation

 KEY FEATURES

ESSENTIALS OF DIAGNOSIS

- Diastolic murmur at the left upper sternal border that increases with inspiration
- Loud pulmonic component of S_2
- Characteristic Doppler echocardiographic findings

GENERAL CONSIDERATIONS

- Pulmonic regurgitation usually occurs with pulmonary hypertension owing to dilatation of the valve ring
- Any cause of pulmonic valve ring enlargement can cause regurgitation such as Marfan syndrome
- Primary valve leaflet disease, such as carcinoid syndrome, rheumatic fever, and endocarditis, can also cause regurgitation
- It can be the result of valvuloplasty for pulmonic stenosis
- Trivial to mild pulmonic regurgitation is frequently seen on routine echocardiography and is a normal variant

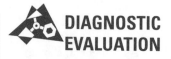 **CLINICAL PRESENTATION**

SYMPTOMS AND SIGNS

- Patients are usually asymptomatic unless right heart failure occurs
- Dyspnea and fatigue with moderate to severe regurgitation can occur

PHYSICAL EXAM FINDINGS

- Prominent jugular venous *a* wave, if pulmonary hypertension is present
- Right ventricular lift if pulmonary hypertension is present
- Loud pulmonic S_2 if pulmonary hypertension is present
- Right ventricular S_3 and S_4 may be heard along the left sternal border
- In normotensive pulmonic regurgitation:
  - The diastolic murmur is heard best in the left second or third interspace
  - It starts after S_2
  - It is medium in pitch
  - It is increased in intensity with inspiration
- With pulmonary hypertension:
  - The diastolic murmur is higher pitched, starts with S_2, and is decrescendo (Graham-Steele murmur)
  - It may be confused with the murmur of aortic regurgitation, but should get louder with inspiration unlike an aortic murmur

DIFFERENTIAL DIAGNOSIS

- Aortic regurgitation
- Tricuspid stenosis
- Right-heart failure from other causes

DIAGNOSTIC EVALUATION

ELECTROCARDIOGRAPHY

- Evidence of right ventricular and atrial hypertrophy

IMAGING STUDIES

- Chest x-ray findings:
  - Enlargement of the right heart chambers
  - Peripheral pulmonary vessel absence with enlarged main pulmonary arteries if pulmonary hypertension is present
- Echocardiography:
  - Enlarged and hypertrophied right heart chambers
  - Dilated main pulmonary artery
  - Possible valve leaflet abnormalities
- Color-flow Doppler:
  - Evidence of pulmonary hypertension by increased tricuspid and pulmonic regurgitant velocities
  - Characteristic regurgitant jet

DIAGNOSTIC PROCEDURES

- Cardiac catheterization is rarely used to assess pulmonic regurgitation, but may be used to quantify pulmonary pressure and assess accompanying lesions

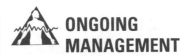

 TREATMENT

CARDIOLOGY REFERRAL

- Moderate to severe pulmonary hypertension
- Moderate to severe regurgitation
- Right heart failure

HOSPITALIZATION CRITERIA

- Right heart failure
- Planned surgery
- Suspected endocarditis

MEDICATIONS

- Diuretics useful for reducing congestion

THERAPEUTIC PROCEDURES

- Percutaneous pulmonic prosthetic valve placement

SURGERY

- Pulmonic valve replacement

MONITORING

- ECG monitoring in the hospital

DIET AND ACTIVITY

- Low-salt diet
- No activity restriction unless heart failure is present

ONGOING MANAGEMENT

HOSPITAL DISCHARGE CRITERIA

- Resolution of right heart failure
- Successful corrective procedure

FOLLOW-UP

- Echocardiogram every 1–3 years, depending on the severity of regurgitation
- Yearly visits

COMPLICATIONS

- Endocarditis
- Right heart failure

PROGNOSIS

- Pulmonary hypertension determines prognosis
- Underlying disease such as endocarditis and carcinoid important for prognosis
- Isolated pulmonary regurgitation carries an excellent prognosis

PREVENTION

- Prevent causative diseases

RESOURCES

PRACTICE GUIDELINES

- Pulmonic regurgitation rarely requires valve replacement
- Usually, treatment of associated conditions determines the patient's course
- If surgery for other conditions is contemplated, then severe pulmonic regurgitation can be addressed with a bioprosthetic valve or a homograft

REFERENCES

- Bonhoeffer P et al: Percutaneous insertion of the pulmonary valve. J Am Coll Cardiol 2002;39:1664.
- Poon LK et al: Pulmonary regurgitation after percutaneous balloon valvuloplasty for isolated pulmonary valvular stenosis in childhood. Cardiol Young 2003;13:444.
- Shively BK: Transesophageal echocardiographic (TEE) evaluation of the aortic valve, left ventricular outflow tract, and pulmonic valve. Cardiol Clin 2000;18:711.
- Warner KG et al: Expanding the indications for pulmonary valve replacement after repair of tetralogy of Fallot. Ann Thorac Surg 2003;76:1066.

INFORMATION FOR PATIENTS

- www.americanheart.org/presenter.jhtml?identifier=4565

WEB SITE

- www.americanheart.org/presenter.jhtml?identifier3002114

Pulmonic Stenosis

 KEY FEATURES

ESSENTIALS OF DIAGNOSIS

- Systolic murmur at the left second intercostal space preceded by a systolic click
- Reduced intensity of pulmonic component of S_2
- Characteristic echocardiographic findings

GENERAL CONSIDERATIONS

- Pulmonic stenosis is almost always congenital and valvular, although supravalvular and subvalvular lesions do occur
- The condition can occur with other congenital lesions/conditions such as tetralogy of Fallot and Noonan's syndrome
- The most commonly acquired form occurs with the carcinoid syndrome
- Rheumatic heart disease rarely involves the pulmonic valve

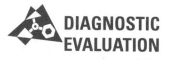 **CLINICAL PRESENTATION**

SYMPTOMS AND SIGNS

- Often asymptomatic
- Fatigue
- Exertional dyspnea

PHYSICAL EXAM FINDINGS

- Prominent *a* wave in the jugular venous pressure
- Right ventricular lift
- Pulmonic ejection sound that gets softer with inspiration
- Reduced pulmonic component of S_2
- Right-sided S_4 along the left sternal border
- Systolic ejection murmur in the pulmonic area that increases with inspiration

DIFFERENTIAL DIAGNOSIS

- Aortic stenosis
- Ventricular septal defect
- Right-heart failure from other causes

DIAGNOSTIC EVALUATION

ELECTROCARDIOGRAPHY

- Evidence of right ventricular and atrial hypertrophy

IMAGING STUDIES

- Chest x-ray: right heart chamber enlargement with dilatation of the main pulmonary artery
- Echocardiography:
  - Thickened, doming, or dysplastic pulmonic valve that has an increased Doppler determined pressure gradient—mild < 40 mm Hg; moderate 41–79; severe ≥ 80
  - Right ventricular hypertrophy and right atrial enlargement common

DIAGNOSTIC PROCEDURES

- Cardiac catheterization: rarely done for diagnosis today, but can confirm the gradient across the valve when echo is unclear

TREATMENT

CARDIOLOGY REFERRAL

• Symptomatic patients

HOSPITALIZATION CRITERIA

• Pre-surgery in patients not treated by balloon valvuloplasty

THERAPEUTIC PROCEDURES

• Percutaneous balloon valvuloplasty is the treatment of choice for symptomatic patients

SURGERY

• If valvuloplasty is unsuccessful or if other lesions need correction, surgical valvuloplasty and rarely valve replacement can be done
• Valve replacement is usually with a homograft or a bioprosthetic valve

MONITORING

• ECG monitoring in the hospital

DIET AND ACTIVITY

• Low-sodium diet

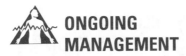

ONGOING MANAGEMENT

HOSPITAL DISCHARGE CRITERIA

• After successful procedure or surgery

FOLLOW-UP

• Depends on severity in asymptomatic patients: 3–12 months with echocardiography every other visit

COMPLICATIONS

• Infective endocarditis—rare
• Right heart failure in severe cases

PROGNOSIS

• Excellent prognosis before and after correction
• Often determined by other associated lesions
• Repeat balloon valvuloplasty rate of 10% over 10 years
• Surgery after valvuloplasty required in 5% over 10 years

PREVENTION

• Bacterial endocarditis prophylaxis

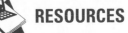

RESOURCES

PRACTICE GUIDELINES

• Corrective procedures:
  – Not indicated for mild cases
  – Indicated for moderate cases only when symptomatic
  – Considered for severe cases regardless of symptoms

REFERENCES

• Fawzy ME et al: Long-term results of pulmonary balloon valvulotomy in adult patients. J Heart Valve Dis 2001;10:812.
• Gupta D et al: Factors influencing late course of residual valvular and infundibular gradient following pulmonary valve balloon dilatation. Int J Cardiol 2001;79:143.
• Sharieff S et al: Short- and intermediate-term follow-up results of percutaneous transluminal balloon valvuloplasty in adolescents and young adults with congenital pulmonic valve stenosis. J Invasive Cardiol 2003;15:484.

INFORMATION FOR PATIENTS

• www.drpen.com/424.3

WEB SITE

• www.emedicine.com/med/topic1965.htm

Radiation Heart Disease

 KEY FEATURES

ESSENTIALS OF DIAGNOSIS

- History of mediastinal radiation therapy, usually for Hodgkin's disease
- Pericarditis early or within 1 year or more after radiation therapy
- Cardiomyopathy, especially if treated with anthracyclines also
- Coronary artery disease after a 3- to 20-year latency period
- Valvular regurgitation; occasionally stenosis
- Heart block; occasionally tachyarrhythmias

GENERAL CONSIDERATIONS

- Heart disease is the leading cause of death not related to cancer in survivors of Hodgkin's disease
- Radiation cardiac injury is a broad spectrum that includes direct effects, indirect effects (lung irradiation) and augmentation of the effects of chemotherapy, such as with anthracyclines
- The initial injury is characterized by neutrophil infiltration and inflammation, which subsides and transitions to a latent phase of progressively increasing fibrosis until clinical disease is evident in the late stage
- Radiation injury can involve any cardiac structure
- The incidence of cardiac injury with anterior mediastium radiation therapy has been estimated at 15–30% over 5–10 years
- Newer techniques have probably lowered this incidence but long-term data are not yet available

 CLINICAL PRESENTATION

SYMPTOMS AND SIGNS

- Pericarditis: pleuritic chest pain, dyspnea
- Cardiomyopathy: dyspnea, fatigue
- Coronary artery disease: angina pectoris, dyspnea
- Valve disease: dyspnea
- Conduction disease: syncope, fatigue, palpitations

PHYSICAL EXAM FINDINGS

- Pericarditis: friction rub, jugular venous distention
- Cardiomyopathy: signs of heart failure
- Valve disease: predominantly mitral regurgitation and mixed aortic valve disease

DIFFERENTIAL DIAGNOSIS

- Pericarditis from other causes, especially hypothyroidism (thyroid in field)
- Cardiomyopathy from other causes, especially anthracyclines
- Coronary artery disease from other causes
- Valvular heart disease from other causes
- Cardiac arrhythmias from other causes

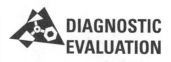 **DIAGNOSTIC EVALUATION**

LABORATORY TESTS

- Thyroid function
- Lipid panel

ELECTROCARDIOGRAPHY

- ST-T-wave changes of acute ischemia or pericarditis
- Q waves of myocardial infarction
- Chamber hypertrophy
- Conduction abnormalities

IMAGING STUDIES

- Chest x-ray: may show cardiomegaly
- Echocardiography: to assess pericardial effusion, myocardial function, and valve pathology

DIAGNOSTIC PROCEDURES

- Ambulatory ECG monitoring to detect arrhythmias
- Exercise of pharmacologic stress testing with echocardiography preferred to detect coronary artery disease
  - Myocardial perfusion imaging may be falsely positive due to radiation fibrosis
- Coronary angiography and cardiac hemodynamic study may be necessary

TREATMENT

CARDIOLOGY REFERRAL

- Suspected cardiac disease
- Syncope

HOSPITALIZATION CRITERIA

- Heart failure
- Acute coronary syndromes
- Significant rhythm disturbances

MEDICATIONS

- Pharmacologic therapy for pericarditis, heart failure, arrhythmias, valve disease and coronary artery disease as appropriate

THERAPEUTIC PROCEDURES

- Coronary artery disease: angioplasty is less successful than bypass surgery
- Heart block: A-V sequential pacing is recommended because the ventricles are often stiff

SURGERY

- The risk of bypass surgery is increased by lung or right ventricular damage
- Sometimes the internal thoracic arteries have been damaged and other conduits are necessary
- Valvular disease: surgery is often complicated by pericardial and coronary artery disease

MONITORING

- ECG monitoring in hospital as appropriate

DIET AND ACTIVITY

- Low-sodium, low-fat diet
- Activity restriction if significant heart disease

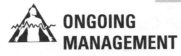 **ONGOING MANAGEMENT**

HOSPITAL DISCHARGE CRITERIA

- Resolution of problem
- Successful procedure or surgery

FOLLOW-UP

- After mediastinal radiation therapy, patients should be seen yearly with an ECG, echocardiogram, ambulatory ECG monitor, and stress test
- Thyroid function, pulmonary function, and lipid profile every 2–3 years if these remain normal

COMPLICATIONS

- Heart failure
- Syncope
- Sudden death
- Acute myocardial infarction
- Constrictive pericarditis

PROGNOSIS

- After the older techniques of radiation therapy, almost all patients had subclinical cardiac disease by 5 years
- Subclinical disease may be progressive, eventually causing morbidity and mortality

PREVENTION

- Modern irradiation techniques reduce the risk of cardiac disease
- Steroids should *not* be used prophylactically to reduce fibrosis—little evidence of benefit and toxicity high

RESOURCES

PRACTICE GUIDELINES

- Continued longitudinal screening for cardiac disease is indicated for all exposed to cardiac irradiation

REFERENCE

- Adams MJ et al: Radiation associated cardiovascular disease. Crit Rev Oncol/Hematol 2003;45:55.

INFORMATION FOR PATIENTS

- www.drpen.com/92.29

Raynaud's Phenomenon

KEY FEATURES

ESSENTIALS OF DIAGNOSIS

- One or more digits blanch with cold exposure or emotional upset and subsequently show hyperemia when warmed
- Nail fold capillaries are normal by microscopy in primary Raynaud's phenomenon
- Focal digital-tip necrosis

GENERAL CONSIDERATIONS

- Primary Raynaud's phenomenon:
  - Is 10 times more common in women than in men
  - Starts around puberty
- Raynaud-type symptoms occur in about 20% of women in northern countries
- Secondary Raynaud's phenomenon:
  - Starts at an older age
  - Is due to vasculitis or coagulopathies
  - Is more likely to result in ischemic digital injury

CLINICAL PRESENTATION

SYMPTOMS AND SIGNS

- Exposure to cold, emotional upset, or smoking causes one or more digits to blanch with subsequent hyperemia on rewarming
- Primary Raynaud's phenomenon usually spares the thumb

PHYSICAL EXAM FINDINGS

- Digital-tip necrosis can be seen in secondary Raynaud's phenomenon
- Physical findings of an autoimmune disease such as arthritis may be found

DIFFERENTIAL DIAGNOSIS

- Primary disease versus secondary causes, such as collagen vascular diseases, vasoactive drugs, and blood viscosity disorders

DIAGNOSTIC EVALUATION
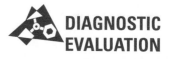

LABORATORY TESTS

- CBC, antinuclear antibody titer, rheumatoid factor, erythrocyte sedimentation rate, von Willebrand factor antigen, cryoglobulins

IMAGING STUDIES

- Capillary microscopy: useful for distinguishing primary from secondary Raynaud's phenomenon:
  - The capillaries are normal in the primary disease
  - Various degrees of capillary loss are seen in the secondary form

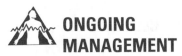

TREATMENT

MEDICATIONS

- Use vasoactive drugs, such as calcium channel blockers, eg, amlodipine 2.5–5 mg PO daily

SURGERY

- Digital sympathectomy in extreme cases

ONGOING MANAGEMENT

COMPLICATIONS

- Digital necrosis

PROGNOSIS

- Excellent in primary disease

PREVENTION

- Stop smoking
- Avoid cold exposure
- Avoid rings on affected digits

RESOURCES

REFERENCE

- Block JA, Sequeira W: Raynaud's phenomenon. Lancet 2001;357:2042.

INFORMATION FOR PATIENTS

- www.emedincine.com/medtopic1993.htm

WEB SITE

- www.emedicine.com/med/topic1993.htm

Renal Dysfunction in Heart Failure

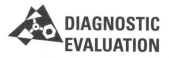 KEY FEATURES

ESSENTIALS OF DIAGNOSIS

- Congestive heart failure with elevated serum creatinine and blood urea nitrogen (BUN)

GENERAL CONSIDERATIONS

- Heart failure is common in patients with chronic renal disease, and signs of renal dysfunction (rising serum creatinine) occur in about 10% of patients with heart failure
- Renal dysfunction with heart failure is directly related to the degree of left ventricular dysfunction and, generally, reduced delivery of cardiac output to the kidney
- Hemodynamically induced renal dysfunction must be differentiated from chronic renal disease (common), the adverse effects of therapy (eg, angiotensin converting enzyme [ACE] inhibitors), and diuretic-induced hypovolemia
- Some patients present with hepatic and renal dysfunction (hepatorenal syndrome)

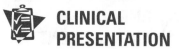 CLINICAL PRESENTATION

SYMPTOMS AND SIGNS

- Symptoms of organ hypoperfusion, such as lethargy and mental confusion

PHYSICAL EXAM FINDINGS

- Evidence of reduced perfusion:
  - Cool extremities
  - Low blood pressure
  - Tachycardia
  - Diffuse neurologic abnormalities
  - Jaundice

DIFFERENTIAL DIAGNOSIS

- Primary renal disease, such as renovascular disease, obstructive uropathy, or urinary tract infection
- Drug-induced renal dysfunction: nonsteroidal anti-inflammatory drugs, allopurinol, ACE inhibitors
- Volume depletion from aggressive use of diuretics

DIAGNOSTIC EVALUATION

LABORATORY TESTS

- Anemia, abnormal liver function tests, increased prothrombin time
- Low serum sodium, high potassium
- Rise in BUN out of proportion to rise in creatinine

ELECTROCARDIOGRAPHY

- Signs of hyperkalemia or hypocalcemia may be present
- Nonspecific ST-T–wave changes are common

IMAGING STUDIES

- Echocardiography usually shows profound left ventricular dysfunction (ejection fraction < 0.20)

DIAGNOSTIC PROCEDURES

- Right heart catheterization may be useful for defining the hemodynamic abnormality and initiating therapy

TREATMENT

CARDIOLOGY REFERRAL

- When renal dysfunction occurs during the treatment of heart failure
- Hypotension or shock

HOSPITALIZATION CRITERIA

- Rising creatinine and BUN in a patient with heart failure
- Hypotension, shock
- Rising potassium levels despite diuretics
- Low serum sodium and signs of heart failure

MEDICATIONS

- Stop unnecessary drugs
- Carefully adjust dosage of ACE inhibitors
- Carefully adjust diuretic dosage
- Maximize beta-blocker therapy for heart failure
- Avoid digoxin if possible

THERAPEUTIC PROCEDURES

- Institute ultrafiltration or hemodialysis if necessary

SURGERY

- Appropriate surgery to improve cardiac function. such as valve repair

MONITORING

- ECG monitoring in hospital

DIET AND ACTIVITY

- As appropriate for the hemodynamic and renal condition

ONGOING MANAGEMENT

HOSPITAL DISCHARGE CRITERIA

- Falling creatinine and BUN with hemodynamic stability
- Resolution of problems

FOLLOW-UP

- Careful follow-up required to maintain stability, such as every 2–6 weeks initially, then every 3 months

COMPLICATIONS

- Persistent marked renal dysfunction requiring dialysis
- Sudden death
- Persistent low output state

PROGNOSIS

- If renal dysfunction is rapidly reversible, prognosis is determined by the severity of left ventricular dysfunction
- Persistent renal dysfunction decreases survival

PREVENTION

- Careful use of diuretics
- Careful follow-up to detect low output syndrome early and intervene

RESOURCES

PRACTICE GUIDELINES

- In general, the beneficial effects of ACE inhibitors outweigh mild adverse effects on the kidney; as long as creatinine is < 2.5 mg/dL and stable, ACE inhibitors should be given
- Other treatable causes of renal dysfunction need to be excluded, such as obstruction and renal artery stenosis

REFERENCES

- Al-Ahmad A et al: Reduced kidney function and anemia as risk factors for mortality in patients with left ventricular dysfunction. J Am Coll Cardiol 2001;38:955.
- Marenzi G et al: Cardiac and renal dysfunction in chronic heart failure: Relation to neurohumoral activation and prognosis. Am J Med Sci 2001;321:359.

INFORMATION FOR PATIENTS

- www.nlm.nih.gov/medlineplus/ency/article/000158.htm

WEB SITE

- www.emedicine.com/med/topic3532.htm

Rheumatic Fever, Acute

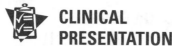 **KEY FEATURES**

ESSENTIALS OF DIAGNOSIS

- Carditis in almost 50% of those with acute rheumatic fever: heart failure, new organic heart murmur (mitral regurgitation), pericarditis
- Evidence of streptococcal infection: throat culture, detection of streptococcal antibodies
- Chorea
- Migratory arthritis
- Typical skin findings: subcutaneous nodules, erythema marginatum

GENERAL CONSIDERATIONS

- Rheumatic fever is the most common cause of cardiac disease worldwide in children and young adults
- The disease is more common in developing countries (100 per 100,000) compared with developed (2 per 100,000) countries
- The rheumatogenic strains of streptococcus have M proteins that share epitopes with cardiac myosin and sarcolemmal membrane proteins
  - Host antibodies against these epitopes cross-react with cardiac tissue, producing an inflammatory disease of all three layers of the heart
- During an outbreak of group A streptococcal pharyngitis, up to 5% get rheumatic fever
- The characteristic lesion in cardiac tissue samples is an aggregation of giant cells called an Aschoff nodule
  - These nodules are seen only in cardiac tissue despite widespread inflammation in other tissues
- Long-term sequelae of rheumatic fever occur only in the heart despite acute involvement of other tissue
- The mitral valve is most commonly affected followed by aortic, tricuspid, and pulmonic
- The valves are thickened from inflammation, and the annuli are dilated producing regurgitation (the most common finding)

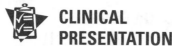 **CLINICAL PRESENTATION**

SYMPTOMS AND SIGNS

- Major manifestations:
  - Polyarthritis
  - Chorea
  - Subcutaneous nodules
  - Erythema margination
  - Carditis (eg, new mitral regurgitation murmur)
- Minor manifestations:
  - Arthralgia
  - Fever
  - Elevated acute-phase reactants (eg, erythrocyte sedimentation rate [ESR])
  - Prolonged PR interval on ECG
- Supporting evidence of antecedent group A streptococcal infection:
  - Positive throat culture
  - Positive rapid streptococcal antibody test
  - Elevated or rising streptococcal antibody titer
- The modified Jones Criteria for the diagnosis of rheumatic fever requires two major criteria or one major and two minor criteria with supporting evidence of streptococcal infection

PHYSICAL EXAM FINDINGS

- Carditis:
  - Apical pansystolic murmur of mitral regurgitation
  - Apical mid-diastolic murmur (Carey Coombs murmur)
  - Basal diastolic decrescendo murmur of aortic regurgitation (50%)
- Polyarthritis: two or more large joints (knees, ankles, elbows, wrists) showing redness, swelling and heat in a migratory pattern for 1 day to 3 weeks
- Chorea (a late manifestation [3 or more months after infection]): involuntary movements while awake
- Erythema margination: pink macular nonpruritic rash on the trunk or extremities (never the face), which appear as rings that may coalesce and look serpiginous (10%)
- Subcutaneous nodules: discrete firm painless mobile nodules (0.5–2 cm) on the extensor surfaces of joints or bony prominences, which occur about 3 weeks after other signs

DIFFERENTIAL DIAGNOSIS

- Juvenile rheumatic arthritis
- Infective endocarditis
- Myocarditis due to other causes
- Pericarditis due to other causes
- Mitral valve prolapse

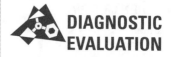 **DIAGNOSTIC EVALUATION**

LABORATORY TESTS

- ESR, CBC, C-reactive protein
- Throat culture
- Streptococcal antibody test

ELECTROCARDIOGRAPHY

- First-degree atrioventricular block
- Tachycardia
- Minor ST-T–wave changes

IMAGING STUDIES

- Chest x-ray finding: cardiac enlargement or venous congestion
- Echocardiography:
  - Increased mitral annular diameter
  - Anterior mitral leaflet prolapse
  - Chordal elongation
  - Mild leaflet thickening
  - Aortic annular dilatation
  - Leaflet prolapse
- Doppler echocardiography: mitral regurgitation or aortic regurgitation

DIAGNOSTIC PROCEDURES

- Endomyocardial biopsy shows Aschoff nodules in < 30% of patients and thus cannot be recommended for diagnostic purposes

TREATMENT

CARDIOLOGY REFERRAL

- If carditis is suspected

HOSPITALIZATION CRITERIA

- Severe valvular regurgitation
- Heart failure

MEDICATIONS

- Benzathine penicillin 1.2 million units IM *or*
- Phenoxymethyl penicillin 250 mg PO every 6 hours for 10 days *or*
- Erythromycin 250 mg PO every 6 hours for 10 days
- Aspirin 100 mg PO per day, divided into 4- to 6-hour doses

SURGERY

- Valve replacement for fulminant rheumatic carditis with severe valve regurgitation
- Valve repair does not hold up in these patients and should be done only when anticoagulation is contraindicated

MONITORING

- ECG monitoring in hospital as appropriate
- Pulse pressure:
  - Widening suggests the development of severe aortic regurgitation
  - Narrowing suggests severe mitral regurgitation

DIET AND ACTIVITY

- Low-sodium diet with carditis
- Bed rest for 8–12 weeks with carditis

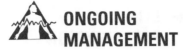 **ONGOING MANAGEMENT**

HOSPITAL DISCHARGE CRITERIA

- Resolution of manifestations of carditis
- Successful surgery

FOLLOW-UP

- After bed rest period, then at 3 months, 6 months, and 1 year

COMPLICATIONS

- Severe valvular regurgitation
- Heart failure
- Infective endocarditis

PROGNOSIS

- After rheumatic fever, < 50% have long-term cardiac sequelae
- Late cardiac disease is more common with multiple episodes of rheumatic fever
- Once valve leaflets are scarred, rheumatic disease is progressive without further episodes of rheumatic fever

PREVENTION

- Benzathine penicillin 1.2 million units IM monthly *or*
- Oral penicillin 125–250 mg PO every 12 hours *or*
- Erythomycin 250 mg PO every 12 hours
- Antibiotic therapy should be continued until age 40 unless the patient has frequent contact with children, such as parent or schoolteacher

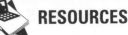 **RESOURCES**

PRACTICE GUIDELINES

- Prompt treatment of infections and prophylactic antibiotics against recurrent rheumatic fever are the mainstays of therapy
- Sporadic antibiotic therapy to prevent endocarditis is not sufficient to prevent rheumatic fever and antibiotics to prevent rheumatic fever are not sufficient for endocarditis prophylaxis

REFERENCE

- Ferrieri P et al: Proceedings of the Jones Criteria workshop. Circulation 2002;106:2521.

INFORMATION FOR PATIENTS

- www.drpen.com/398.90

WEB SITE

- www.emedicine.com/med/topic3435.htm

Rheumatoid Arthritis and the Heart

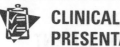

KEY FEATURES

ESSENTIALS OF DIAGNOSIS

- Clinical evidence of rheumatoid arthritis
- Pericarditis and myocarditis with characteristic granuloma on biopsy
- Granulomatous heart valve disease, predominantly of the mitral and aortic valves

GENERAL CONSIDERATIONS

- Rheumatoid arthritis (RA) is a chronic inflammatory disease characterized by specific distal extremity arthritis and arthralgias
- RA affects women more than men (2–4:1) and occurs in about 1% of the adult population
- Cardiopulmonary complications are the second leading cause of death after articular complications
- The characteristic cardiac lesion consists in granulomas involving all parts of the heart
- Clinically, cardiac disease is seen in about one-third of patients and involves all parts of the heart and blood vessels (vasculitis)
- Cardiovascular disease is more commonly found in older male patients with evidence of active inflammation
- RA also predisposes patients to atherosclerotic cardiovascular disease

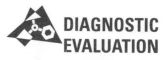

CLINICAL PRESENTATION

SYMPTOMS AND SIGNS

- Characteristic chest pain of pericarditis or myocardial ischemia
- Dyspnea on exertion, fatigue
- Palpitation

PHYSICAL EXAM FINDINGS

- Pericardial friction rub
- Murmurs of valvular heart disease
- Evidence of heart failure
- Evidence of pulmonary hypertension

DIFFERENTIAL DIAGNOSIS

- Other causes of acute pericarditis or myocarditis
- Other causes of valvular heart disease
- Other connective tissue diseases
- Other causes of pulmonary hypertension

DIAGNOSTIC EVALUATION

LABORATORY TESTS

- Positive rheumatoid factor, high erythrocyte sedimentation rate (> 55 mm/hour)
- Pericardial fluid is exudative with high protein, lactic dehydrogenase and rheumatoid factor, but low glucose
- Cardiac biomarkers: elevated myocardial creatine kinase and troponins

ELECTROCARDIOGRAPHY

- Diffuse nonspecific ST-T–wave changes are most common
- ST elevation may be seen in pericarditis and myocardial infarction
- Conduction disturbances in some
- Right ventricular hypertrophy if pulmonary pressures are elevated

IMAGING STUDIES

- Chest x-ray:
  – Cardiomegaly may be seen
- Echocardiography:
  – Pericardial effusion with pericarditis
  – Valve thickening (diffuse and nodular)
  – Valve regurgitation
  – Left ventricular dysfunction
  – Segmental wall motion abnormalities
  – Evidence of pulmonary hypertension

DIAGNOSTIC PROCEDURES

- Lung biopsy may be necessary to diagnose pulmonary vasculopathy as the cause of pulmonary hypertension
- Cardiac biopsy may be required to diagnose myocarditis
- Stress myocardial imaging studies to evaluate possible coronary artery disease
- Coronary angiography in selected cases
- Holter ambulatory ECG monitoring may be needed to diagnose significant conduction abnormalities or arrhythmias

TREATMENT

CARDIOLOGY REFERRAL

- Acute pericarditis
- Acute myocardial ischemia or infarction
- Significant valve disease
- Left ventricular dysfunction or heart failure
- Significant conduction abnormalities or arrhythmias

HOSPITALIZATION CRITERIA

- Acute pericarditis
- Heart failure
- Third-degree heart block
- Acute myocardial ischemia or infarction

MEDICATIONS

- Anti-inflammatory pharmacotherapy
- Appropriate therapy for valvular heart disease
- Lipid-lowering therapy as appropriate

THERAPEUTIC PROCEDURES

- Pericardiocentesis as necessary
- Pacemaker
- Tachycardia ablation
- Coronary artery revascularization

SURGERY

- Coronary artery bypass surgery
- Valve replacement surgery

MONITORING

- ECG monitoring in hospital as appropriate
- Inflammatory markers

DIET AND ACTIVITY

- Low-calorie, low-fat, low-sodium diet
- Activity restrictions as appropriate for condition

ONGOING MANAGEMENT

HOSPITAL DISCHARGE CRITERIA

- Resolution of problem
- Pacemaker placement
- Successful procedure/surgery

FOLLOW-UP

- Predicated on type and severity of cardiac disease

COMPLICATIONS

- Pericardial tamponade
- Heart failure
- Heart block
- Pulmonary hypertension
- Acute myocardial infarction
- Tachyarrhythmias

PROGNOSIS

- The presence of cardiac disease worsens the prognosis of rheumatoid arthritis

PREVENTION

- Coronary artery disease risk factor reduction
- Antibiotic prophylaxis for endocarditis in selected cases

RESOURCES

PRACTICE GUIDELINES

- In addition to effective anti-inflammatory and anti-immune therapy, careful attention to controlling risk factors for coronary artery disease must be taken because cardiac involvement is common and is the second leading cause of death

REFERENCES

- Nossent H: Risk of cardiovascular events and effect on mortality in patients with rheumatoid arthritis. J Rheumatol 2000;27:2282.
- Solomon DH et al: Cardiovascular morbidity and mortality in women diagnosed with rheumatoid arthritis. Circulation 2003;107:1303.
- Wolfe F et al: Increase in cardiovascular and cerebrovascular disease prevalence in rheumatoid arthritis. J Rheumatol 2003;30:36.
- Wolfe F, Michand K: Heart failure in rheumatoid arthritis: rates, predictors, and the effect of anti-tumor necrosis factor therapy. Am J Med 2004;116:305.

INFORMATION FOR PATIENTS

- www.drpen.com/714.0

WEB SITE

- www.emedicine.com/med/topic2024.htm

Scleroderma and the Heart

 KEY FEATURES

ESSENTIALS OF DIAGNOSIS

- Sclerotic skin, esophageal dysfunction, Raynaud's phenomenon
- Heart failure
- Multisegmental myocardial perfusion abnormalities
- Cor pulmonale

GENERAL CONSIDERATIONS

- Scleroderma or progressive systemic sclerosis is characterized by excessive accumulation of connective tissue and fibrosis of the skin, skeletal muscles, joint, blood vessels, kidneys, lung, gastrointestinal tract, and heart
- Scleroderma occurs in 10–20 per million people per year, is more common in women (3:1), and usually occurs in people between ages 30 and 50 years
- Ninety percent of patients with scleroderma have Raynaud's phenomenon, esophageal dysfunction, and sclerotic skin changes in a focal (80%) or a diffuse pattern (20%)
  - The more common focal type is associated with the CREST syndrome (calcinosis, Raynaud's, esophageal, sclerodactyly and telangiectasia)
  - Skin changes are often limited to the face and fingers
  - The diffuse type more frequently involves the abdominal and thoracic organs
- The diffuse type has a worse prognosis than the focal type
- The major causes of mortality are pulmonary hypertension, renal dysfunction, and heart disease
- The cardiac diseases most commonly associated with scleroderma include coronary artery disease, myocarditis, and pulmonary hypertension

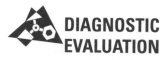 CLINICAL PRESENTATION

SYMPTOMS AND SIGNS

- Chest pain is common, but is more often due to pericarditis or esophageal reflux than to myocardial ischemia
- Dyspnea, orthopnea, and edema

PHYSICAL EXAM FINDINGS

- Typical skin findings of scleroderma, telangiectasia, subcutaneous calcified nodules
- Signs of heart failure, such as cardiomegaly, S_3, jugular venous distention, pulmonary rales, and edema
- Pericardial friction rub, pulsus paradoxus, fever
- Right ventricular lift, loud pulmonic component of S_2 with pulmonary hypertension

DIFFERENTIAL DIAGNOSIS

- Typical coronary artery disease
- Other causes of myopericarditis and heart failure
- Other causes of pulmonary hypertension and cor pulmonale

DIAGNOSTIC EVALUATION

LABORATORY TESTS

- Elevated cardiac biomarkers in myocarditis or infarction
- Exudative pericardial effusion

ELECTROCARDIOGRAPHY

- Septal Q waves usually due to fibrosis rather than infarction
- Signs of acute pericarditis
- Conduction abnormalities
- Nonspecific ST-T–wave changes
- Right ventricular hypertrophy

IMAGING STUDIES

- Chest x-ray: enlarged cardiac silhouette
- Echocardiography may show the following common findings:
  - Diffuse left ventricular dysfunction or segmental wall motion abnormalities
  - Left ventricular hypertrophy
  - Left atrial enlargement
  - Doppler evidence of diastolic dysfunction
  - Nonspecific valve thickening and regurgitation
  - Also seen are pericardial effusion and signs of tamponade, and right ventricular and atrial hypertrophy
- Rest or exercise radionuclide myocardial perfusion imaging may show multisegmental perfusion defects
- CT or MRI is useful for evaluating pericardial thickness

DIAGNOSTIC PROCEDURES

- Myocardial biopsy may be useful to diagnose scleroderma involvement in selected patients
- Electrophysiologic studies may be useful to define the severity of conduction disease and arrhythmias

TREATMENT

CARDIOLOGY REFERRAL

- Suspected cardiac disease
- Syncope
- Pulmonary hypertension

HOSPITALIZATION CRITERIA

- Syncope
- Myocardial ischemia/infarction
- Pericarditis/tamponade
- Heart failure

MEDICATIONS

- Specific anti-inflammatory pharma-cotherapy
- Calcium channel blockers for Raynaud's phenomenon and pulmonary hypertension, eg, amlodipine 2.5–10 mg PO daily
- Specific therapy for pulmonary hypertension, eg, Flolan, Bosentan

THERAPEUTIC PROCEDURES

- Pericardiocentesis as necessary
- Coronary revascularization
- Pacemaker

SURGERY

- Pericardial stripping
- Valve repair/replacement

MONITORING

- ECG monitoring in hospital as appropriate

DIET AND ACTIVITY

- Low-sodium diet in heart failure
- Low-fat diet in coronary disease

ONGOING MANAGEMENT

HOSPITAL DISCHARGE CRITERIA

- Resolution of acute problem
- Successful procedures or surgery

FOLLOW-UP

- Depends on the cardiac problem and its severity

COMPLICATIONS

- Pericardial tamponade/constriction
- Heart failure
- Myocardial infarction
- Syncope

PROGNOSIS

- Cumulative survival rate in scleroderma is about 50% at 10 years
- Heart failure markedly reduces survival in scleroderma
- Cardiac arrhythmias and conduction abnormalities portend a poor prognosis
- Pericarditis reduces survival perhaps because it is associated with chronic renal disease severity

PREVENTION

- There are no known preventive measures for scleroderma

RESOURCES

PRACTICE GUIDELINES

- Most cardiac disease seen with scleroderma is secondary to pulmonary and systemic hypertension due to pulmonary fibrosis and renovascular disease, respectively
- Selected patients may benefit from lung or kidney transplantation

REFERENCE

- Steen V: The heart in systemic sclerosis. Curr Rheumatol Rep 2004;6:137.

INFORMATION FOR PATIENTS

- www.hlm.nih.gov/medlineplus/scleroderma.html
- www.drpen.com/710.1

WEB SITE

- www.emedicine.com/med/topic2076.htm

Sexual Dysfunction in Cardiac Disease

KEY FEATURES

ESSENTIALS OF DIAGNOSIS

- Erectile dysfunction is more prevalent in patients with cardiovascular disease
- Leriche syndrome and vascular impotence occasionally cause erectile dysfunction
- Sexual activity is a form of exercise and can precipitate angina or acute coronary syndromes

GENERAL CONSIDERATIONS

- Erectile dysfunction can be primary or secondary to risk factors, such as hypertension, diabetes, cigarette smoking, and hypercholesterolemia
- Little is known about female sexual dysfunction in cardiovascular disease
- Erectile dysfunction increases with age
- New pharmacologic treatments for erectile dysfunction have exposed sexually inactive men to the risks of sexual activities
- Sexual intercourse increases oxygen demand by about 3–5 metabolic equivalents
- Any patient who is free of ischemia on submaximal exercise test can safely engage in sexual activity

CLINICAL PRESENTATION

SYMPTOMS AND SIGNS

- Erectile dysfunction
- Dizziness, syncope after sexual activity
- Angina with sexual activity

PHYSICAL EXAM FINDINGS

- Hypotension
- Tachycardia
- S_4

DIFFERENTIAL DIAGNOSIS

- Psychogenic impotence
- Medication-induced sexual dysfunction
- Autonomic neuropathy
- Severe ischemia heart disease
- Hypogonadism

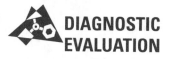 DIAGNOSTIC EVALUATION

LABORATORY TESTS

- Low serum testosterone in some

ELECTROCARDIOGRAPHY

- ECG: may show signs of myocardial ischemia/infarction

IMAGING STUDIES

- Echocardiography: may show left ventricular hypertrophy or dysfunction

DIAGNOSTIC PROCEDURES

- Coronary angiography may be necessary

TREATMENT

CARDIOLOGY REFERRAL

- Presence of cardiac disease

HOSPITALIZATION CRITERIA

- Acute coronary syndromes
- Syncope
- Persistent hypotension

MEDICATIONS

- Oral sildenafil 25–100 mg PO, vardenofil, and tadalafil are effective for erectile dysfunction (caution with concurrent nitroglycerin use)
- Give transurethral or cavernosal alprostadil (prostaglandin E1) if nitrates cannot be stopped
- Testosterone may help some

THERAPEUTIC PROCEDURES

- Percutaneous revascularization may be necessary

SURGERY

- Coronary bypass surgery may be indicated

MONITORING

- ECG monitoring in hospital as appropriate

DIET AND ACTIVITY

- Low-fat diet
- Activity predicted by cardiac disease
- In general, a negative exercise stress test permits sexual intercourse

ONGOING MANAGEMENT

HOSPITAL DISCHARGE CRITERIA

- Resolution of problem
- Successful revascularization

FOLLOW-UP

- Predicated by cardiac disease status

COMPLICATIONS

- Erectile dysfunction drugs can precipitate dangerous hypotension in certain circumstances, such as concomitant nitroglycerin use
- Sexual activity can lead to acute coronary syndromes

PROGNOSIS

- Myocardial ischemia caused by sexual activity suggests severe coronary artery disease, since sexual activity with a familiar partner is a low-intensity exercise
- Erectile dysfunction can often be safely managed with the phosphodiesterase 5 inhibitors, such as sildenafil

PREVENTION

- Acute ischemic events during sexual intercourse can be prevented by pretreatment with nitrates if erectile dysfunction drugs are not necessary for sexual activity
- Revascularization or effective anti anginal therapy may permit sexual activity without precipitating myocardial ischemia
- Erectile dysfunction drugs should be used with caution in patients on multiple vasodilator drugs for hypertension or heart failure or cytochrome P450 3A4 inhibitors, such as erythromycin
- Erectile dysfunction can be improved by stopping certain antihypertensive drugs, such as thiazide diuretics

RESOURCES

PRACTICE GUIDELINES

- Erectile dysfunction drug plus nitrate-induced hypotension should be treated with volume infusion and vasoconstrictor drugs such as dopamine
- Acute myocardial ischemia after use of an erectile dysfunction drug should be treated with IV beta blockers or diltiazem

REFERENCE

- Solomon H et al: Relation of erectile dysfunction to angiographic coronary artery disease. Am J Cardiol 2003;91:230.

INFORMATION FOR PATIENTS

- www.my.webmd.com/medical_information/condition_centers/default.htm (select Men's Health - erectile dysfunction)

Sinus Arrhythmia

KEY FEATURES

ESSENTIALS OF DIAGNOSIS

- Cyclic heart rate variation with respiration
- Nonrespiratory form may be related to sick sinus syndrome or digitalis intoxication
- Variability of P-P cycle length at least 160 ms or 10% of the minimum cycle length
- P-wave morphology identical to normal sinus rhythm

GENERAL CONSIDERATIONS

- Sinus arrhythmia is seen in young patients or those treated with digitalis or morphine
- It is rarely associated with increased intracranial pressure
- The respiratory form is common in young people because of enhanced vagal tone
- The respiratory form becomes less pronounced with advancing age and in autonomic dysfunction such as diabetes
- The nonrespiratory form is seen in diseased hearts
- Sinus arrhythmia with bradycardia can develop during recovery from acute illness or 2–3 days after inferior myocardial infarction
- P-P intervals that contain a QRS complex are shorter than those that do not (ventriculophasic sinus arrhythmia); this may be secondary to vagal influence responding to changes in stroke volume
- Loss of sinus rhythm variability is a marker for sudden cardiac death

CLINICAL PRESENTATION

SYMPTOMS AND SIGNS

- Usually causes no symptoms
- The nonrespiratory form with sick sinus syndrome may cause features of cerebral hypoperfusion such as lightheadedness

PHYSICAL EXAM FINDINGS

- Normal exam in most patients

DIFFERENTIAL DIAGNOSIS

- Sinoatrial exit block
- Sinus pause
- Nonconducted premature atrial beats

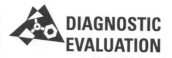 DIAGNOSTIC EVALUATION

LABORATORY TESTS

- None required

ELECTROCARDIOGRAPHY

- ECG with a rhythm strip to diagnose and document rhythm disorder

IMAGING STUDIES

- Usually none required

DIAGNOSTIC PROCEDURES

- Electrophysiology study rarely indicated

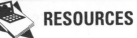

TREATMENT

CARDIOLOGY REFERRAL

- Not required in most situations

HOSPITALIZATION CRITERIA

- Not required in most situations

MEDICATIONS

- Treat underlying cause
- Withdraw offending drug

THERAPEUTIC PROCEDURES

- None required

SURGERY

- None required

MONITORING

- None required in the respiratory form
- In nonrespiratory form, ECG monitoring in hospital may be useful

DIET AND ACTIVITY

- General healthy life style

ONGOING MANAGEMENT

FOLLOW-UP

- Not required except for the nonrespiratory form
- In the nonrespiratory form, patients should be reevaluated once there are symptoms of cerebral hypoperfusion

COMPLICATIONS

- Usually none

PROGNOSIS

- Very good

RESOURCES

PRACTICE GUIDELINES

- This is benign arrhythmia
- Reassurance may be needed in some patients

REFERENCES

- Blomstrom-Lundqvist C, Scheinman MM, Aliot EM et al: ACC/AHA/ESC guidelines for the management of patients with supraventricular arrhythmias: executive summary. A report of the American College of Cardiology/American Heart Association Task Force on Practice Guidelines and the European Society of Cardiology Committee for Practice Guidelines (writing committee to develop guidelines for the management of patients with supraventricular arrhythmias) developed in collaboration with NASPE-Heart Rhythm Society. J Am Coll Cardiol 2003;42:1493.

INFORMATION FOR PATIENTS

- www.nlm.nih.gov/medlineplus/arrhythmia.html

WEB SITES

- www.acc.org
- www.hrsonline.org

Sinus Bradycardia

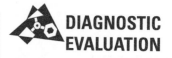

KEY FEATURES

ESSENTIALS OF DIAGNOSIS

- Sinus rate is less than 60 bpm
- P waves have normal contour with a constant PR interval
- PR interval exceeds 120 ms
- Sinus arrhythmia often coexists

GENERAL CONSIDERATIONS

- May be a manifestation of sick sinus syndrome
- High vagal tone (young adults and athletes) or medications (eg, beta blockers) are possible causes
- Increased intracranial pressure and myxedema are among several other causes
- Acute myocardial infarction (particularly inferior) is associated with sinus bradycardia
- Patients with anorexia nervosa may have sinus bradycardia
- Not uncommon in cardiac transplant recipients
- During sleep, the heart rate can fall to 35–40 bpm especially in young adults; pauses ≥ 2 sec are not uncommon
- Hypothermia, severe hypoxia, coronary angiography, eye surgery, mediastinal tumors, and convalescence from infection are possible causes
- Obstructive jaundice is a possible cause
- Eye drops containing beta blockers is an easily overlooked cause
- Bradycardia after resuscitation from cardiac arrest carries a poor prognosis

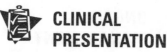

CLINICAL PRESENTATION

SYMPTOMS AND SIGNS

- Generally asymptomatic

PHYSICAL EXAM FINDINGS

- Rarely causes hemodynamic decompensation in acute myocardial infarction

DIFFERENTIAL DIAGNOSIS

- Ectopic atrial bradycardia

DIAGNOSTIC EVALUATION

LABORATORY TESTS

- Depends on clinical situation
- Thyroid-stimulating hormone

ELECTROCARDIOGRAPHY

- ECG to document rhythm
- Rhythm strip to define mechanism

IMAGING STUDIES

- Usually none required

DIAGNOSTIC PROCEDURES

- ECG and clinical examination are sufficient for diagnosis

TREATMENT

CARDIOLOGY REFERRAL

- If part of sick sinus syndrome, referral to an electrophysiologist is required for evaluation of permanent pacemaker

HOSPITALIZATION CRITERIA

- Does not require hospitalization by itself
- Hospitalization may be for concomitant illness

MEDICATIONS

- Usually no specific treatment is needed
- If patients are symptomatic acutely, atropine may be used to increase the sinus rate
- Medications such as theophylline and ephedrine may be used cautiously without overshooting to sinus tachycardia

THERAPEUTIC PROCEDURES

- Patients with recurrent symptoms are treated with a pacemaker

SURGERY

- None required

MONITORING

- ECG monitoring if hospitalized

DIET AND ACTIVITY

- General healthy life style

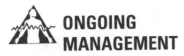 **ONGOING MANAGEMENT**

HOSPITAL DISCHARGE CRITERIA

- Depends on concomitant illness

FOLLOW-UP

- Usually none required except when symptoms are suggestive of sick sinus syndrome

COMPLICATIONS

- Syncope secondary to sick sinus syndrome

PROGNOSIS

- Generally very good
- A benign condition in most patients

PREVENTION

- Avoid negative chronotropic medications in patients with baseline heart rate that is bordering on sinus bradycardia

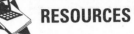 **RESOURCES**

PRACTICE GUIDELINES

- Pacemaker is rarely necessary
- Symptoms must correlate with bradycardia before a pacemaker is inserted
- It is usually a benign condition

REFERENCES

- Blomstrom-Lundqvist C, Scheinman MM, Aliot EM et al: ACC/AHA/ESC guidelines for the management of patients with supraventricular arrhythmias: executive summary. A report of the American College of Cardiology/ American Heart Association Task Force on Practice Guidelines and the European Society of Cardiology Committee for Practice Guidelines (writing committee to develop guidelines for the management of patients with supraventricular arrhythmias) developed in collaboration with NASPE-Heart Rhythm Society. J Am Coll Cardiol 2003;42:1493.
- Mangrum JM, DiMarco JP: The evaluation and management of bradycardia. N Engl J Med 2000;342:703.

INFORMATION FOR PATIENTS

- www.nlm.nih.gov/medlineplus/ arrhythmia.html

WEB SITE

- www.hrsonline.org

Sinus Node Dysfunction

 KEY FEATURES

ESSENTIALS OF DIAGNOSIS

- Sinus bradycardia with rate < 50 bpm
- Sinoatrial exit block type I: progressively shorter P-P intervals followed by failure of occurrence of a P wave
- Sinoatrial exit block type II: pauses in sinus rhythm that are multiples of basic sinus rate
- First-degree and third-degree sinoatrial exit blocks are difficult to diagnose
- Sinus arrest or pause: failure of occurrence of P waves at expected times

GENERAL CONSIDERATIONS

- Usually caused by a degenerative process associated with aging
- Negative chronotropic drugs may cause a similar problem
- Tachycardia–bradycardia syndrome (bradycardia secondary to sinus node dysfunction coupled with supraventricular arrhythmia such as atrial fibrillation)
- Differentiation between sinus arrest and high-grade exit block is not possible without direct recordings of sinus node discharge
- Myocardial infarction (MI), digitalis toxicity, stroke or excessive vagal tone all may cause this problem

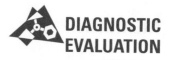 **CLINICAL PRESENTATION**

SYMPTOMS AND SIGNS

- Syncope
- Lightheadedness
- Dizziness
- Symptoms of concomitant illness such as MI

PHYSICAL EXAM FINDINGS

- Bradycardia
- Irregular heart sounds
- Other findings depend on precipitating cause

DIFFERENTIAL DIAGNOSIS

- Blocked premature atrial contraction may resemble sinoatrial exit block
- Marked sinus arrhythmia
- Conditions with high vagal tone (eg, young athletic individual, cough, micturition)

DIAGNOSTIC EVALUATION

LABORATORY TESTS

- Depends on suspected concomitant illness or precipitating causes
- CBC, basic metabolic panel, thyroid-stimulating hormone

ELECTROCARDIOGRAPHY

- ECG to document rhythm disturbance

IMAGING STUDIES

- None required for the rhythm alone
- Echocardiogram may be done if the precipitating cause is MI or myocarditis

DIAGNOSTIC PROCEDURES

- Electrophysiologic study rarely indicated

TREATMENT

CARDIOLOGY REFERRAL

- If associated with syncope or symptoms of cerebral hypoperfusion, then referral to an electrophysiologist is required

HOSPITALIZATION CRITERIA

- Syncope
- Usually hospitalized for precipitating cause

MEDICATIONS

- Avoid or eliminate negative chronotropic drugs

THERAPEUTIC PROCEDURES

- Symptomatic patients without reversible cause need a pacemaker
- Although atrial pacing may be sufficient because most patients subsequently develop atrioventricular nodal disease, dual-chamber pacemakers are recommended

SURGERY

- None required

MONITORING

- ECG monitoring for hospitalized patients

DIET AND ACTIVITY

- General healthy life style
- Depends on underlying medical illness

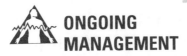

ONGOING MANAGEMENT

HOSPITAL DISCHARGE CRITERIA

- After pacemaker implantation
- Stabilization of precipitating cause

FOLLOW-UP

- Two weeks after discharge from the hospital
- Depends on comorbid conditions
- After pacemaker implantation, long-term follow up with primary care physician

COMPLICATIONS

- Syncope and associated trauma

PROGNOSIS

- Generally very good
- Depends on comorbid conditions

PREVENTION

- Avoid negative chronotropic drugs if possible in patients with sinus bradycardia

RESOURCES

PRACTICE GUIDELINES

- Indications for pacemaker insertion:
  - Sinus node dysfunction with documented symptomatic bradycardia, including frequent sinus pauses that produce symptoms
  - Iatrogenic bradycardia occurring as a consequence of essential long-term medication
  - Symptomatic chronotropic incompetence

REFERENCES

- Adan V, Crown LA: Diagnosis and treatment of sick sinus syndrome. Am Fam Physician 2003;67:1725.

INFORMATION FOR PATIENTS

- www.nlm.nih.gov/medlineplus/arrhythmia.html

WEB SITE

- www.hrsonline.org

Sinus Node Reentry

 KEY FEATURES

ESSENTIALS OF DIAGNOSIS

- Heart rate 100–160 bpm
- Each QRS preceded by a P wave identical with the P wave of normal sinus rhythm
- Abrupt onset and termination
- Organic heart disease in many patients

GENERAL CONSIDERATIONS

- Accounts for less than 5% of supraventricular tachycardia
- Reentry uses the sinus node or perinodal tissue
- Heart rate similar to that in sinus tachycardia
- Longitudinal dissociation as seen in atrioventricular node may be substrate for reentry in the sinoatrial node
- This tachycardia is not physiologic unlike sinus tachycardia
- Tachycardia is precipitated by an ectopic beat and exhibits characteristics of a reentry circuit
- The arrhythmia can be acutely terminated by adenosine, verapamil, or carotid sinus massage
- The tachycardia may be induced in the electrophysiologic lab with premature atrial stimuli or burst pacing
- May be an incidental arrhythmia during a study for another diagnosis

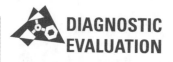 **CLINICAL PRESENTATION**

SYMPTOMS AND SIGNS

- Palpitations
- Dyspnea

PHYSICAL EXAM FINDINGS

- Depends on precipitating cause
- Elevated jugular venous pressure
- S_3

DIFFERENTIAL DIAGNOSIS

- Sinus tachycardia
- Inappropriate sinus tachycardia
- Atrial tachycardia

DIAGNOSTIC EVALUATION

LABORATORY TESTS

- CBC, brain natriuretic peptide
- Thyroid-stimulating hormone

ELECTROCARDIOGRAPHY

- ECG to document rhythm disorder
- Holter monitoring to determine frequency

IMAGING STUDIES

- None required
- Echocardiogram for underlying myocardial disease

DIAGNOSTIC PROCEDURES

- Electrophysiologic study to confirm mechanism and determine suitability for ablation

TREATMENT

CARDIOLOGY REFERRAL

- If the tachycardia is precipitating recurrent heart failure, then electrophysiology referral recommended

HOSPITALIZATION CRITERIA

- Symptomatic patients may require hospitalization for control with medications or ablation

MEDICATIONS

- Digoxin and calcium channel blockers are the most useful drugs
- Beta blockers may not be very useful

THERAPEUTIC PROCEDURES

- Radiofrequency ablation is usually curative

SURGERY

- Generally not required

MONITORING

- ECG monitoring if hospitalized

DIET AND ACTIVITY

- Depends on underlying heart disease

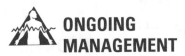

ONGOING MANAGEMENT

HOSPITAL DISCHARGE CRITERIA

- Symptomatic stability

FOLLOW-UP

- Depends on underlying heart disease

COMPLICATIONS

- Exacerbations of heart failure

PROGNOSIS

- Depends on underlying heart disease

RESOURCES

PRACTICE GUIDELINES

- Indications for electrophysiologic study:
  - Frequent and poorly tolerated tachycardia that does not adequately respond to medications and exact nature of the tachycardia is uncertain

REFERENCE

- Cossu SF, Steinberg JS: Supraventricular tachyarrhythmias involving the sinus node: clinical and electrophysiologic characteristics. Prog Cardiovasc Dis 1998;41:51.

INFORMATION FOR PATIENTS

- www.nlm.nih.gov/medlineplus/ arrhythmia.html

WEB SITES

- www.hrsonline.org
- www.acc.org

Sinus of Valsalva Aneurysm

KEY FEATURES

ESSENTIALS OF DIAGNOSIS

- Diverticulum of a coronary sinus of the aortic valve

GENERAL CONSIDERATIONS

- Rare congenital cardiac defect due to a defect in the aortic media that leads to aortic root dilation and usually including the right aortic sinus
- Acquired sinus of Valsalva aneurysm may be due to Marfan syndrome or syphilitic aortitis or is a function of aging
- Other generalized disorders such as Ehlers-Danlos, Turner, and Williams syndromes, osteogenesis imperfecta, and traumatic injury may be associated with aortic root dilation and/or distortion
- Associated with a ventricular septal defect (usually supracristal) in 40% of patients
- Often associated with aortic insufficiency
- Leads to progressive dilation of the aorta usually over many years
- Rupture into any chamber (usually the right ventricle followed by the right atrium) possible
- Compression of the coronary arteries and/or the conduction system may lead to ischemia and/or heart block, respectively

CLINICAL PRESENTATION

SYMPTOMS AND SIGNS

- Chest and/or epigastric pain similar to that in acute myocardial infarction, which occurs suddenly after strenuous exertion due to sudden rupture of the aneurysm
- Progressive exertional dyspnea and/or chest pain in patients with advancing heart failure related to smaller insidious ruptures
- Patients with unruptured aneurysms may be asymptomatic or have angina from coronary artery compression or symptoms of heart block related to compression of the conduction system

PHYSICAL EXAM FINDINGS

- Patients without aneurysm rupture often have normal exam findings
- An ejection murmur may be present at the left base radiating into the back with an unruptured aneurysm partially obstructing the right ventricular outflow tract
- Bounding pulses, aortic regurgitation in patients with rupture into the left ventricle
- Loud continuous murmur with the diastolic component best heard along the sternal border in patients with rupture into the right cardiac chambers
- Pulmonary rales may be present

DIFFERENTIAL DIAGNOSIS

- Aortic dissection
- Aortic regurgitation with aortic root dilatation
- Aorta to pulmonary artery fistula (anterior-posterior window)
- Ventricular septal defect
- Coronary artery aneurysm with fistula to right heart
- Rupture may simulate other causes of acute chest pain or heart failure

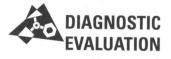 DIAGNOSTIC EVALUATION

LABORATORY TESTS

- No specific serologic or genetic markers have been identified

ELECTROCARDIOGRAPHY

- Biventricular hypertrophy by voltage in patients with ruptured aneurysm
- ST-T depression caused by myocardial ischemia
- Second- or third-degree heart block in patients with conduction system involvement

IMAGING STUDIES

- Echocardiography:
  - Provides an accurate description of the aortic root, proximal aorta, aortic valve, and surrounding structures
  - Doppler findings can provide an accurate indication of the shunt location and magnitude
- Chest x-ray:
  - Cardiomegaly—right heart enlargement in the setting of rupture into the right ventricle
  - Pulmonary congestion may be present
- MRI: identifies ruptured and unruptured sinus Valsalva aneurysms and detects shunt flow
- Transesophageal echocardiography:
  - May be helpful to depict the exact point of rupture and more detailed diagnosis of anatomy and shunt description

DIAGNOSTIC PROCEDURES

- Cardiac catheterization with coronary and aortic angiography:
  - Allows magnification of shunts, cardiac outputs, and hemodynamics

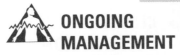

 TREATMENT

CARDIOLOGY REFERRAL

- Ruptured or unruptured sinus of Valsalva aneurysm
- Heart failure
- Dysrhythmias

HOSPITALIZATION CRITERIA

- Rupture or suspected rupture of sinus of Valsalva aneurysm
- Congestive heart failure
- Dysrhythmia

MEDICATIONS

- Diuretics, digitalis, and angiotensin-converting enzyme inhibitors as indicated for heart failure
- Nitrates and beta blocker for myocardial ischemia
- Endocarditis prophylaxis is recommended
- Antihypertensives as needed

THERAPEUTIC PROCEDURES

- Catheter-based device closure for ruptured aneurysms may be performed in some cases based on the anatomy and shunt severity

SURGERY

- Prompt surgical therapy is recommended for ruptured sinus of Valsalva aneurysm with closure of a ventricular septal defect and/or aortic valve replacement, if necessary
- Repair of a known unruptured sinus of Valsalva aneurysm is recommended at the time of surgical repair of any intracardiac shunt or defect

MONITORING

- ECG monitoring in hospital

DIET AND ACTIVITY

- Avoidance of vigorous exertion and contact sports for patients with unruptured aneurysms
- Activity as tolerated for patients with ruptured aneurysms awaiting surgery

ONGOING MANAGEMENT

HOSPITAL DISCHARGE CRITERIA

- After surgical repair of ruptured aneurysm

FOLLOW-UP

- For unruptured aneurysms: serial echo or MRI to document size of aneurysm

COMPLICATIONS

- Congestive heart failure and infective endocarditis in patients with ruptured aneurysms
- Heart block
- Angina and myocardial ischemia
- Aortobronchial fistula or aortopulmonary artery fistula (rare)

PROGNOSIS

- Morbidity and mortality are related to rupture and the size and location of the shunt
- Mortality rate within the first year after rupture is high in those who do not have surgery
- Prognosis after surgical repair is excellent

PREVENTION

- No known preventive measures other than endocarditis prophylaxis

RESOURCES

PRACTICE GUIDELINES

- Prompt surgical repair of ruptured sinus of Valsalva aneurysms with aortic valve replacement and/or closure of a ventricular septal defect, if necessary, is recommended
- No consensus exists as to when to electively repair incidentally discovered unruptured sinus of Valsalva aneurysms
- Affected patients should be counseled to avoid contact sports and other strenuous activities, and they should be monitored with serial imaging studies using echo or MRI

REFERENCES

- Harkness JR: A 32-year experience with surgical repair of sinus of Valsalva aneurysms. J Card Surg 2005;20:198.
- Hijazi ZM: Ruptured sinus of Valsalva aneurysm: management options. Catheter Cardiovasc Interv 2003;58:135.

INFORMATION FOR PATIENTS

- http://www.heartcenteronline.com/ myheartdr/common/ articles.cfm?ARTID=551

WEB SITE

- http://www.emedicine.com/ped/ topic2106.htm

Sinus Tachycardia

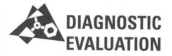 KEY FEATURES

ESSENTIALS OF DIAGNOSIS

- Heart rate 100–160 bpm
- Each QRS is preceded by a P wave identical to the P wave of normal sinus rhythm
- Physiologic response to exercise or adrenergic response to disease

GENERAL CONSIDERATIONS

- Common causes:
  – Blood loss
  – Volume depletion
  – Hyperthyroidism
  – Fever
  – Sepsis
  – Pulmonary embolism
  – Hypotension
- Heart rate achieved is proportional to the intensity of the stimulus
- Rate changes result from a shift of pacemaker activity within sinus node
- Carotid sinus massage or Valsalva maneuver may temporarily slow the heart rate, and the rate returns to baseline upon cessation of the maneuver
- Common in infancy and early childhood
- Thyroid medication excess, alcohol, nicotine, and caffeine may cause sinus tachycardia
- Sinus tachycardia after heart transplantation carries adverse prognosis
- Persistent sinus tachycardia may be a manifestation of heart failure
- May be appropriate response to stimuli, or inappropriate without any provocation

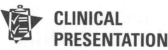 CLINICAL PRESENTATION

SYMPTOMS AND SIGNS

- Palpitations
- Depends on precipitating cause

PHYSICAL EXAM FINDINGS

- Other than tachycardia, findings depends on underlying precipitating cause

DIFFERENTIAL DIAGNOSIS

- Sinus node reentry
- Atrial tachycardia

DIAGNOSTIC EVALUATION

LABORATORY TESTS

- Thyroid-stimulating hormone
- CBC, basal metabolic panel
- Depending on clinical suspicion

ELECTROCARDIOGRAPHY

- ECG

IMAGING STUDIES

- If heart failure is suspected, then echocardiogram to evaluate left ventricular function

DIAGNOSTIC PROCEDURES

- None required

TREATMENT

CARDIOLOGY REFERRAL

• Generally not required

HOSPITALIZATION CRITERIA

• Depends on underlying precipitating cause

MEDICATIONS

• Treat underlying cause

THERAPEUTIC PROCEDURES

• None required

SURGERY

• None required

MONITORING

• Depends on precipitating cause

DIET AND ACTIVITY

• General healthy life style

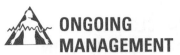

ONGOING MANAGEMENT

HOSPITAL DISCHARGE CRITERIA

• Depends on underlying clinical illness

FOLLOW-UP

• Depends on precipitating cause

COMPLICATIONS

• Usually none
• If tachycardia is inappropriate and persistent, it may lead to cardiomyopathy

PROGNOSIS

• Depends on precipitating cause
• Tachycardia resolves with the cure of the inciting condition

RESOURCES

PRACTICE GUIDELINES

• Management:
  – Identify a secondary cause and treat
  – Beta blockade is very useful for emotional stress and anxiety-related tachycardia

REFERENCE

• Cossu SF, Steinberg JS: Supraventricular tachyarrhythmias involving the sinus node: clinical and electrophysiologic characteristics. Prog Cardiovasc Dis 1998;41:51.

INFORMATION FOR PATIENTS

• www.nlm.nih.gov/medlineplus/arrhythmia.html

WEB SITE

• www.hrsonline.org

Sinus Tachycardia, Inappropriate

 KEY FEATURES

ESSENTIALS OF DIAGNOSIS

- Heart rates > 100 bpm at rest or with minimal exertion
- P waves identical or nearly identical to sinus P wave
- Chronic duration of symptoms
- Exclusion of other causes of sinus tachycardia

GENERAL CONSIDERATIONS

- Frequently seen in young female health care workers
- May occur transiently after ablation of other supraventricular arrhythmias
- The arrhythmia is nonparoxysmal and not associated with underlying cardiac pathologic process
- Alteration in autonomic tone with increase in sympathetic output or reduction in parasympathetic tone is likely to be the primary abnormality
- Primary problem of the sinus node itself and beta-adrenergic hypersensitivity suggested in some studies
- May cause tachycardia cardiomyopathy if untreated

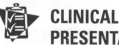 **CLINICAL PRESENTATION**

SYMPTOMS AND SIGNS

- Chest pain
- Palpitations
- Dyspnea
- Near syncope

PHYSICAL EXAM FINDINGS

- Tachycardia

DIFFERENTIAL DIAGNOSIS

- Appropriate sinus tachycardia
- Sinus node reentry
- Atrial tachycardia
- Postural orthostatic tachycardia syndrome (POTS)

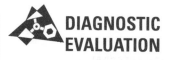 **DIAGNOSTIC EVALUATION**

LABORATORY TESTS

- Serum thyroid-stimulating hormone
- CBC, basal metabolic panel

ELECTROCARDIOGRAPHY

- ECG to document rhythm disorder

IMAGING STUDIES

- Echocardiogram if there are features of heart failure

DIAGNOSTIC PROCEDURES

- Electrophysiologic study may be necessary to establish mechanism of arrhythmia and determine suitability for ablation

TREATMENT

CARDIOLOGY REFERRAL

- Electrophysiology referral is required if heart rate cannot be controlled with adequate doses of beta blockers

HOSPITALIZATION CRITERIA

- Usually not required except in tachycardia cardiomyopathy

MEDICATIONS

- High doses of beta blockers (atenolol 100–200 mg/day) or propranolol 320 mg/day
- Rate-lowering calcium channel blockers

THERAPEUTIC PROCEDURES

- Radiofrequency modification of sinoatrial node (high recurrence rate of 20–30%)
- Intracoronary ethanol ablation may be tried in selected patients

SURGERY

- Surgery rarely done
- Surgical exclusion of right atrium
- Intraoperative cryoablation

MONITORING

- Monitor heart rate and symptoms of cardiomyopathy

DIET AND ACTIVITY

- General healthy life style

ONGOING MANAGEMENT

HOSPITAL DISCHARGE CRITERIA

- After control of heat failure

FOLLOW-UP

- Frequent follow-up may be needed to titrate medications
- Follow-up 2–4 weeks after radiofrequency ablation

COMPLICATIONS

- Cardiomyopathy
- Complications of radiofrequency ablation include:
  - Need for a pacemaker
  - Superior vena cava syndrome

PROGNOSIS

- Patient may remain symptomatic but mortality is uncommon except when associated with advanced heart failure

RESOURCES

PRACTICE GUIDELINES

- Diagnosis:
  - Nonparoxysmal tachycardia
  - Increases with activity
  - Normalizes nocturnally
  - Endocardial activation sequence identical to sinus rhythm and secondary causes excluded
- Management:
  - Beta blockers
  - Non-dihydropyridine calcium channel blockers
  - Exclude POTS before ablation attempts

REFERENCE

- Kanjwal MY, Kosinski DJ, Grubb BP: Treatment of postural orthostatic tachycardia syndrome and inappropriate sinus tachycardia. Curr Cardiol Rep 2003;5:402.

INFORMATION FOR PATIENTS

- www.nlm.nih.gov/medlineplus/ arrhythmia.html

WEB SITE

- www.hrsonline.org

Subclavian Coronary Artery Steal Syndrome

KEY FEATURES

ESSENTIALS OF DIAGNOSIS

- Post–coronary artery bypass grafting (CABG) using an internal thoracic artery pedicle graft
- Angina with unilateral arm exercise
- Subclavian artery stenosis demonstrated by imaging, proximal to the internal thoracic artery used for the coronary graft in the affected upper arm

GENERAL CONSIDERATIONS

- The internal thoracic artery is the preferred conduit for proximal left anterior descending CABG because of its relative resistance to atherosclerosis and demonstrated excellent long-term patency
- Unfortunately, the subclavian artery, from which the internal thoracic is a branch, is a common site of atherosclerotic plaque build-up
- When the subclavian is obstructed proximal to the origin of the internal thoracic, coronary blood flow can be compromised, especially during arm exercise

CLINICAL PRESENTATION

SYMPTOMS AND SIGNS

- Angina pectoris with unilateral arm exercise
- Vertebrobasilar symptoms with unilateral arm exercise

PHYSICAL EXAM FINDINGS

- Systolic blood pressure > 20 mm Hg difference between right and left arm
- Reduced pulse in affected arm

DIFFERENTIAL DIAGNOSIS

- Progressive native coronary artery disease
- Technical problems with the internal thoracic artery graft
- Disease in vein grafts to other coronary arteries

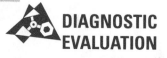 DIAGNOSTIC EVALUATION

ELECTROCARDIOGRAPHY

- ST-T changes of ischemia

IMAGING STUDIES

- Stress myocardial imaging demonstrates ischemia

DIAGNOSTIC PROCEDURES

- Catheterization and angiography demonstrate the subclavian obstruction proximal to the internal thoracic artery origin

TREATMENT

CARDIOLOGY REFERRAL

- Recurrent angina after bypass surgery

HOSPITALIZATION CRITERIA

- Acute coronary syndrome
- Significant resting arm ischemia (rare)

MEDICATIONS

- Standard antianginal drugs, such as beta blockers

THERAPEUTIC PROCEDURES

- Angioplasty and stenting of the subclavian artery

SURGERY

- Extrathoracic surgical approach:
  - Conduit from carotid to the subclavian distal to the stenosis or distal subclavian to carotid anastomosis
- Intrathoracic surgical approach:
  - Subclavian endarterectomy or aorto-subclavian grafting

MONITORING

- ECG monitoring in hospital as appropriate

DIET AND ACTIVITY

- Restrict arm exercise until problem corrected
- Low-fat diet

ONGOING MANAGEMENT

HOSPITAL DISCHARGE CRITERIA

- Resolution of symptoms
- After successful procedure or surgery

FOLLOW-UP

- Three months, 6 months, then yearly if stable

COMPLICATIONS

- Ischemic digits due to emboli
- Myocardial infarction

PROGNOSIS

- Good, with correction of subclavian stenosis

PREVENTION

- Because the incidence of significant asymptomatic subclavian artery disease is low (< 5%), routine angiography of this vessel at the time of cardiac catheterization is not recommended
- The blood pressure in both arms should always be measured before catheterization
  - A difference > 20 mm Hg indicates the appropriateness of subclavian angiography

RESOURCES

PRACTICE GUIDELINES

- Although the overall incidence of significant subclavian artery disease is low in patients undergoing CABG surgery, in patients with known peripheral vascular disease it can be as high as 20%
- Patients with peripheral vascular disease may also benefit from preoperative angiography of the subclavian if internal thoracic grafting is planned

REFERENCE

- Osborn LA et al: Screening for subclavian artery stenosis in patients who are candidates for coronary bypass surgery. Catheter Cardiovasc Interv 2002;56:162.

INFORMATION FOR PATIENTS

- www.drpen.com/4439

Sudden Cardiac Death (SCD)

KEY FEATURES

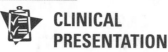

ESSENTIALS OF DIAGNOSIS

- Unexpected death within 1 hour of onset of symptoms; if a patient is successfully resuscitated, it is called a sudden-death episode
- Primary electrical mechanisms include:
  - Ventricular fibrillation (VF)
  - Ventricular tachycardia (VT)
  - Asystole
  - Pulseless electrical activity
- May also be due to massive pulmonary embolism, rupture of an aortic aneurysm, or massive stroke

GENERAL CONSIDERATIONS

- Each year, 300,000 individuals in the United States die suddenly from cardiovascular disease
- Associated diseases include:
  - Coronary artery disease
  - Dilated cardiomyopathy
  - Hypertrophic cardiomyopathy
  - Arrhythmogenic right ventricular dysplasia
  - Primary electrophysiologic disorders such as long QT syndrome, Brugada syndrome, and idiopathic ventricular arrhythmia
- Patients with ischemic heart disease are the largest single group at risk for sudden death
- Myocardial infarction (MI)–related scar is the substrate, and the triggering event may be ischemia, electrolyte imbalance, autonomic dysfunction, or drug toxicity
- Ejection fraction (EF) is an important predictor of survival in those who survive an episode of sudden death
  - EF is also an important tool in assessing the risk for sudden death
  - The lower the EF (< 0.35), the higher the risk and maximal benefit from primary prevention therapy (implantable cardioverter-defibrillator [ICD])
- Sudden cardiac death is rare among patients with structurally normal hearts

CLINICAL PRESENTATION

SYMPTOMS AND SIGNS

- Cardiac arrest
- Patients may arrive at the hospital after successful resuscitation

PHYSICAL EXAM FINDINGS

- Assess hemodynamic stability
- Many patients are on ventilatory support
- Shock, cold clammy extremities, and pulmonary edema are not uncommon
- Features of neurologic insult may be primary or secondary to prolonged resuscitation and anoxic encephalopathy
- Aortic regurgitation murmur secondary to dissection of the aorta
- Gray Turner's or Cullen's sign secondary to intraperitoneal hemorrhage secondary to rupture of aortic aneurysm

DIFFERENTIAL DIAGNOSIS

- Syncope
- In young patients, consider coronary artery anomalies, with intermittent ischemia giving rise to ventricular arrhythmia
- Drug-induced torsades de pointes

DIAGNOSTIC EVALUATION

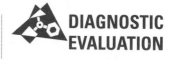

LABORATORY TESTS

- CBC, comprehensive metabolic panel including thyroid-stimulating hormone
- Cardiac biomarkers
- Arterial blood gas analysis

ELECTROCARDIOGRAPHY

- ECG to evaluate for acute MI, ischemia or arrhythmia such as VT, evidence of preexcitation, long QT syndrome, or Brugada-type ECG

IMAGING STUDIES

- Both transthoracic and transesophageal echocardiogram:
  - To evaluate left ventricular function
  - To assess the aorta for dissection, valvular function, right ventricular dilatation (suggests pulmonary embolism), and hemodynamic status
- Spiral CT of the chest
- CT of the head

DIAGNOSTIC PROCEDURES

- Depends on the suspected cause, but electrophysiology study may be indicated
- Coronary angiography to assess for coronary artery disease and acute MI if the clinical situation permits

TREATMENT

CARDIOLOGY REFERRAL

- All patients should be seen by a cardiologist
- Cardiologist may request evaluation by an electrophysiologist

HOSPITALIZATION CRITERIA

- All patients must be hospitalized until risk stratification and subsequent management plans are complete

MEDICATIONS

- Antiarrhythmic drugs as a group are not effective, but beta blockers and amiodarone may play a role

THERAPEUTIC PROCEDURES

- ICD in patients with cardiac disease because recurrence rates are high
- Radiofrequency ablation of ventricular arrhythmia focus may be required
- Percutaneous revascularization when appropriate

SURGERY

- Surgery for dissection or aortic aneurysm rupture

MONITORING

- ECG monitoring in hospital

DIET AND ACTIVITY

- Depends on precipitating cause

ONGOING MANAGEMENT

HOSPITAL DISCHARGE CRITERIA

- When the precipitating cause is adequately treated and secondary prevention issues are complete

FOLLOW-UP

- Depends on precipitating cause
- Most patients require a 2-week and a 3-month follow-up

COMPLICATIONS

- Anoxic brain damage
- Recurrence of sudden death
- Complications of operative procedures

PROGNOSIS

- Depends on precipitating cause
- In cardiac conditions, prognosis depends on EF—the better the EF, the better the prognosis
- Ischemic cause carries a worse prognosis than nonischemic causes

PREVENTION

- Implantation of ICD in high-risk cardiac patients
- All patients with EF ≤ 0.35 must be considered for ICD implantation

RESOURCES

PRACTICE GUIDELINES

- Indications for ICD implantation:
  - Cardiac arrest due to VF or VT not due to a potentially reversible cause
- Spontaneous sustained VT in patients with structural heart disease
- Syncope of undetermined origin with hemodynamically significant sustained VT or VF induced at electrophysiologic study
- Nonsustained VT in patients with coronary disease, prior MI, left ventricular dysfunction, or inducible VF or sustained VT at electrophysiologic study
- Spontaneous sustained VT in patients without structural heart disease not amenable to other treatments

REFERENCES

- Huikuri HV et al: Sudden death due to cardiac arrhythmias. N Engl J Med 2001;345:1473.
- Oseroff O, Retyk E, Bochoeyer A: Subanalyses of secondary prevention implantable cardioverter-defibrillator trials: antiarrhythmics versus implantable defibrillators (AVID), Canadian Implantable Defibrillator Study (CIDS), and Cardiac Arrest Study Hamburg (CASH). Curr Opin Cardiol.2004;19:26.

INFORMATION FOR PATIENTS

- www.nlm.nih.gov/medlineplus/arrhythmia.html

WEB SITE

- www.hrsonline.org

Sudden Death in Athletes

 KEY FEATURES

ESSENTIALS OF DIAGNOSIS

- Sudden unexplained death or cardiovascular arrest in a trained athlete is rare
- Incidence increases with age because of concomitant coronary artery disease
- Occurrence is unrelated to athletic performance or level of training
- Incidence is higher if the athlete has symptoms or a family history of sudden death at a young age

GENERAL CONSIDERATIONS

- Sudden death in athletes is usually due to underlying cardiovascular disease
- The most common underlying cardiac disease in young athletes is hypertrophic cardiomyopathy, followed by congenital coronary anomalies, Marfan syndrome, aortic stenosis, arrhythmogenic right ventricle, pre-excitation, and prolonged QT
- Coronary artery disease predominates in older athletes
- Athletic sudden death generally occurs during or shortly after exercise
- Sudden death in athletes is rare (about 1 per year for every 18,000 to 750,000 male athletes, depending on age (range 18–75 years)
- Little data exist on women athletes

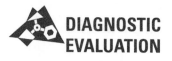 **CLINICAL PRESENTATION**

SYMPTOMS AND SIGNS

- A family history of sudden death or congenital heart disease is important
- Symptoms are related to the underlying disease: chest pain, dyspnea, syncope, palpitations
- Signs of importance would be those of Marfan syndrome or those of other syndromes known to have cardiovascular disease, such as Williams syndrome

PHYSICAL EXAM FINDINGS

- A systolic murmur heard in the upright position (standing) is of critical importance because an innocent flow murmur (common in athletes supine) would be expected to disappear upright
- An ejection sound suggests aortic valve abnormalities
- S_4 suggests left ventricular hypertrophy, but some highly trained athletes have S_4

DIFFERENTIAL DIAGNOSIS

- Distinguish congenital and acquired heart disease from cardiac trauma, which can result in arrhythmias (commotio cordis), rupture of cardiac structures, or dissection of great vessels

DIAGNOSTIC EVALUATION

LABORATORY TESTS

- Those pertinent to underlying condition, eg, genetic profiles

ELECTROCARDIOGRAPHY

- Extensive physical training can lead to ECG evidence of chamber hypertrophy and even myocardial infarction patterns
- Prolonged QT interval and pre-excitation are important findings not caused by training

IMAGING STUDIES

- Echocardiography is important for detecting structural abnormalities of the heart such as hypertrophic cardiomyopathy and valvular disease
  - Transesophageal echo can help evaluate suspected diseases of the aorta
- CT or MRI may be needed to further evaluate conditions such as arrhythmogenic right ventricular dysplasia

DIAGNOSTIC PROCEDURES

- Exercise testing is useful for evaluating symptoms that occur during exercise
- Holter ambulatory ECG monitoring, event recorders, or implanted loop recorders may be useful for detecting arrhythmias in symptomatic athletes

TREATMENT

CARDIOLOGY REFERRAL

- Cardiac symptoms in an athlete
- Suspected cardiac disease, such as loud systolic murmur standing
- Abnormal ECG in an athlete

HOSPITALIZATION CRITERIA

- Those of underlying disease, such as suspected myocardial ischemia
- Syncope

MEDICATIONS

- As appropriate for underlying disease

THERAPEUTIC PROCEDURES

- As appropriate for underlying disease, such as coronary revascularization

SURGERY

- As appropriate for underlying disease, such as valve replacement

MONITORING

- ECG monitoring in hospital as appropriate

DIET AND ACTIVITY

- As appropriate for underlying disease

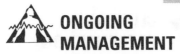 **ONGOING MANAGEMENT**

HOSPITAL DISCHARGE CRITERIA

- Resolution of problem or definitive treatment

FOLLOW-UP

- As appropriate for underlying disease, such as every 3 months if implanted defibrillator

COMPLICATIONS

- Syncope and resuscitated sudden death may result in injuries

PROGNOSIS

- The physical conditioning required for athletic activities improves the prognosis of any underlying cardiovascular disease

PREVENTION

- Recognize the underlying disease and restrict activities as appropriate
- Perform history and physical examination in all athletes at least every 2 years
- The prevalence of hypertrophic cardiomyopathy in young athletes is too low to warrant routine echocardiography
- Any cardiovascular symptoms should prompt an evaluation
- A family history of sudden death should prompt an evaluation

RESOURCES

PRACTICE GUIDELINES

- Individuals with cardiovascular disease can often participate in some type of athletic activities
- Guidelines for which sports are appropriate for each type of disease are available

REFERENCES

- Biffi A et al: Long-term clinical significance of frequent and complex ventricular tachyarrhythmias in trained athletes. J Am Coll Cardiol 2002;40:446.
- Maron BJ et al: The young competitive athlete with cardiovascular abnormalities: causes of sudden death, detection by preparticipation screening and standards for disqualification. Card Electrophysiol Rev 2002;6:100.
- Spirito P et al: Magnitude of LVH and risk of sudden death in hypertrophic cardiomyopathy. N Engl J Med 2000;342:1778.

INFORMATION FOR PATIENTS

- www.nlm.nihigov/medlineplus/exerciseandphysicalfitness.htm

WEB SITE

- www.americanheart.org/presenter.jhtml?identifier=3004574

Superficial Thrombophlebitis

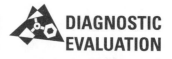 KEY FEATURES

ESSENTIALS OF DIAGNOSIS

- Redness, swelling, and pain, usually in a preexisting varicose vein
- Duplex ultrasound detection of thrombosis in a superficial vein

GENERAL CONSIDERATIONS

- Common in the elderly and usually benign
- Less common in the upper extremities, where it usually occurs in association with venipuncture, catheter insertion, or chemical phlebitis

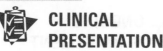 CLINICAL PRESENTATION

SYMPTOMS AND SIGNS

- Redness and pain in an extremity superficial vein
- Swelling of the affected extremity suggests deep venous involvement

PHYSICAL EXAM FINDINGS

- Tender, red, warm chord beneath the skin that follows the course of the vein

DIFFERENTIAL DIAGNOSIS

- Cellulitis
- Insect bite
- Trauma

DIAGNOSTIC EVALUATION

IMAGING STUDIES

- Although the diagnosis is usually based on the physical examination, confirmation can be done by venous ultrasonography

DIAGNOSTIC PROCEDURES

- Contrast venography can be used if the ultrasound results are equivocal, especially in upper extremity venous thrombosis

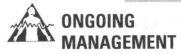
 TREATMENT

HOSPITALIZATION CRITERIA

- Suspected deep venous thrombosis accompanying superficial thrombophlebitis:
  - Occurs in 10–20% of cases of lower extremity thrombophlebitis

MEDICATIONS

- Warm compresses
- Nonsteroidal anti-inflammatory agents
- Limb elevation

THERAPEUTIC PROCEDURES

- Heparin for refractory cases only

DIET AND ACTIVITY

- Exercise should be curtailed until the inflammation has abated

ONGOING MANAGEMENT

FOLLOW-UP

- One visit in 2 weeks to check resolution

COMPLICATIONS

- Extension to deep venous thrombosis

PROGNOSIS

- Excellent

PREVENTION

- Meticulous care with intravenous injections and catheters

RESOURCES

PRACTICE GUIDELINES

- Care must be taken not to miss possible underlying deep venous thrombosis, which requires anticoagulation, especially in the lower extremities; extremity swelling is a tip-off
- Recurrent superficial thrombophlebitis without obvious trauma should prompt a search for underlying malignancy or inherited thrombophilia

REFERENCES

- Neher JO et al: Clinical inquiries. What is the best therapy for superficial thrombophlebitis? J Fam Pract 2004;53:583.
- Schonauer V et al: Superficial thrombophlebitis and risk for recurrent venous thromboembolism. J Vasc Surg 2003;37:834.

INFORMATION FOR PATIENTS

- www.drpen.com/451.0

WEB SITE

- www.emedicine.com/med/topic3201.htm

Superior Vena Cava Syndrome

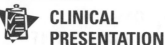

KEY FEATURES

ESSENTIALS OF DIAGNOSIS

- Facial swelling, headache, and arm edema
- Prominent venous pattern may be seen over the anterior chest wall
- Associated conditions may aid in the diagnosis, such as lung cancer, lymphoma, and indwelling catheter or pacemaker
- Venography is diagnostic
  - Magnetic resonance imaging, ultrasound, and CT may be alternates

GENERAL CONSIDERATIONS

- A relatively rare condition in which the thin-walled superior vena cava is compressed extrinsically by neoplasms, fibrosis due to pulmonary infections or drug toxicity, aneurysm of the aortic arches; or it may be thrombosed owing to extension from tributary vein thrombosis or indwelling catheters
- Causative factors are changing (from lung cancer) with increased use of indwelling catheters

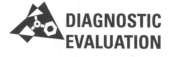

CLINICAL PRESENTATION

SYMPTOMS AND SIGNS

- Acute or subacute symptoms
- Headache, dizziness, visual disturbances, stupor
- Symptoms accentuated by bending over or lying down

PHYSICAL EXAM FINDINGS

- Swelling and flushing of the neck and face progressing to cyanosis
- Dilated cutaneous veins of the upper chest and neck
- Eventually, brawny edema of the face, neck, and arms developing
- Laryngeal edema leads to respiratory insufficiency

DIFFERENTIAL DIAGNOSIS

- Differential diagnosis of causes of superior vena cava syndrome includes:
  - Lung cancer
  - Lymphoma
  - Indwelling catheters and pacemaker leads
  - Fibrosing mediastinitis
  - Thoracic outlet syndrome
  - Retrosternal goiter

DIAGNOSTIC EVALUATION

IMAGING STUDIES

- Chest x-ray: localizes the site of obstruction
- CT scan or MRI: delineates the anatomy
- Phlebography: outlines the venous pattern and collaterals

DIAGNOSTIC PROCEDURES

- Venous pressure measurements in the neck or arm (greater than in the leg)

TREATMENT

CARDIOLOGY REFERRAL

- If syndrome is believed to be due to pacemaker catheters

HOSPITALIZATION CRITERIA

- Marked symptoms
- Need for corrective procedure such as pacemaker lead change

MEDICATIONS

- Cautious use of diuretics
- Heparin or thrombolysis with thrombosis

THERAPEUTIC PROCEDURES

- Mediastinal irradiation for neoplasm
- Removal of venous catheters or pacemaker leads
- Balloon venoplasty and stent placement for thrombosed pacemaker leads

SURGERY

- If mediastinal fibrosis is present, surgical excision may be necessary
- Some catheters need to be removed surgically

MONITORING

- Chest x-ray to assess response to therapy

DIET AND ACTIVITY

- Low-sodium diet until obstruction is resolved

ONGOING MANAGEMENT

HOSPITAL DISCHARGE CRITERIA

- Resolution of the obstruction
- Transfer to comfort care

FOLLOW-UP

- Depends on the cause of the obstruction

COMPLICATIONS

- Death from increased intracranial pressure and cerebral hemorrhage
- Pulmonary embolus from thrombosis
- Endocarditis of thrombosed pacemaker lead

PROGNOSIS

- Depends on the cause of the obstruction

PREVENTION

- Attention to the neck veins in patients with mediastinal or upper lobe lung neoplasms

RESOURCES

PRACTICE GUIDELINES

- Since thoracotomy carries increased risk, percutaneous pacemaker lead extraction followed by venoplasty, stenting, and pacemaker lead replacement is the treatment of choice for superior vena cava syndrome due to thrombosed pacemaker leads

REFERENCES

- Chan AW et al: Percutaneous treatment for pacemaker associated superior vena cava syndrome. Pacing Clin Electrophysiol 2002;25:1628.
- Otten TR et al: Thromboembolic disease involving the superior vena cava and brachiocephalic veins. Chest 2003;123:809.

INFORMATION FOR PATIENTS

- www.nlm.nih.gob/medlineplus/ency/article/001097.htm

WEB SITE

- www.emedicine.com/med/topic2208.htm

Syncope

 KEY FEATURES

ESSENTIALS OF DIAGNOSIS

- Sudden, unexpected, and transient loss of consciousness and postural tone
- Spontaneous and full recovery

GENERAL CONSIDERATIONS

- The loss of consciousness resolves spontaneously without intervention
- Common pathophysiologic mechanism is secondary to reduction in cerebral blood flow and cerebral hypoperfusion
- Common condition experienced by 5–20% of adults by age 75
- Responsible for 3% of hospital admissions and 6% of emergency room visits
- In general, syncope carries a benign prognosis
- Important causes include:
  – Valvular stenosis
  – Hypertrophic cardiomyopathy
  – Pulmonary emboli
  – Bradyarrhythmias such as complete heart block
  – Tachyarrhythmias such as ventricular tachycardia
  – Neurocardiogenic syncope
  – Situational syncope such as cough or micturition syncope
- Iatrogenic causes include:
  – Medications with negative chronotropic activity such as beta blockers
  – Orthostatic hypotension secondary to vasodilators
  – Pacemaker malfunction
- History establishes the cause of syncope or suggests the necessary diagnostic test in up to 85% of patients

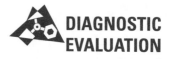 **CLINICAL PRESENTATION**

SYMPTOMS AND SIGNS

- History and symptoms depend on precipitating causes
- Relevant information includes:
  – Details of precipitating factors (micturition, cough, exertion)
  – Associated symptoms (palpitations, chest pain)
  – Position (standing, sitting, changing position)
  – Details about the episode (injury, incontinence, rapid recovery versus postictal state

PHYSICAL EXAM FINDINGS

- Orthostatic blood pressure must be assessed (orthostatic hypotension within 3 minutes on standing)
- Carotid sinus massage may be useful to elicit carotid hypersensitivity with a marked fall in heart rate
- Other findings depend on the cause of syncope

DIFFERENTIAL DIAGNOSIS

- Seizures
- Glossopharyngeal neuralgia
- Metabolic states such as hypoglycemia
- Cerebrovascular disease such as vertebrobasilar insufficiency
- Psychiatric disorder with hyperventilation
- Akinetic falling spells of the aged

DIAGNOSTIC EVALUATION

LABORATORY TESTS

- CBC
- Basal metabolic panel

ELECTROCARDIOGRAPHY

- ECG to detect cardiac disease
- Ambulatory ECG, event recorder, or implantable ECG loop recorder, to diagnose either marked bradycardia or tachycardia

IMAGING STUDIES

- Echocardiography is done to exclude valvular heart disease, hypertrophic cardiomyopathy and other hemodynamically significant changes (should be done only if clinical examination is suggestive)
- Spiral CT or pulmonary angiogram may be done to diagnose pulmonary embolism or dissection of the aorta

DIAGNOSTIC PROCEDURES

- Head-up tilt testing to evaluate neurocardiogenic syncope
- Electrophysiologic studies to evaluate for life-threatening ventricular arrhythmia

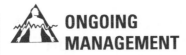

 TREATMENT

CARDIOLOGY REFERRAL

- If a cardiac cause is likely or suggested by initial evaluation, then referral is recommended

HOSPITALIZATION CRITERIA

- Patients with known structural heart disease and syncope
- Definite diagnosis is obvious that could be treated in the hospital (acute myocardial infarction [MI], pulmonary embolism, and gastrointestinal bleeding)

MEDICATIONS

- Treatment depends on the cause
- If possible, withdraw offending or exacerbating agents
- Treat neurocardiogenic syncope with beta blockers, volume expansion, vasoconstrictors such as midodrine, and a selective serotonin reuptake inhibitor such as sertraline (patient response may vary; tilt-table test may assist with treatment choice)

THERAPEUTIC PROCEDURES

- Depends on the cause
- Implant pacemaker for bradyarrhythmias and use radiofrequency ablation or implantable cardioverter-defibrillator for tachyarrhythmia
- If the cause is acute MI, then percutaneous coronary intervention is indicated

SURGERY

- Depending on the cause, surgery may be required

MONITORING

- In-hospital ECG telemetry

DIET AND ACTIVITY

- No dietary restrictions are generally required
- Activity may have to restricted depending on underling cause and occupation of the patient
- Most states restrict driving for at least 1 week or up to 3 months

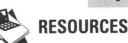 **ONGOING MANAGEMENT**

HOSPITAL DISCHARGE CRITERIA

- When patient is stable
- When all immediate life-threatening conditions have been addressed
- Conditions such as neurocardiogenic syncope may be investigated on an outpatient basis

FOLLOW-UP

- A return visit in 2–4 weeks, depending on underling cause
- Further follow-up usually not required in most patients unless structural heart disease or arrhythmias identified

COMPLICATIONS

- Trauma from fall
- Accidents secondary to loss of consciousness during a critical time

PROGNOSIS

- Cardiac causes of syncope (underlying structural heart disease): mortality rate ranging from 18% to 33% at 1 year
- Noncardiac cause: mortality ranging from 0% to 12%
- Best prognosis for syncope of unknown origin after clinical assessment and work-up: mortality rate of 6% at 1 year

PREVENTION

- Depends on underlying cause

RESOURCES

PRACTICE GUIDELINES

- Indications for referral to an electrophysiologist:
  - Neurocardiogenic syncope not responding to avoidance of triggers, medication, and long pauses in rhythm
- Identified supraventricular arrhythmia or ventricular tachycardia
- Structural heart disease
- Syncope during exercise, congenital long QT syndrome, and Brugada syndrome

REFERENCES

- Kapoor WN: Current evaluation and management of syncope. Circulation 2002;106:1606.
- Weimer LH: Syncope and orthostatic intolerance for the primary care physician. Prim Care 2004;31:175.

INFORMATION FOR PATIENTS

- www.drpen.com/780.2
- www.hlm.nih.gov/medlineplus/arrhythmia.html

WEB SITES

- www.hrsonline.org
- www.americanheart.org
- www.acc.org

Systemic Lupus Erythematosus and the Heart

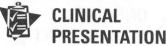 **KEY FEATURES**

ESSENTIALS OF DIAGNOSIS

- Musculoskeletal and mucocutaneous manifestations of systemic lupus erythematosus
- Acute pericarditis with antinuclear antibodies detected in the pericardial fluid
- Libman-Sacks vegetations and atrioventricular valve regurgitation
- Myocarditis and vascular thrombotic disease

GENERAL CONSIDERATIONS

- Systemic lupus erythematosis (SLE) is a multisystem chronic or recurrent inflammatory disease that mainly involves the musculoskeletal and mucocutaneous systems
- SLE is seen mainly in women (10:1) and is more common in those of African origin (3:1); it is rare, occurring in 4 to 250 per 100,000 people (varies with age, sex, and race of population)
- SLE-related cardiovascular disease is the third most common cause of death from SLE after infectious and renal disease
- Clinically important cardiovascular manifestations:
  - Valvulopathy
  - Pericarditis
  - Myocarditis
  - Vascular thrombosis
- Valvular disease is characterized by Libman-Sacks vegetations and leaflet thickening and regurgitation
  - The incidence of valve disease increases with age, duration of SLE, and treatment with corticosteroids
  - Aortic and mitral valve disease predominate

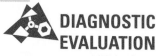 **CLINICAL PRESENTATION**

SYMPTOMS AND SIGNS

- Valvular disease and myocarditis are usually mild and often asymptomatic; severe disease can lead to dyspnea and fatigue
- Pericarditis often presents with SLE flare-ups and is manifested by typical chest pain and dyspnea
- Tamponade is uncommon and constriction is rare
- Vascular thrombosis can present as deep venous thrombosis with pulmonary emboli
- Acute arterial thrombosis can present as acute myocardial infarction or stroke

PHYSICAL EXAM FINDINGS

- Murmurs of mitral or aortic regurgitation are found in a minority of those with valve disease
- Fever, tachycardia, tachypnea, and a pericardial friction rub are often seen in those with acute pericarditis
- Signs of tamponade can occur:
  - Elevated jugular pressure
  - Pulsus paradoxus
- Those with myocarditis may have cardiomegaly, gallop sounds, pulmonary rales, and edema
- Often findings vary according to which blood vessels are involved with thrombosis or emboli

DIFFERENTIAL DIAGNOSIS

- Other causes of acute pericarditis or myocarditis
- Other causes of valvular heart disease
- Other causes of vascular thrombosis
- Other connective tissue diseases

DIAGNOSTIC EVALUATION

LABORATORY TESTS

- Blood tests: low white blood cell count, elevated antiphospholipid antibodies, and a low C-reactive protein suggest an acute SLE flare-up
- Pericardial fluid is usually exudative and positive for antinuclear antibodies

ELECTROCARDIOGRAPHY

- Chamber enlargement is seen with chronic, more severe valve disease or hypertension associated with renal disease
- Typical ST changes of pericarditis can be seen
- Nonspecific ST-T–wave changes are seen with myocarditis

IMAGING STUDIES

- Chest x-ray: may show cardiomegaly from valve disease or pericardial effusion
- Echocardiography detects:
  - Valvular thickening, regurgitation, or stenosis (less reliable for Libman-Sacks vegetations) and pericardial fluid or tamponade
- Myocarditis usually shows no abnormalities unless severe, then abnormal systolic function my be seen
  - Some young individuals demonstrate abnormal diastolic function
  - Left ventricular hypertrophy may be seen if hypertension is present
  - Doppler techniques can detect pulmonary hypertension
- Transesophageal echocardiography is indicated for patients with focal neurologic defects to exclude a cardioembolic source or infective endocarditis and to detect Libman-Sacks vegetations
  - These findings must not be confused with infective vegetations, which can be difficult
- CT scanning can be useful to detect pulmonary emboli or deep venous thromboses and to define pericardial thickening

DIAGNOSTIC PROCEDURES

- Cardiac catheterization may be required if myocardial infarction or constrictive pericarditis is suspected
- Myocardial biopsy may be necessary to confirm myocarditis

TREATMENT

CARDIOLOGY REFERRAL

- Evidence of significant valve disease
- Pericarditis or tamponade
- Myocarditis or infarction
- Thromboembolic disease

HOSPITALIZATION CRITERIA

- Heart failure
- Stroke
- Acute pericarditis or tamponade
- Myocardial infarction or myocarditis suspected
- Pulmonary embolism suspected

MEDICATIONS

- Anti-inflammatory pharmacotherapy
- Pericardiocentesis as necessary
- Appropriate therapy for valvular heart disease, eg, vasodilators for severe aortic regurgitation
- Anticoagulation for thromboembolic disease

THERAPEUTIC PROCEDURES

- Pericardiocentesis for large effusions or tamponade
- Percutaneous coronary interventions have been done successfully

SURGERY

- Valve replacement may be needed in selected cases
- Pericardial stripping may be needed for chronic constriction
- Coronary bypass surgery has been done in selected cases

MONITORING

- ECG monitoring in hospital as appropriate

DIET AND ACTIVITY

- Low-sodium diet, especially if hypertension is present
- Activity restriction if significant valve, pericardial, or myocardial disease is present

ONGOING MANAGEMENT

HOSPITAL DISCHARGE CRITERIA

- Resolution of acute problem
- Successful procedure or surgery

FOLLOW-UP

- Patients with significant cardiovascular disease need careful follow-up with repeat testing as appropriate

COMPLICATIONS

- Infective endocarditis
- Heart failure
- Pulmonary emboli
- Cardiac tamponade
- Myocardial infarction
- Stroke
- Pulmonary hypertension

PROGNOSIS

- Cardiovascular disease decreases survival rate, which overall is 75% over 10 years

PREVENTION

- Endocarditis prophylaxis is indicated with or without clinical evidence of valvular disease because of the high prevalence of mild valve disease

RESOURCES

PRACTICE GUIDELINES

- Anti-inflammatory therapy is indicated for acute pericarditis, myocarditis or arteritis, but no evidence that anti-inflammatory or immunosuppressive therapy is useful for SLE valve disease
- Steroids are contraindicated in SLE patients with myocardial infarction
- Chronic anticoagulation in patients with antiphospholipid antibodies is controversial

REFERENCES

- AsanumaY et al: Premature coronary-artery atherosclerosis in systemic lupus erythematosus. N Engl J Med 2003;349:2407.
- Cauduro SA et al: Clinical and echocardiographic characteristics of hemodynamically significant pericardial effusions in patients with systemic lupus erythematosus. Am J Cardiol 2003;92:1370.
- Tanaka E et al: Pulmonary hypertension in systemic lupus erythematosus: evaluation of clinical characteristics and response to immunosuppressive treatment. J Rheumatol 2002;29:282.

INFORMATION FOR PATIENTS

- www.americanheart.org/ presenter.jhtml?identifier=4459

WEB SITE

- www.emedicine.com/med/ topic2228.htm

Takayasu's Arteritis

 KEY FEATURES

ESSENTIALS OF DIAGNOSIS

- A severe inflammatory vascular disorder involving the aorta, its major branches, and the pulmonary artery
- Predominantly found in Asian women < 40 years old
- Evidence of diffuse vascular disease (coronary, cerebral, peripheral), especially involving the upper extremities (pulseless disease)
- Elevated erythrocyte sedimentation rate

GENERAL CONSIDERATIONS

- An uncommon vasculitis of the thoracic aorta and its major branches
- Aneurysms and occlusions found
- Half of those affected have a systemic illness
- More common in Asian women aged 15–35 years

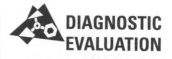 **CLINICAL PRESENTATION**

SYMPTOMS AND SIGNS

- Fever, lymphodenopathy, arthralgias or arthritis
- Weakness of the arms or, less commonly, the legs
- Chest or abdominal pain
- Many are asymptomatic

PHYSICAL EXAM FINDINGS

- Absent or diminished pulses in the upper extremities

DIFFERENTIAL DIAGNOSIS

- Diffuse atherosclerosis
- Other vasculitides (eg, Buerger's disease)

DIAGNOSTIC EVALUATION

LABORATORY TESTS

- Elevated erythrocyte sedimentation rate

IMAGING STUDIES

- MR or CT angiography is usually diagnostic

DIAGNOSTIC PROCEDURES

- Invasive angiography is the reference standard

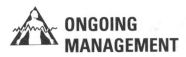

TREATMENT

CARDIOLOGY REFERRAL

• Suspected cardiac disease
• Severe hypertension

HOSPITALIZATION CRITERIA

• Acute coronary syndromes

MEDICATIONS

• Corticosteroid: Prednisone 5–60 mg PO daily

THERAPEUTIC PROCEDURES

• Percutaneous transluminal revascularization procedures

SURGERY

• Vascular surgery for occlusion not amenable to angioplasty

MONITORING

• ECG monitoring in hospital as appropriate

DIET AND ACTIVITY

• Restricted activity until disease controlled

ONGOING MANAGEMENT

HOSPITAL DISCHARGE CRITERIA

• Resolution of problem
• Successful revascularization

FOLLOW-UP

• Depends on the severity and extent of disease

COMPLICATIONS

• Hypertension due to renal artery involvement
• Myocardial infarction
• Stroke
• Intestinal ischemia
• Critical limb ischemia

PROGNOSIS

• Generally good with treatment
• Mortality rate is low

RESOURCES

PRACTICE GUIDELINES

• The diagnosis of this disease is difficult because the clinical presentation depends on the location and severity of the aortic branch lesions
• Once the diagnosis is made, many respond well to anti-inflammatory therapy or revascularization

REFERENCE

• Creager MA: Takayasu's arteritis. Rev Cardiovasc Med 2001;2:211.

INFORMATION FOR PATIENTS

• www.clevelandclinic.org/arthritis/treat/facts/takayasu.htm

Tetralogy of Fallot

KEY FEATURES

ESSENTIALS OF DIAGNOSIS

- Neonate, infant, or child with cyanosis (typically a neonate) or heart failure (infant or child)
- Central cyanosis, mildly prominent right ventricular (RV) impulse, murmur of pulmonic stenosis (with sufficient pulmonary blood flow), and absent pulmonic component of S_2
- Echocardiogram shows RV hypertrophy, overriding aorta, large perimembranous ventricular septal defect (VSD), and obstruction of the RV outflow tract (subvalvular, valvular, supravalvular, or in the pulmonary arterial branches)

GENERAL CONSIDERATIONS

- RV outflow tract obstruction is often at multiple levels
- Associated cardiac anomalies occur in approximately 40% of patients including: right-sided aortic arch, coronary artery anomalies, systemic to pulmonary collateral vessels, patent ductus arteriosus, multiple ventricular defects, atrioventricular septal defects, and aortic cusp prolapse and regurgitation
- Fifteen percent of patients have extracardiac anomalies, including Down's syndrome, Alagille syndrome, and DiGeorge and velocardiofacial syndromes
- Physiologic manifestations depend on the degree of RV outflow tract obstruction
  - More severely obstructed RV outflow tract leads to greater shunting right to left across the VSD and into the aorta, resulting in cyanosis and polycythemia
- Women without severe hemodynamic abnormalities before pregnancy who have had corrective surgery generally have good maternal and infant outcomes

CLINICAL PRESENTATION

SYMPTOMS AND SIGNS

- Symptoms depend on the degree of RV outflow tract obstruction
- Children may present with profound cyanosis at birth, dyspnea related to heart failure due to increased pulmonary blood flow, or no symptoms
- Infants may have spells with profound cyanosis

PHYSICAL EXAM FINDINGS

- Central cyanosis
- Digital clubbing
- Single S_2
- Early systolic click along the left sternal border due to flow into a dilated ascending aorta
- Harsh systolic ejection murmur along the left mid to upper sternal border that radiates posteriorly owing to the RV outflow tract obstruction
- A murmur from the VSD is not usually appreciated

DIFFERENTIAL DIAGNOSIS

- Truncus arteriosus
- VSD and pulmonic stenosis
- Transposition of the great vessels
- Other causes of cyanosis with exercise intolerance

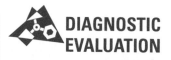 DIAGNOSTIC EVALUATION

LABORATORY TESTS

- No specific laboratory tests
- Arterial blood gases consistent with hypoxia
- Erythrocytosis in cyanotic patients

ELECTROCARDIOGRAPHY

- Right atrial enlargement and RV hypertrophy with right-axis deviation, prominent anterior R waves and posterior S waves, upright T wave in V1, a qR in the right chest leads

IMAGING STUDIES

- Chest x-ray findings: classic boot-shaped heart with an upturned apex and concave main pulmonary artery segment; normal heart size; normal or decreased pulmonary flow pattern; 25% of patients have a right aortic arch
- Echocardiography: demonstrates all essential features of tetralogy of Fallot for the diagnosis and preoperative evaluation

DIAGNOSTIC PROCEDURES

- Transesophageal echocardiography: usually not necessary
- Cardiac catheterization: helpful for assessing levels of RV outflow tract obstruction, branch pulmonary artery stenosis, or hypoplasia, coronary artery anatomy and the presence of aorta to pulmonary artery collaterals and accessory VSDs

TREATMENT

CARDIOLOGY REFERRAL

- Atypical murmur in an asymptomatic child
- Cyanosis
- Congestive heart failure
- Tachyarrhythmias

HOSPITALIZATION CRITERIA

- Cyanosis
- Congestive heart failure
- Atrial or ventricular tachyarrhythmias
- Cardiac arrest

MEDICATIONS

- Severely cyanotic newborns may require IV prostaglandin to maintain ductal patency pending more definitive therapy
- Digoxin and diuretics for infants with congestive heart failure due to pulmonary overcirculation
- Supplemental oxygen and knee-chest position for infants with hypercyanotic spells
  - Intramuscular morphine and IV beta blockers may be administered to improve RV filling and reduce the heart rate
  - IV phenylephrine is sometimes used to increase the systemic afterload

THERAPEUTIC PROCEDURES

- Percutaneous pulmonary balloon valvuloplasty may be performed in some infants or children to improve RV outflow tract obstruction and delay or avoid surgery

SURGERY

- Palliative systemic to pulmonary artery shunts, such as the Blalock-Taussig shunt, are reserved for patients who are not acceptable candidates for definitive surgical repair
- Patch closure of the VSD and enlargement of the RV outflow tract with resection of the subinfundibular muscle bundles and placement of an interpositioned patch

MONITORING

- ECG monitoring during hospitalization
- Pulse oximetry
- Fluid balance for patients with congestive heart failure

DIET AND ACTIVITY

- High-energy, low-sodium diet for patients with congestive heart failure
- Restricted activity for cyanotic patients

ONGOING MANAGEMENT

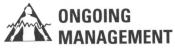

HOSPITAL DISCHARGE CRITERIA

- Stable cardiac rhythm
- After successful percutaneous or surgical repair

COMPLICATIONS

- Chronic pulmonary valvular regurgitation most common late complication
- Residual RV outflow tract and/or branch pulmonary artery stenosis
- Atrial tachyarrhythmias
- Ventricular tachyarrhythmias or sudden cardiac death
- Subclavian steal—potential complication of the Blalock-Taussig shunt

PROGNOSIS

- Low preoperative mortality with intercardiac repair in neonates or young infants
- Some infants require a second surgical procedure owing to pulmonary artery branch stenosis and residual RV outflow tract obstruction
- Atrial tachyarrhythmias are common after surgical repair and are an important cause of morbidity and mortality due to heart failure, reoperation, and the subsequent development of ventricular tachycardia (VT), stroke, or death
- VT and late sudden cardiac death occur in approximately 9% of patients over 25 years

PREVENTION

- Offspring of parents with congenital heart disease are at increased risk for congenital heart disease (these patients should undergo genetic counseling)
- Endocarditis prophylaxis is recommended
- Patients with moderate-to-severe pulmonic regurgitation and RV volume overload and/or RV systolic dysfunction should be considered for pulmonary valve replacement

RESOURCES

PRACTICE GUIDELINES

- Nearly all patients with tetralogy of Fallot should undergo definitive surgical repair in the neonatal or infant period
- After surgery, patients should be monitored for residual or recurrent RV outflow tract obstruction, pulmonic regurgitation, and atrial or ventricular tachyarrhythmias
- Patients with moderate-to-severe pulmonic regurgitation and RV volume overload should be considered for pulmonary valve replacement to prevent progressive RV enlargement, right heart failure, and tachyarrhythmias and sudden death
- Patients with palpitations, syncope, or other signs and symptoms suggestive of arrhythmias should have an aggressive hemodynamic and electrophysiologic workup

REFERENCES

- Davlouros PA: Timing and type of surgery for severe pulmonary regurgitation after repair of tetralogy of Fallot. Int J Cardiol 2004;97(suppl 1):91.
- Giannopoulos NM: Tetralogy of Fallot: influence of right ventricular outflow tract reconstruction on late outcome. Int J Cardiol 2004;97(suppl 1):87.

INFORMATION FOR PATIENTS

- http://www.americanheart.org/presenter.jhtml?identifier=11071
- http://www.nhlbi.nih.gov/health/dci/Diseases/tof/tof_what.html
- http://www.heartcenteronline.com/myheartdr/common/articles.cfm?Artid=60&startpage=1&#1

WEB SITE

- http://www.emedicine.com/radio/topic685.htm

Thoracic Aortic Aneurysm

KEY FEATURES

ESSENTIALS OF DIAGNOSIS

- Ascending aortic diameter > 4 cm on imaging study
- Descending aortic diameter > 3.5 cm on imaging study

GENERAL CONSIDERATIONS

- Ascending aortic aneurysms usually fall into one of three patterns:
  1. Supracoronary sinus dilatation
  2. Annuloaortic ectasia (Marfan syndrome)
  3. Diffuse tubular enlargement
- Descending aortic aneurysm are classified into four types:
  1. Thoracic and upper abdominal aorta
  2. Entire thoracic and abdominal aorta
  3. Lower thoracic and abdominal
  4. Predominantly abdominal
- Aortic aneurysms are often familial (eg, Marfan's syndrome)
- Aortic aneurysms grow about 1 mm/year, faster in the descending aorta compared with the ascending aorta
- As the aorta enlarges, rupture becomes more likely in an exponential fashion with the rapid acceleration point of the curve at 6 cm for the ascending aorta and 7 cm for the descending aorta

CLINICAL PRESENTATION

SYMPTOMS AND SIGNS

- Generally no symptoms until rupture or dissection occurs
- Deep visceral pain in upper anterior chest or back
- Possible dysphagia or stridor

PHYSICAL EXAM FINDINGS

- Possible aortic regurgitation murmur
- Signs of Marfan's syndrome
- Rarely, anterior upper chest wall pulsations

DIFFERENTIAL DIAGNOSIS

- Aortic dissection
- Aortic rupture with contained hematoma
- Mediastinal or thoracic tumor

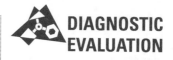

DIAGNOSTIC EVALUATION

IMAGING STUDIES

- Chest x-ray: thoracic aortic aneurysms are almost always visible
- CT or MRI: defines the aortic anatomy very well

DIAGNOSTIC PROCEDURES

- Aortography is rarely used today

TREATMENT

CARDIOLOGY REFERRAL

- Significant aortic regurgitation
- Suspected cardiac disease

HOSPITALIZATION CRITERIA

- Pain likely from aneurysm
- Planned surgery

THERAPEUTIC PROCEDURES

- Endoluminal stent grafts are an alternative under investigation (long-term results not yet known)

SURGERY

- Surgical replacement with a synthetic graft is considered in asymptomatic patients at the following diameters:

	Non-Marfan	Marfan
Ascending	5.5 cm	5.0 cm
Descending	6.5 cm	6.0 cm

- Symptomatic aneurysms (pain, impingement on other structures) need immediate replacement

MONITORING

- ECG monitoring in hospital as appropriate

DIET AND ACTIVITY

- Restricted activity in symptomatic patients until surgery is completed
- Asymptomatic patients should not do major weight lifting

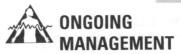

ONGOING MANAGEMENT

HOSPITAL DISCHARGE CRITERIA

- Resolution of problem
- Successful surgery

FOLLOW-UP

- Stable, asymptomatic patients should have repeat imaging every 2 years
- New patients with moderately large aneurysms should be imaged in 3–6 months; if stable in 1 year, then every 2 years

COMPLICATIONS

- Dissection
- Rupture

PROGNOSIS

- Good with elective surgery; not as good with emergency surgery

PREVENTION

- Screen adult family members (women > 50 years, all men) with CT scanning
- Screen children and women < 50 years with transthoracic echocardiogram and abdominal ultrasound

RESOURCES

PRACTICE GUIDELINES

- Since elective surgery is preferable, it is advisable to operate earlier in younger healthy patients (5.0 cm non-Marfan; 4.5 cm Marfan syndrome) and delay in those with considerable co-morbidity that would increase the risk of surgery (7 cm non-Marfan; 6.5 cm Marfan syndrome)

REFERENCE

- Davis RR et al: Yearly rupture/dissection rates for thoracic aortic aneurysms: simple prediction based on size. Ann Thorac Surg 2002;73:291.

INFORMATION FOR PATIENTS

- www.drpen.com/441.9

WEB SITE

- www.emedicine.com/med/topic2783htm

Thoracic Aortic Dissection

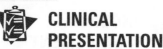 KEY FEATURES

ESSENTIALS OF DIAGNOSIS

- Acute upper chest or back pain
- Widened mediastinum on chest x-ray
- Confirmatory aortic imaging study

GENERAL CONSIDERATIONS

- Usually occurs in middle-aged or elderly hypertensive men
  - Occasionally occurs in young patients with history of Marfan syndrome or other connective tissue disorder
  - Rarely occurs in young women in late pregnancy or during labor
- Pathology usually an internal tear that permits dissection of the media to create a false and true channel
- May present as one of two precursors to frank dissection: intramural hematoma or penetrating aortic ulcer
- Usually classified into two types:
  - Type A: Tear in ascending aorta
  - Type B: Tear in arch or more commonly the descending aorta
- Hypertension and Marfan syndrome—the two main predisposing conditions
- Bicuspid aortic valve and coarctation of the aorta also associated with aortic dissection

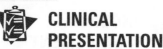 CLINICAL PRESENTATION

SYMPTOMS AND SIGNS

- Sudden, unremitting chest or back pain
- Syncope may occur
- Paralysis may occur

PHYSICAL EXAM FINDINGS

- High or low blood pressure
- Diminished or absent pulses possible
- Aortic regurgitation murmur in some
- Pericardial rub in a few
- Neurologic findings:
  - Horner's syndrome
  - Paraplegia
  - Stroke

DIFFERENTIAL DIAGNOSIS

- Acute myocardial infarction
- Angina pectoris
- Acute pericarditis
- Pneumothorax
- Pulmonary embolism
- Boerhaave's syndrome
- Cerebrovascular accident
- Acute surgical abdomen
- Peripheral embolism
- Neurologic disease causing paraplegia, Horner's syndrome

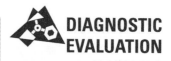 DIAGNOSTIC EVALUATION

LABORATORY TESTS

ELECTROCARDIOGRAPHY

- Left ventricular hypertrophy may be seen if hypertensive
- Myocardial ischemia can occur

IMAGING STUDIES

- Chest x-ray:
  - Widened upper mediastinum
  - Double shadow of aortic wall
  - Disparity in size of ascending and descending aorta
- Transthoracic echocardiography: occasionally demonstrates an ascending tear and dissection; less commonly a descending dissection
- Transesophageal echocardiography: excellent for detecting dissection of the ascending and descending aorta, but less so with the arch
- CT and MRI: excellent for detecting aortic dissection and intramural hematoma

DIAGNOSTIC PROCEDURES

- Aortography is rarely used today, but demonstrates penetrating aortic ulcers well
- Coronary arterography may be required in some patients and is accomplished at some increase in risk

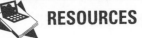

 TREATMENT

CARDIOLOGY REFERRAL

- Suspected aortic dissection
- Hypotension, shock
- Acute aortic regurgitation

HOSPITALIZATION CRITERIA

- Suspected aortic dissection
- Hypotension, shock

MEDICATIONS

Acute management

- Transfer to intensive care unit of tertiary care hospital without waiting for confirmatory imaging studies
- Sodium nitroprusside IV to lower blood pressure acutely to the lowest level compatible with normal organ perfusion
- Adjunctive IV beta blockade to reduce aortic dP/dt
- Uncomplicated type B dissection: continued medical management

Long-term management

- Effective control of blood pressure and aortic dP/dt by appropriate drugs

THERAPEUTIC PROCEDURES

- Complicated type B dissection: endovascular stent graft placed percutaneously

SURGERY

- Surgery in type A dissection to prevent aortic rupture, reestablish blood flow to occluded arteries, and correct aortic regurgitation if present

MONITORING

- ECG monitoring in hospital as appropriate

DIET AND ACTIVITY

- Restricted activity until blood pressure is controlled or surgery is completed

ONGOING MANAGEMENT

HOSPITAL DISCHARGE CRITERIA

- Type B: control of pain and blood pressure or after stent graft
- Type A: after successful surgery

FOLLOW-UP

- Exam and chest x-ray every 3 months for 1 year, then every 6 months thereafter
- Aortic imaging at 3 and then 6 months
  - If aorta dilation continues, at 3 to 6-month intervals, if not every year

COMPLICATIONS

- Rupture into mediastinum, pericardium, or pleura
- Persistent paraplegia
- Other organ compromise, such as kidneys

PROGNOSIS

- Untreated: 15% die in 15 minutes, 50% in 48 hours, and 25% in 3 months for a 3-month survival rate of 10%
- Treated patients: have a good long-term prognosis, but reoperation is necessary in 25% over 10 years

PREVENTION

- Control of hypertension indefinitely
- Early recognition and correction of coarctation of the aorta
- Genetic counseling

RESOURCES

PRACTICE GUIDELINES

- All patients who survive aortic dissection should be followed up carefully for life

REFERENCE

- Sabik JF et al: Long-term effectiveness of operations for ascending aortic dissections. J Thorac Cardiovasc Surg 2000;119:946.

INFORMATION FOR PATIENTS

- www.nlm.nih.gov/medlineplus/ency/article/000181.htm

WEB SITE

- www.emedicine.com/med/topic2784.htm

Torsades de Pointes

 KEY FEATURES

ESSENTIALS OF DIAGNOSIS

- Pause-dependent polymorphic ventricular tachycardia occurs in the presence of a prolonged QT interval (ECG pattern often resembles twisting around a point, hence the name)
- Torsades de pointes in congenital long QT syndrome (LQTS) is not pause dependent:
  - It is referred to as adrenergic torsades de pointes
  - It is secondary to delayed after depolarizations

GENERAL CONSIDERATIONS

- Lengthening of the pause-dependent action potential provides the substrate for the arrhythmia
- QT prolongation may be induced by:
  - Medications such as class IA and III antiarrhythmic drugs
  - Antibiotics such as erythromycin (macrolides)
  - The phenothiazine group of drugs
  - Metabolic states such as hypokalemia and hypomagnesemia
- Antihistamines such as terfenadine can cause QT prolongation (avoid in combination with macrolide antibiotic)

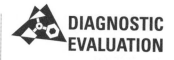 **CLINICAL PRESENTATION**

SYMPTOMS AND SIGNS

- Family history of LQTS in some
- Syncope
- Lightheadedness
- Palpitations
- Sudden cardiac death

PHYSICAL EXAM FINDINGS

- Deafness as part of congenital LQTS

DIFFERENTIAL DIAGNOSIS

- Polymorphic ventricular tachycardia secondary to acute ischemia (QT interval may be normal)
- Catecholamine-dependent polymorphic ventricular arrhythmia

DIAGNOSTIC EVALUATION

LABORATORY TESTS

- Serum potassium
- Serum magnesium
- Cardiac biomarkers
- Metabolic panel

ELECTROCARDIOGRAPHY

- ECG usually shows prolonged QT interval
- Telemetry for arrhythmia detection
- Holter monitoring if patient complains of palpitations or syncope but has no documented arrhythmia

IMAGING STUDIES

- Echocardiogram to evaluate left ventricular function and evaluate for structural heart disease

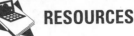

Torsades de Pointes

TREATMENT

CARDIOLOGY REFERRAL

- All patients should be evaluated by a cardiologist and preferably by an electrophysiologist at the cardiologist's discretion

HOSPITALIZATION CRITERIA

- All patients must remain hospitalized until the problem resolves and secondary prevention is addressed

MEDICATIONS

- Patients with hemodynamic collapse require emergent electrical countershock
- Stable patients can start with IV magnesium
- For frequent pauses, consider temporary pacing or IV isoproterenol
- Eliminate medications that prolong the QT interval
- Beta blockers for congenital LQTS

THERAPEUTIC PROCEDURES

- Implantable cardioverter-defibrillator (ICD) in patients with congenital LQTS

MONITORING

- ECG monitoring in the hospital

DIET AND ACTIVITY

- No long-term restrictions recommended

ONGOING MANAGEMENT

HOSPITAL DISCHARGE CRITERIA

- Once the acute symptoms and arrhythmia resolves
- After an ICD implantation in patients with LQTS

FOLLOW-UP

- Two weeks after hospital discharge
- Holter monitor to document arrhythmia control in medically treated patients

COMPLICATIONS

- Death

PROGNOSIS

- In medication-induced torsades de pointes, prognosis is generally good
- In LQTS, prognosis is variable

PREVENTION

- Avoiding combinations of medications that are dangerous such as erythromycin and terfenadine
- Family screening and risk stratification in congenital LQTS

RESOURCES

PRACTICE GUIDELINES

- Drug-induced torsades de pointes is more common than congenital LQTS
- Drug interaction may prolong the QT interval (eg, erythromycin and antihistamines)
- Family history is critical in recognizing LQTS

REFERENCES

- Roden DM: Drug-induced prolongation of the QT interval. N Engl J Med 2004;350:1013.
- Walker BD et al: Congenital and acquired long QT syndromes. Can J Cardiol 2003;19:76.

INFORMATION FOR PATIENTS

- www.nlm.nih.gov/medlineplus/arrhythmia.html

WEB SITES

- www.hrsonline.org
- www.americanheart.org

Total Anomalous Pulmonary Venous Drainage

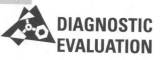

KEY FEATURES

ESSENTIALS OF DIAGNOSIS

- Infant with cyanosis or congestive heart failure, depending on the size of the interatrial communication and whether the pulmonary venous channel is obstructed
- Hyperdynamic right ventricular impulse with wide fixed split S_2 and an S_3; systolic ejection murmur along the left sternal border and a diastolic flow rumble across the tricuspid valve
- Right-heart chamber enlargement on ECG
- Right-heart enlargement and pulmonary vascular engorgement on chest x-ray

GENERAL CONSIDERATIONS

- Congenital anomaly in which all pulmonary veins drain into the right atrium
- Condition is incompatible with life unless a large atrial septal defect (ASD), patent foramen ovale, patent ductus arteriosus, or ventricular septal defect exists
- Severity depends on whether the pulmonary veins are obstructed
- Pulmonary veins may drain into the superior vena cava (most common), right atrium, coronary sinus, portal vein, sinus venosus; or they may have multiple connections

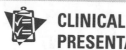

CLINICAL PRESENTATION

SYMPTOMS AND SIGNS

- Infant with cyanosis, lethargy, poor feeding, tachypnea, frequent respiratory infections

PHYSICAL EXAM FINDINGS

- Cyanosis
- Hyperdynamic right ventricular impulse
- Wide fixed split S_2 and S_3
- Systolic ejection murmur along the left sternal border
- Diastolic and loud rumble across the tricuspid valve

DIFFERENTIAL DIAGNOSIS

- ASD
- Pentalogy of Fallot (tetralogy plus ASD)
- Other causes of cyanosis and heart failure

DIAGNOSTIC EVALUATION

LABORATORY TESTS

- No specific tests

ELECTROCARDIOGRAPHY

- Right atrial enlargement
- Right ventricular enlargement

IMAGING STUDIES

- Chest x-ray:
  - Right atrial and ventricular enlargement
  - Pulmonary vascular engorgement
- Echocardiography:
  - Right heart enlargement
  - Absence of pulmonary venous flow into the left atrium
  - Associated lesions such as an atrial septal defect or ventricular septal defect may be visualized
- Transesophageal echocardiography may disclose the site of anomalous drainage of all four pulmonary veins leading to right-sided structures

DIAGNOSTIC PROCEDURES

- Cardiac catheterization:
  - Oxygen saturation step-up usually in the superior vena cava
  - Contrast dye reveals the pulmonary veins draining into the right-sided structures instead of the left atrium

TREATMENT

CARDIOLOGY REFERRAL

- Infants are often cyanotic and seen by a cardiologist immediately

HOSPITALIZATION CRITERIA

- Infants are often cyanotic and critically ill in the hospital after birth

MEDICATIONS

- Aggressive medical therapy for palliation

THERAPEUTIC PROCEDURES

- Balloon atrial septostomy for palliation

SURGERY

- Early complete surgical repair with reimplantation of all four pulmonary veins into the left atrium recommended

MONITORING

- ECG monitoring in the hospital
- Fluid intake and output during hospitalization

ONGOING MANAGEMENT

HOSPITAL DISCHARGE CRITERIA

- After successful surgery

FOLLOW-UP

- Within 2 weeks after hospital discharge
- Regular follow-up with pediatric cardiologist every 6–12 months

COMPLICATIONS

- Heart failure
- Breathing difficulties
- Lung infections
- Late pulmonary vein stenosis at anastomic sites
- Atrial arrhythmias, including sick sinus syndrome

PROGNOSIS

- Normal life expectancy if complete surgical correction is performed in the absence of other congenital defects
- Late pulmonary venous obstruction after surgical correction occurs in approximately 10% and often requires reoperation

PREVENTION

- No known preventive measures

RESOURCES

PRACTICE GUIDELINES

- Pulmonary vein stenosis usually occurs within 6–12 months after repair
- Patients who develop atrial arrhythmias, including sick sinus syndrome, are treated with medications and/or a pacemaker as indicated

REFERENCES

- Kung GC et al: Total anomalous pulmonary venous return involving drainage above, below and to the heart: a mixed bag. J Am Soc Echocardiogr 2004;17:91.
- Ricci M et al: Management of pulmonary venous obstruction after correction of TAPVC: risk factors for adverse outcome. Eur J Cardiothorac Surg 2003;24:28.

INFORMATION FOR PATIENTS

- http://www.pediheart.org/parents/defects/TAPVR.htm
- http://www.americanheart.org/presenter.jhtml?identifier=1315

WEB SITE

- http://www.emedicine.com/ped/topic2540.htm

Transposition of the Great Arteries, Congenitally Corrected

KEY FEATURES

ESSENTIALS OF DIAGNOSIS

- Prominent left parasternal impulse, soft S_1, loud single S_2 along the upper left sternal border
- Absence of left-sided aortic knob on chest x-ray
- Ventricular inversion (ie, ventriculoarterial and ventriculoatrial discordance) apparent on cardiac imaging
- Atria in normal position

GENERAL CONSIDERATIONS

- Rare condition with male predominance
- Usually associated with other abnormalities such as:
  - Ventriculoseptal defects
  - Pulmonic stenosis
  - Tricuspid valve abnormalities
- When a ventricular septal defect is present, there is a risk of developing pulmonary vascular disease in the absence of pulmonary stenosis because of increased pulmonary blood flow

CLINICAL PRESENTATION

SYMPTOMS AND SIGNS

- May be asymptomatic until the third or fourth decade of life
- Patients who develop systemic ventricular failure may experience fatigue, dyspnea, orthopnea, paroxysmal nocturnal dyspnea, and edema
- Patients with heart block or tachyarrhythmias may have palpitations and/or syncopal episodes

PHYSICAL EXAM FINDINGS

- Prominent right ventricular impulse
- Loud single S_2 along the upper left sternal border
- Murmurs caused by associated defects (ventricular septal defect, pulmonic stenosis)
- Adults who develop systemic right ventricular failure may have a gallop and/or pulmonary rales

DIFFERENTIAL DIAGNOSIS

- Other causes of complete heart block
- Other causes of heart failure

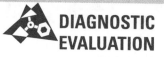 DIAGNOSTIC EVALUATION

LABORATORY TESTS

- No specific tests

ELECTROCARDIOGRAPHY

- Right atrial enlargement
- P-R prolongation
- Variable degrees of atrioventricular (AV) block
- Right ventricular hypertrophy
- Right axis deviation
- Q waves in the right precordial leads

IMAGING STUDIES

- Chest x-ray findings:
  - Absence of left-sided aortic knob
  - Prominent right atrium and right ventricle
- Echocardiography:
  - Atria are in the normal position with the morphologic left ventricle situated between the right atrium and pulmonary artery, and the morphologic right ventricle between the left atrium and aorta
  - The systemic right ventricle is hypertrophied and may be dilated with reduced contractile function
  - Associated abnormalities may be present, such as a ventriculoseptal defect, abnormalities of the tricuspid valve with variable degrees of tricuspid regurgitation, and/or pulmonary valve stenosis

DIAGNOSTIC PROCEDURES

- In the adult with associated ventricular septal defect, cardiac catheterization may be indicated to determine pulmonary vascular resistance or severity of pulmonic stenosis

Transposition of the Great Arteries, Congenitally Corrected

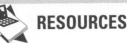

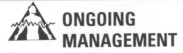

TREATMENT

CARDIOLOGY REFERRAL

- All patients with transposition of the great arteries should be followed up regularly by a cardiologist who specializes in congenital heart disease

HOSPITALIZATION CRITERIA

- Atrial or ventricular tachyarrhythmias
- Symptomatic bradycardia
- High-grade AV block
- Heart failure

MEDICATIONS

- Endocarditis prophylaxis for patients with a ventriculoseptal defect or valvular abnormalities
- Drugs to control atrial tachyarrhythmias
- Appropriate drugs for left ventricular dysfunction or heart failure
- Furosemide for congestion or edema

THERAPEUTIC PROCEDURES

- Pacemaker for heart block

SURGERY

- Pulmonary valve repair or replacement when indicated for pulmonic stenosis
- Ventricular septal defect repair
- Tricuspid valve repair or replacement when indicated
- Cardiac transplantation

MONITORING

- ECG monitoring in the hospital

DIET AND ACTIVITY

- Low-sodium diet for patients with heart failure
- Activity as tolerated

ONGOING MANAGEMENT

HOSPITAL DISCHARGE CRITERIA

- Stable cardiac medications
- Stable cardiac rhythm

FOLLOW-UP

- Cardiologist within 2 weeks of hospital discharge

COMPLICATIONS

- Sick sinus syndrome
- Atrial and ventricular tachyarrhythmias
- Heart block
- Systemic ventricular dysfunction

PROGNOSIS

- Near-normal life expectancy for patients with isolated transposition and no associated defects
- Systemic ventricular dysfunction by age 50 years in over 50% of patients

PREVENTION

- Early closure of moderate- to large-sized ventriculoseptal defects may prevent the development of pulmonary vascular disease

RESOURCES

PRACTICE GUIDELINES

- Surgery may be indicated for associated lesions, such as ventricular septal defect, tricuspid regurgitation, and pulmonary valve stenosis
- Patients who develop systemic ventricular failure unresponsive to medical therapy may be candidates for cardiac transplantation

REFERENCES

- Graham TP Jr et al: Long-term outcome in congenitally corrected transposition of the great arteries: a multi-institutional study. J Am Coll Cardiol 2000;36:255.
- Hraska V et al: Long-term outcome of surgically treated patients with corrected transposition of the great arteries. J Thorac Cardiovasc Surg 2005;124:182.

INFORMATION FOR PATIENTS

- http://www.heartcenteronline.com/ myheartdr/common/articles.cfm? ARTID=418
- http://www.americanheart.org/ presenter.jhtml?identifier=11074
- http://www.pediheart.org/parents/ defects/TGA.htm

WEB SITE

- http://www.emedicine.com/ped/ topic2831.htm

Transposition of the Great Arteries

 KEY FEATURES

ESSENTIALS OF DIAGNOSIS

- History of cyanosis that worsens shortly after birth at the time of ductal closure
- Prominent right ventricular impulse, palpable and delayed A_2
- Murmurs from associated defects (eg, ventricular septal defect, pulmonic stenosis)
- Chest x-ray shows narrowing at base of heart in region of great vessels; prominent pulmonary vascularity unless pulmonary vascular resistance is increased
- Discordant ventriculoarterial connections such that the aorta arises from the right ventricle and the pulmonary artery arises from the left ventricle
- Right atrial enlargement, right ventricular hypertrophy; occasionally biventricular hypertrophy (with an associated ventricular septal defect) visualized with echocardiography

GENERAL CONSIDERATIONS

- Most common cyanotic congenital heart lesion
- Survival of patients with transposition of the great arteries (D-TGA) after birth depends on mixing saturated and desaturated blood via a patent ductus arteriosus or atrial septal defect or ventricular septal defect
- When a ventricular septal defect is present, there is a risk of developing pulmonary vascular disease in the absence of pulmonary stenosis because of increased pulmonic blood flow
- Virtually all surviving adults with transposition of the great arteries have had corrective surgeries, such as the Mustard or Senning (atria switch), the Jatene (arterial switch), or combined atrial and arterial switch operations

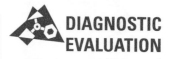 **CLINICAL PRESENTATION**

SYMPTOMS AND SIGNS

- Male predominance (3:1)
- History of cyanosis at birth that worsens after the ductus closes
- Adults who have had corrective surgeries are acyanotic, although they may develop signs and symptoms of heart failure due to systemic right ventricular dysfunction or atrial baffle obstruction or leaks

PHYSICAL EXAM FINDINGS

- Prominent right ventricular impulse
- Accentuated S_2 with soft or inaudible pulmonic component
- Murmurs caused by associated defects (ventricular septal defect, pulmonic stenosis)
- Adults who develop systemic right ventricular failure may have a gallop and/or pulmonary rales

DIFFERENTIAL DIAGNOSIS

- Truncus arteriosus
- Tetralogy of Fallot
- Eisenmenger syndrome
- Other causes of cyanosis

DIAGNOSTIC EVALUATION

ELECTROCARDIOGRAPHY

- Right atrial enlargement
- P-R prolongation
- Variable degrees of atrioventricular (AV) block
- Right ventricular hypertrophy
- Right axis deviation
- Q waves in the right precordial leads

IMAGING STUDIES

- Chest x-ray:
  - Absence of left-sided aortic knob, prominent right atrium and right ventricle
- Echocardiography:
  - Atria and ventricles in the normal position with severe right ventricular hypertrophy and some degree of right ventricular enlargement with or without right ventricular systolic dysfunction
  - In patients with atrial switch procedures, baffle leaks or obstruction can be detected with color-flow Doppler and contrast injection
  - Arterial switch procedures may show neoaortic valve regurgitation or neopulmonary valve stenosis
- MRI:
  - May be helpful in determining the anatomy of the vena cavae and pulmonary veins

DIAGNOSTIC PROCEDURES

- Cardiac catheterization: In the adult with associated ventricular septal defect, cardiac catheterization may be indicated to determine pulmonary vascular resistance or severity of pulmonic stenosis

TREATMENT

CARDIOLOGY REFERRAL

- All patients with transposition of the great arteries should be followed up regularly by a cardiologist who specializes in congenital heart disease

HOSPITALIZATION CRITERIA

- Atrial or ventricular tachyarrhythmias
- Symptomatic bradycardia
- High-grade AV block
- Heart failure

MEDICATIONS

- Endocarditis prophylaxis
- Drugs to control atrial tachyarrhythmias (eg, beta blockers and calcium channel blockers)
- Appropriate drugs for ventricular dysfunction
- Furosemide for congestion or edema

THERAPEUTIC PROCEDURES

- Pacemaker for heart block

SURGERY

- Surgical correction involves switching the great vessels (Jatene repair)
- The atrial switch operations (Mustard, Senning) are less favored today because of the high incidence of late complications and the need for the anatomic right ventricle to supply the systemic circulation
- Pulmonary valve repair or replacement when indicated for pulmonic stenosis
- Ventricular septal defect repair
- Tricuspid valve repair or replacement when indicated
- Cardiac transplantation

MONITORING

- ECG monitoring in the hospital

DIET AND ACTIVITY

- Low sodium diet for patients with heart failure
- Activity as tolerated

ONGOING MANAGEMENT

HOSPITAL DISCHARGE CRITERIA

- Stable cardiac medications
- Stable cardiac rhythm

FOLLOW-UP

- Cardiologist within 2 weeks of hospital discharge

COMPLICATIONS

- Sick sinus syndrome
- Atrial and ventricular tachyarrhythmias
- Heart block
- Atrial baffle obstruction or leaks
- Systemic ventricular dysfunction

PROGNOSIS

- Ninety percent or greater mortality rate in first year of life without treatment for transposition of the great arteries
- Loss of sinus rhythm at rate of 2–3% per year
- Thirty-year mortality rate approximately 20% (mostly sudden death)
- Survival rates of 1, 5, 10, and 15 years are approximately 84%, 75%, 68%, and 61%, respectively, after surgical treatment
- Many patients require procedures or re-operation for late postoperative complications

PREVENTION

- In patients with transposition of the great arteries and ventricular septal defect, surgical placement of a pulmonary artery band may prevent the development of pulmonary vascular disease

RESOURCES

PRACTICE GUIDELINES

- Adults who have had corrective surgeries should be monitored for evidence of:
  - Baffle obstruction or leaks
  - Systemic right ventricular failure
  - Heart block or tachyarrhythmias
- Surgery may be indicated for associated lesions such as ventricular septal defect, tricuspid regurgitation, and pulmonary valve stenosis
- Patients who develop systemic ventricular failure unresponsive to medical therapy may be candidates for cardiac transplantation

REFERENCE

- Losasy J et al: Late outcome after arterial switch operation for transposition of the great arteries. Circulation 2001;104:121I

INFORMATION FOR PATIENTS

- http://www.heartcenteronline.com/myheartdr/common/articles.cfm?ARTID=418
- http://www.americanheart.org/presenter.jhtml?identifier=11074
- http://www.pediheart.org/parents/defects/TGA.htm

WEB SITE

- http://www.emedicine.com/ped/topic2548.htm

Tricuspid Atresia

KEY FEATURES

ESSENTIALS OF DIAGNOSIS

- History of either cyanosis (70%) or congestive heart failure (30%)
- Cyanotic patient with absent right ventricular impulse and prominent left ventricular impulse
- Oligemic lung fields, right atrial and left ventricular prominence without right ventricular enlargement in retrosternal air space on chest radiograph
- Evidence of left ventricular hypertrophy, absent or atretic tricuspid valve, atrial septal defect (ASD), small right ventricle

GENERAL CONSIDERATIONS

- Includes a spectrum of morphologic tricuspid valve abnormalities:
- Survival requires the presence of an interatrial communication, such as a patent foramen ovale or ASD
- Other associated cardiac defects:
  - Ventricular septal defects (VSDs) may result in right ventricular outflow tract obstruction)
  - Patent ductus arteriosus
  - Transposition of the great arteries
  - Truncus arteriosus
  - Double-outlet right or left ventricle
  - Anomalous entry of the coronary sinus into the left atrium
  - Coarctation of the aorta
- The left ventricle functions as a univentricle and receives the entire systemic, coronary, and pulmonary venous return
- Congestive heart failure may develop in the setting of increased pulmonary blood flow

CLINICAL PRESENTATION

SYMPTOMS AND SIGNS

- The clinical presentation depend on the magnitude of pulmonary blood flow
- Neonates with reduced pulmonary blood flow present early with profound cyanosis
- Infants with increased pulmonary blood flow may present later with symptoms of congestive heart failure (dyspnea, fatigue, and difficulty feeding); cyanosis may or may not be present
- Other symptoms:
  - Recurrent respiratory tract infections
  - Failure to thrive

PHYSICAL EXAM FINDINGS

Reduced pulmonary blood flow:

- Tachypnea
- Central cyanosis
- Normal pulses
- Holosystolic murmur of a VSD at the lower sternal border
- Systolic ejection murmur (or no murmur) and single S_2 in patients with pulmonary atresia

Increased pulmonary blood flow:

- Minimal or absent cyanosis
- Elevated jugular venous pressure
- Hyperdynamic precordial impulse
- Single or split S_2
- S_3 may be present
- Pansystolic murmur of a VSD at the lower sternal border
- Mid-diastolic rumble at the apex due to increased flow across the mitral valve
- Pulmonary rales and/or peripheral edema may be present

DIFFERENTIAL DIAGNOSIS

- Ebstein anomaly with intermittent cyanosis
- Pulmonary atresia with intact ventricular septum
- Transposition of the great arteries
- Other causes of cyanosis and heart failure

DIAGNOSTIC EVALUATION

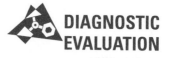

LABORATORY TESTS

- Arterial blood gases and pulse oximetry: demonstrate oxygen desaturation
- Polycythemia in cyanotic patients
- Microcytic anemia in patients who have had chronic phlebotomy without iron replacement
- Coagulation abnormalities
- Hyperuricemia

ELECTROCARDIOGRAPHY

- Right atrial enlargement
- Abnormal superior QRS vector (usually left axis deviation in the frontal plane); or, less commonly, normal axis or right axis deviation
- Left ventricular hypertrophy
- Decreased right ventricular forces
- Atrial arrhythmias occasionally seen in older patients

IMAGING STUDIES

- Chest x-ray:
  - Pulmonary oligemia or plethora
  - Normal heart size in pulmonary oligemia; moderate to severely enlarged cardiac silhouette in pulmonary plethora
- Echocardiography:
  - Small right ventricle
  - Enlarged left and right atria
  - The left ventricular systolic dysfunction may develop with chronic volume-overload
  - Thick, linear echo-density at the usual site of the tricuspid valve without Doppler evidence of flow from right atrium to right ventricle
  - Atrial and/or ventricular septal communications may be detected by two-dimensional and color Doppler imaging
  - Injection of agitated saline contrast demonstrates sequential opacification of the right atrium, left atrium, left ventricle, and right ventricle

DIAGNOSTIC PROCEDURES

- Cardiac catheterization
  - Rarely needed for diagnosis in neonates

TREATMENT

CARDIOLOGY REFERRAL

- Referral to a pediatric cardiologist upon diagnosis
- Any patient with a history of TA and who have a change in clinical status

HOSPITALIZATION CRITERIA

- Hypoxia/cyanosis
- Congestive heart failure
- Syncope
- Infective endocarditis or brain abscess
- Atrial or ventricular arrhythmias
- Stroke

MEDICATIONS

- Oxygen for cyanotic patients
- IV prostaglandin E_1 infusion for neonates with hypoxia and ductal-dependent pulmonary blood flow
- Therapy for congestive heart failure, including digoxin, diuretics, and afterload reduction

THERAPEUTIC PROCEDURES

- Percutaneous atrial septostomy for interatrial obstruction
- Balloon pulmonary valvuloplasty of valvular pulmonic stenosis
- Aortic balloon dilatation for significant aortic coarctation
- Balloon angioplasty with or without intravascular stenting for branch pulmonary artery stenosis

SURGERY

- Palliative surgery to increase pulmonary blood flow, such as creation of an aortopulmonary connection (eg, Blalock-Taussig shunt)
- The procedure of choice for patients with increased pulmonary blood flow or after improvement in pulmonary blood flow following aortopulmonary shunt surgery is the Fontan operation with total cavopulmonary connection
- Occasionally, resection of conoseptal muscle is needed to relieve outflow tract obstruction related to the VSD

MONITORING

- ECG monitoring
- Fluid balance
- Pulse oximetry

DIET AND ACTIVITY

- Fluid and salt restriction for patients with heart failure
- High-calorie formulas for infants with heart failure and failure to thrive
- Activity as tolerated
- Postoperative patients restricted from professional sports or activities with extreme exertion

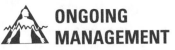

ONGOING MANAGEMENT

HOSPITAL DISCHARGE CRITERIA

- After successful percutaneous or surgical therapy
- Stable cardiac rhythm
- Stable arterial oxygenation

FOLLOW-UP

- Frequent follow-up every few weeks to months after surgical correction is recommended, followed by lifelong annual or semiannual clinical examination
- Serial echocardiography on an annual basis or more often if clinical status is unstable

COMPLICATIONS

- Vascular stenosis at anastomotic sites
- Aortic or pulmonary outflow tract obstruction due to muscular overgrowth related to a VSD
- Stroke
- Bacterial endocarditis
- Right atrial thrombosis with or without thromboembolic events
- Atrial arrhythmias
- Chronic systemic venous congestion with or without protein-losing enteropathy
- Obstructed Fontan pathways
- Residual shunts from ASDs and/or Fontan fenestrations can lead to arterial hypoxemia
- Systemic ventricular dysfunction and congestive heart failure, which is poorly tolerated in Fontan patients

PROGNOSIS

- Prognosis is dismal without treatment
- Survival beyond the second decade of life is improving with widespread use of a staged Fontan operation

PREVENTION

- Antibiotics to prevent bacterial endocarditis
- Anticoagulation with warfarin recommended to prevent right atrial thrombosis and thrombotic events after the classic Fontan procedure; antiplatelet agents (or warfarin) recommended for those with total cavopulmonary connection

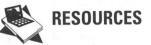

RESOURCES

PRACTICE GUIDELINES

- Upon disease recognition, the neonate should be transferred to a specialized pediatric cardiology center
- Palliative surgeries should be performed and medical therapy instituted to normalize pulmonary blood flow and maintain normal ventricular function, so that corrective surgery can be safely performed when the infant reaches an optimal age and weight
- For infants 6 months to 1 year, the modified Blalock-Taussig shunt and bidirectional Glenn are procedures of choice, followed by a Fontan conversion at ages 1–2 years

REFERENCE

- Mair DD et al: The Fontan procedure for tricuspid atresia: early and late results of a 25-year experience with 216 patients. J Am Coll Cardiol 2001;37:933.

Information for PATIENTs

- http://www.heartcenteronline.com/myheartdr/common/articles.cfm?ARTID=311
- http://www.americanheart.org/presenter.jhtml?identifier=1310

WEB SITE

- http://www.emedicine.com/ped/topic2550.htm

Tricuspid Regurgitation

KEY FEATURES

ESSENTIALS OF DIAGNOSIS

- Prominent *v* wave in jugular venous pulse
- Systolic murmur at left lower sternal border that increases with inspiration
- Characteristic Doppler echocardiographic findings

GENERAL CONSIDERATIONS

- Tricuspid regurgitation usually occurs with a structurally normal valve; this type of functional regurgitation is often due to right ventricular dilatation or pressure overload
- Functional tricuspid regurgitation is due to:
  - Left ventricular dysfunction or mitral valve disease (usually)
  - Pulmonary disease leading to pulmonary hypertension (less commonly)
  - Right ventricular dysplasia (rarely)
- Organic tricuspid regurgitation is due to:
  - Rheumatic heart disease or bacterial endocarditis (most often)
  - Carcinoid involvement, tricuspid valve prolapse, or Ebstein's anomaly (less commonly)
  - Deceleration trauma, which can damage the tricuspid valve (rarely)

CLINICAL PRESENTATION

SYMPTOMS AND SIGNS

- Symptoms of the underlying disease often predominate
- Abdominal distention, jaundice, and inanition due to hepatic engorgement
- Peripheral edema and ascites

PHYSICAL EXAM FINDINGS

- Elevated jugular venous pulse with an early *v* wave and rapid *y* descent, both of which are augmented by inspiration
- Right ventricular lift along the left sternal border
- Findings at auscultation:
  - Right-sided S_3 sound that increases in intensity with inspiration
  - Early, mid, late, or holosystolic murmur at the lower left sternal border that increases with inspiration
  - Mid diastolic flow rumble in severe cases
- Pulsatile enlarged liver in severe cases
- Ascites and peripheral edema in severe cases

DIFFERENTIAL DIAGNOSIS

- Mitral regurgitation
- Other causes of elevated jugular veins

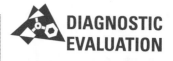 DIAGNOSTIC EVALUATION

LABORATORY TESTS

- Liver function tests and prothrombin time: may be elevated in severe cases

ELECTROCARDIOGRAPHY

- ECG findings:
  - Right atrial enlargement with or without evidence of right ventricular hypertrophy
  - Right ventricular hypertrophy, which usually indicates pulmonary hypertension
  - Possible atrial fibrillation

IMAGING STUDIES

- Chest x-ray:
  - Right heart chamber enlargement
  - Pleural effusions if right heart failure is present
  - Pulmonary vascular markings possibly reduced if pulmonary hypertension is present
- Echocardiography:
  - Dilated right heart chambers
  - Paradoxical septal motion with flattening if pulmonary hypertension is present
  - Color-flow Doppler: for visualizing the regurgitant jet
  - Systolic reversal of hepatic vein flow on color Doppler suggests severe regurgitation
  - Continuous-wave Doppler: for estimating pulmonary artery pressure

DIAGNOSTIC PROCEDURES

- Cardiac catheterization:
  - Right ventricular angiography can demonstrate tricuspid regurgitation into the right atrium
  - Elevated right atrial and ventricular pressures may be found
  - Right atrial pressure becomes "ventricularized"
  - Severe regurgitation may result in Kussmaul's sign, a rise or no fall in right atrial pressure with inspiration

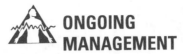

TREATMENT

CARDIOLOGY REFERRAL

- Evidence of elevated jugular venous pulse, pulsatile liver or heart failure
- Evidence of pulmonary hypertension
- Suspicion of infective endocarditis

HOSPITALIZATION CRITERIA

- Heart failure
- Infective endocarditis

MEDICATIONS

- Diuretics for venous congestion
- Drugs to reduce pulmonary hypertension, eg, epoprostenol, bosentan, or sildenafil

THERAPEUTIC PROCEDURES

- Percutaneous tricuspid valve procedures are being perfected

SURGERY

- Surgical repair or replacement for severe regurgitation in symptomatic patients
- Tricuspid valve repair is preferred whenever possible

MONITORING

- ECG in the hospital
- Weight in outpatients on diuretic therapy

DIET AND ACTIVITY

- Low-sodium diet
- Restricted activity in heart failure and pulmonary hypertension

ONGOING MANAGEMENT

HOSPITAL DISCHARGE CRITERIA

- Resolution of heart failure
- Effective treatment for pulmonary hypertension
- After successful surgery

FOLLOW-UP

- Presurgery patients: severe, every 3 months; moderate, every 6–12 months; mild, every 1–2 years
- Postsurgery patients: 3 months, 6 months, then yearly

COMPLICATIONS

- Right heart failure
- Hepatic dysfunction
- Endocarditis
- Atrial fibrillation
- Sudden death

PROGNOSIS

- Depends on the underlying cause
- Natural history of primary tricuspid regurgitation is unknown

PREVENTION

- Antibiotic prophylaxis for bacterial endocarditis

EVIDENCE

PRACTICE GUIDELINES

- In severe tricuspid regurgitation in association with pulmonary hypertension due to mitral valve disease, the tricuspid valve should be repaired, if possible, or replaced at the time of mitral valve surgery
- In severe tricuspid regurgitation with symptoms not responsive to diet and diuretics, tricuspid repair should be considered unless pulmonary artery systolic pressure is > 60 mm Hg

REFERENCE

- Shatapathy P et al: Tricuspid valve repair: a rational alternative. J Heart Valve Dis 2000;9:276.

INFORMATION FOR PATIENTS

- www.americanheart.org/presenter.jhtml?identifier=45

WEB SITE

- www.emedicine.com/med/topic2314.htm

Tricuspid Stenosis

KEY FEATURES

ESSENTIALS OF DIAGNOSIS

- Almost always accompanies rheumatic mitral stenosis, but can be due to carcinoid heart disease
- Prominent *a* wave and reduced *y* descent in jugular venous pulse
- Diastolic murmur at left lower sternal border that increases with inspiration
- Characteristic Doppler echocardiographic findings

GENERAL CONSIDERATIONS

- An uncommon lesion, tricuspid stenosis almost always is due to rheumatic heart disease and accompanies mitral stenosis
- Occasionally congenital in origin
- Infrequently the predominant lesion in Ebstein's anomaly
- Rarely, carcinoid can cause tricuspid stenosis along with pulmonic stenosis
- Another unusual cause is methysergide therapy

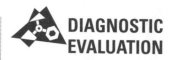 CLINICAL PRESENTATION

SYMPTOMS AND SIGNS

- Abdominal distention, jaundice, and wasting
- Fatigue
- Symptoms of the underlying or associated disease, such as exertional dyspnea with mitral stenosis

PHYSICAL EXAM FINDINGS

- Elevated jugular venous pulse with a slow *y* descent and a prominent *a* wave
- Auscultation:
  - Tricuspid opening snap and diastolic rumble along the lower left sternal border that increases with inspiration
  - May be difficult to distinguish from associated mitral stenosis

DIFFERENTIAL DIAGNOSIS

- Mitral stenosis
- Right atrial myxoma
- Metastatic tumors to right heart
- Pulmonary hypertension with right-heart failure

DIAGNOSTIC EVALUATION

LABORATORY TESTS

- Liver function tests: abnormal

ELECTROCARDIOGRAPHY

- ECG findings:
  - Right atrial enlargement without right ventricular hypertrophy
  - Atrial fibrillation common

IMAGING STUDIES

- Chest x-ray:
  - Right atrial enlargement
  - Reduced pulmonary vasculature
  - Pleural effusions
- Echocardiography:
  - Thickened, domed tricuspid valve with restricted motion
  - Dilated right atrium
- Continuous-wave Doppler estimates the pressure gradient across the valve, which determines severity of obstruction

DIAGNOSTIC PROCEDURES

- Cardiac catheterization:
  - Elevated right atrial pressure with a dominant *a* wave and a slow *y* descent
  - Diastolic gradient between right atrium and ventricle—often small—so calculation of tricuspid valve area is unreliable

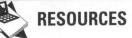

Tricuspid Stenosis

TREATMENT

CARDIOLOGY REFERRAL

- Right heart failure
- Symptoms due to underlying or accompanying disease

HOSPITALIZATION CRITERIA

- Heart failure
- Atrial fibrillation

MEDICATIONS

- Treatment of underlying or associated diseases such as carcinoid
- Diuretics for right heart failure, eg, furosemide 20–80 mg bid

THERAPEUTIC PROCEDURES

- Percutaneous balloon valvuloplasty feasible in some cases

SURGERY

- Repair or replacement, usually with a bioprosthetic valve

MONITORING

- ECG in hospital

DIET AND ACTIVITY

- Low-salt diet
- Activity restricted if evidence of heart failure

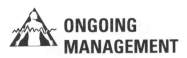

ONGOING MANAGEMENT

HOSPITAL DISCHARGE CRITERIA

- Alleviation of heart failure
- Successful surgery

FOLLOW-UP

- After surgery: 3 months, then 6 months, then yearly
- Asymptomatic patients with mild to moderate stenosis: yearly
- Severe stenosis: every 3–6 months

COMPLICATIONS

- Right heart failure
- Atrial fibrillation
- Infective endocarditis
- Sudden death
- Prosthetic valve thrombosis

PROGNOSIS

- Often determined by the underlying or accompanying disease
- Although thrombosis is lower with bioprosthetic valves, tricuspid prosthetic valves have the highest incidence of thrombosis compared with that of other valves

PREVENTION

- Antibiotic prophylaxis for bacterial endocarditis
- Prevention of rheumatic fever with antibiotics

RESOURCES

PRACTICE GUIDELINES

- Tricuspid stenosis is rarely present as an isolated condition, but when it is, correction by balloon valvuloplasty or surgical replacement should be considered if symptoms cannot be managed medically
- Usually, the condition is addressed at the time of mitral valve surgery for mitral stenosis
- Tricuspid valve replacement should be considered when the mean pressure gradient across the tricuspid valve is > 3 mm Hg

REFERENCES

- Kawano H et al: Tricuspid valve replacement with the St. Jude Medical valve: 19 years of experience. Eur J Cardiothorac Surg 2000;18:565.
- Mangoni AA et al: Outcome following isolated tricuspid valve replacement. Eur J Cardiothorac Surg 2001;19:68.
- Staicu I et al: Tricuspid stenosis: a rare cause of heart failure in the United States. Congest Heart Fail 2002;8:281.

INFORMATION FOR PATIENTS

- www.americanheart.org/ presenter.jhtml?identifier=45

WEB SITE

- www.emedicine.com/med/ topic2315.htm

Tricyclic Antidepressants, Cardiac Effects

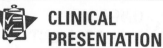 KEY FEATURES

ESSENTIALS OF DIAGNOSIS

- QT interval prolongation
- QRS prolongation (>100 ms) is a sign of toxicity
- Rightward deviation of terminal 40 ms of the QRS is the most sensitive marker of toxicity (rightward terminal R wave in aVR)
- Ventricular arrhythmias

GENERAL CONSIDERATIONS

- Properties are similar to those of class I antiarrhythmic agents
- Orthostatic hypotension secondary to alpha-1-adrenergic receptor blockade may cause frequent falls, particularly in the elderly
- Ventricular proarrhythmia may occur in patients with serious structural heart disease
- Tricyclic antidepressant overdose carries a mortality rate of 2–3% secondary to cardiac complications

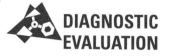 CLINICAL PRESENTATION

SYMPTOMS AND SIGNS

- Dizziness, syncope
- Dry mouth
- Urinary hesitancy
- Muscle rigidity
- Incoordination
- Drowsiness
- Blurred vision

PHYSICAL EXAM FINDINGS

- Orthostatic hypotension
- Irregular pulse
- Low blood pressure

DIFFERENTIAL DIAGNOSIS

- Overdose of anticholinergic agents
- Brugada syndrome

DIAGNOSTIC EVALUATION

LABORATORY TESTS

- Drug screen

ELECTROCARDIOGRAPHY

- QT, ORS prolongation
- Terminal R wave in aVR
- Ventricular arrhythmias

TREATMENT

CARDIOLOGY REFERRAL

- Ventricular arrhythmias
- Syncope
- Suspected tricylic toxicity

HOSPITALIZATION CRITERIA

- Syncope
- Serious ventricular arrhythmias
- Suspected overdose

MEDICATIONS

- Aggressive supportive measures, such as gastric lavage, airway maintenance, and activated charcoal
- Alkalinization with IV bicarbonate for cardiac arrest, hypotension, arrhythmias, acidosis, and QRS prolongation

MONITORING

- ECG monitoring in hospital

DIET AND ACTIVITY

- Restricted activities until adverse effects are gone

ONGOING MANAGEMENT

HOSPITAL DISCHARGE CRITERIA

- Resolution of drug effects

COMPLICATIONS

- Sudden death

PROGNOSIS

- Excellent with early recognition and appropriate treatment

PREVENTION

- Patient education about drugs

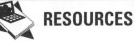

RESOURCES

PRACTICE GUIDELINES

- Tricyclic antidepressant overdose almost always requires hospitalization

REFERENCE

- Witchel HJ et al: Psychotropic drugs, cardiac arrhythmia, and sudden death. J Clin Psychopharmacol 2003;23:58.

INFORMATION FOR PATIENTS

- www.nlm.nih.gov/medlineplus/ency/article/002631.htm

WEB SITE

- www.emedicine.com/med/topic1983.htm

Truncus Arteriosus

KEY FEATURES

ESSENTIALS OF DIAGNOSIS

- Thirty percent of patients have DiGeorge syndrome and chromosome 22q11 deletion
- Clinical presentation is congestive heart failure or cyanosis, depending on pulmonary blood flow and associated lesions
- Imaging studies show a single great vessel arising from the heart and a single semilunar valve that gives rise to the aorta, the pulmonary, and the coronary arteries

GENERAL CONSIDERATIONS

- Truncus arteriosus is an uncommon congenital anomaly, characterized by a single arterial trunk with a single semiluminar valve (truncal valve) arising from normally formed ventricles
- The defect arises from a failure of the single truncus in the embryo to divide into pulmonary and aortic vessels
- The pulmonary artery, aorta, and coronary arteries arise from a single main trunk
- In one-third of patients, the truncal valve is bicuspid or quadricuspid
- Truncal valve regurgitation occurs in 50% of patients
- Associated anomalies include:
  - Coronary artery anomalies
  - Interrupted aortic arch
  - Persistent left superior vena cava
  - A barren subclavian artery
  - Atrial septal defect
  - Atrioventricular septal defect
- Combined ventricular output is directed into the common arterial trunk, and the magnitude of pulmonary blood flow is determined by the ratio of resistances to flow in the pulmonary and systemic vascular beds
- Because of mixing of the systemic and pulmonary venous blood, subnormal systemic arterial oxygen saturation is common

CLINICAL PRESENTATION

SYMPTOMS AND SIGNS

- Young infants may present with pseudosepsis and shock from high-output failure as a result of significant pulmonary overcirculation
- Poor feeding
- Diaphoresis
- Congestive heart failure symptoms

PHYSICAL EXAM FINDINGS

- Cyanosis
- Tachypnea
- Elevated jugular venous pulsation
- Pulmonary rales
- Single S_2 systolic flow murmur
- Diastolic murmur along the left sternal border from truncal valve regurgitation
- An S_3 gallop may be present
- Crescendo/decrescendo murmurs in the lung fields may be due to branch pulmonary stenosis

DIFFERENTIAL DIAGNOSIS

- Tetralogy of Fallot with pulmonary atresia (pseudotruncus)
- Aortopulmonary septal defect or window
- Origin of the right pulmonary artery from the aorta
- Other causes of cyanosis or heart failure

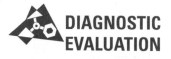 DIAGNOSTIC EVALUATION

LABORATORY TESTS

- Arterial blood gases: reveal arterial oxygen desaturation of varying degrees

ELECTROCARDIOGRAPHY

- Normal QRS axis or minimal right axis deviation
- Biventricular hypertrophy
- Left atrial enlargement and increased left ventricular forces in patients with substantial pulmonary overcirculation

IMAGING STUDIES

- Chest x-ray:
  - Cardiomegaly and increased pulmonary vascular marking
  - A plethoric single truncal root may be detected
  - A right aortic arch in some patients
- Echocardiography is sufficient to confirm diagnosis; characteristic findings—a single arterial trunk arising from the ventricles with variable override of the ventricular septum
  - Two-dimensional imaging can determine the number, thickness, mobility, and competency of the truncal valve leaflets, the pulmonary arterial origin (s) from the common trunk and the origins and course of the proximal coronary arteries
  - Color Doppler can detect ventricular septal defect (VSD) and truncal regurgitation
- MRI rarely necessary, but excellent for characterizing the anatomy

DIAGNOSTIC PROCEDURES

- Cardiac catheterization:
  - Angiographic images from the truncal root can define the anatomy of the pulmonary and coronary arteries

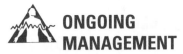
 TREATMENT

CARDIOLOGY REFERRAL

- Upon diagnosis, the patient should be seen immediately by a pediatric cardiologist and a pediatric cardiothoracic surgeon

HOSPITALIZATION CRITERIA

- Cyanosis
- Congestive heart failure
- Failure to thrive
- Shock
- Endocarditis

MEDICATIONS

- Digitalis and diuretics for congestive heat failure
- Inotropic medications as needed for heart failure and hypertension
- Anti-arrhythmics in some cases

THERAPEUTIC PROCEDURES

- No specific therapeutic procedures have been identified
- Balloon dilatation of stenosed pulmonary arteries or pulmonary outflow conduit

SURGERY

- Complete primary repair with closure of the VSD, committal of the common arterial trunk to the left ventricle, and reconstruction of the pulmonary outflow tract connection to the pulmonary arteries to be determined by the anatomy

MONITORING

- Pulse oximetry
- Fluid balance
- ECG monitoring

DIET AND ACTIVITY

- Sodium- and fluid-restricted diet for infants with congestive heart failure
- High-calorie diet for infants with failure to thrive
- No specific activity restrictions

ONGOING MANAGEMENT

HOSPITAL DISCHARGE CRITERIA

- Stable cardiac rhythm and vital signs
- Successful surgical repair

FOLLOW-UP

- Frequent follow-up with pediatric cardiologists over the following months
- Annual or semi-annual clinical and echocardiographic follow-up care is sufficient to monitor most patients who have recovered from surgery

COMPLICATIONS

- Right ventricle to pulmonary arterial conduit regurgitation or obstruction
- Truncal valve regurgitation
- Recurrent arch obstruction or compression of the bronchial tree in patients with a history of interrupted aortic arch after repair
- Pulmonary hypertension in some patients with delayed surgical repairs
- Branch pulmonary artery stenosis

PROGNOSIS

- Without surgery, survival is poor
- Early postoperative mortality rate is less than 10% in patients undergoing complete repair in the neonatal or early infant periods
- Mortality rate among patients who undergo early repair is minimal
- Most patients outgrow the right ventricle to pulmonary artery conduit after 5–6 years and require conduit replacement, revision, or dilatation
- Some patients require early reintervention for truncal valve regurgitation

PREVENTION

- Antibiotic prophylaxis against endocarditis recommended

RESOURCES

PRACTICE GUIDELINES

- After stabilization in the pediatric intensive care unit, early complete surgical repair is recommended for all patients with truncus arteriosus
- Patients beyond the first few months of life should have a preoperative cardiac catheterization to exclude pulmonary vascular obstructive disease
- Regular clinical and echocardiographic follow-up should be performed because these patients often require reintervention

INFORMATION FOR PATIENTS

- http://www.heartcenteronline.com/ myheartdr/common/articles.cfm? ARTID=438
- http://www.nlm.nih.gov/medlineplus/ ency/article/001111.htm

WEB SITE

- http://www.emedicine.com/ped/ topic2316.htm

Tumors to the Heart, Metastatic

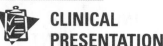 **KEY FEATURES**

ESSENTIALS OF DIAGNOSIS

- Evidence of tumors elsewhere in the body, especially bronchogenic carcinoma, breast cancer, lymphoma, and leukemia
- Positive imaging study for characteristic cardiac masses
- Positive biopsy of cardiac masses

GENERAL CONSIDERATIONS

- Metastatic tumors are the most common type of cardiac tumors
- Bronchogenic and breast cancers spread to the heart by direct extension and usually involve the pericardium
- Lymphoma and leukemia reach the heart by hematogeneous spread and usually involve the myocardium
- Malignant melanoma is an unusual tumor, but has a predilection for cardiac involvement
- Endocardial metastases most often occur with renal cell and adenocarcinoma from abdominal organs
- Renal cell carcinoma can extend from the renal vein up the inferior vena cava and appear in the right atrium

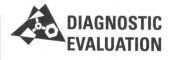 **CLINICAL PRESENTATION**

SYMPTOMS AND SIGNS

- Symptoms and signs of the primary tumor usually predominate
- The most common cardiac presentation is pericardial tamponade due to tumor involvement of the pericardium
- Patients with myocardial and endocardial metastases may present with signs of heart failure due to ventricular dysfunction
- Chest pain and arrhythmias are common

PHYSICAL EXAM FINDINGS

- Findings related to the primary tumor predominate
- Evidence of pericardial involvement with a pericardial friction rub or signs of tamponade such as elevated jugular venous pressure and pulsus paradoxus
- Findings of heart failure may occur

DIFFERENTIAL DIAGNOSIS

- Primary cardiac tumors: metastatic tumors are 50 times more common
- Thrombus: renal cell carcinoma may grow up the inferior vena cava and mimic thrombus in the right atrium
- Vegetations; flail or prolapsing cardiac valves
- Pericardial cysts
- Giant aneurysm of the coronary artery
- Diaphragmatic hernia can mimic left atrial mass on transthoracic echocardiography
- Lipomatous infiltration
- Normal anatomic variants:
  - Chiari network
  - Eustachian valve
  - Septum spurium
  - Thebesian valve
  - Left superior pulmonary vein
  - Atrial septal aneurysm

DIAGNOSTIC EVALUATION

LABORATORY TESTS

- Characteristic findings of neoplasia, such as anemia

ELECTROCARDIOGRAPHY

- Findings depend on the structures involved
  - Loss of myocardium may appear as infarction-like Q waves
  - Pericarditis can result in classic diffuse ST elevation
  - The most common finding is nonspecific ST-T–wave abnormalities

IMAGING STUDIES

- Echocardiography is not particularly good at defining myocardial involvement
  - Visualization of pericardial metastases is limited, although it can readily detect pericardial fluid and tamponade
- X-ray or electron-beam CT or MRI are superior for defining myocardial, pericardial, and paracardiac tumors
  - MRI can characterize tissue, especially fat, which is valuable for distinguishing the former from tumors

DIAGNOSTIC PROCEDURES

- Biopsy of metastases can be useful in undiagnosed metastatic cancer, but the risk of cardiac biopsy usually outweighs the diagnostic benefit unless surgery is indicated for other reasons

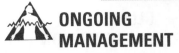

TREATMENT

CARDIOLOGY REFERRAL

- Cardiac functional abnormalities, such as pericardial tamponade and heart failure, in the presence of suspected or known cardiac metastases

HOSPITALIZATION CRITERIA

- Pericardial tamponade
- Heart failure
- Significant arrhythmias

MEDICATIONS

- Pharmacologic chemotherapy is usually disappointing

THERAPEUTIC PROCEDURES

- Radiation therapy can prolong life
- Pericardiocentesis, percutaneous pericardiostomy, and partial pericardiectomy may be required because of pericardial tamponade
- If surgery is not feasible, sclerosing agents such as doxycycline can be instilled into the pericardium by needle to prevent recurrences of cardiac tamponade

SURGERY

- Surgery is definitive therapy, but is rarely considered unless cure of the primary tumor is highly likely

MONITORING

- ECG monitoring in hospital as appropriate

DIET AND ACTIVITY

- Predicated by primary tumor
- Low-sodium diet and fluids if heart failure

ONGOING MANAGEMENT

HOSPITAL DISCHARGE CRITERIA

- Resolution or control of cardiac complications

FOLLOW-UP

- Careful follow-up is usually required because recurrences are common unless definitive therapy was possible

COMPLICATIONS

- Significant arrhythmias
- Pericardial tamponade
- Heart failure

PROGNOSIS

- Cardiac metastases usually portend a poor prognosis

PREVENTION

- Cancer preventive measures

RESOURCES

PRACTICE GUIDELINES

- Cardiac procedures and surgery should be applied as appropriate to the whole picture
- Often cardiac involvement occurs in the terminal phases of metastatic cancer, and aggressive therapy is not indicated
- Pericardial procedures are the most likely to provide symptom relief at relatively low risk

REFERENCES

- Keefe DL: Cardiovascular emergencies in the cancer patient. Semin Oncol 2000;27:244.
- Kirkpatrick JN et al: Differential diagnosis of cardiac masses using contrast echocardiographic perfusion imaging. J Am Coll Cardiol 2004;43:1412.
- Rannikko A et al: Cavoatrial extension of renal cell cancer: results of operative treatment in Helsinki University Hospital between 1990 and 2000. Scand J Surg 2004;93:213.

INFORMATION FOR PATIENTS

- www.nlm.nih.gov/medlineplus/ency/article/002260.htm

WEB SITE

- www.emedicine.com/med/topic1463.htm

Tumors of the Heart, Primary (excluding Myxoma)

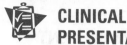 **KEY FEATURES**

ESSENTIALS OF DIAGNOSIS

- Positive imaging study for characteristic cardiac masses
- Positive biopsy of cardiac masses

GENERAL CONSIDERATIONS

- Primary tumors of the heart (excluding myxomas) are rare (see *Left Atrial Myxoma*):
- Metastatic tumors to the heart occur 40 times more frequently than primary tumors
- Most primary cardiac tumors are benign:
  - Fibromas
  - Lipomas
  - Papillary fibroelastomas
  - Rhabdomyomas
- Malignant tumors include:
  - Lymphomas
  - Sarcomas
- Most benign cardiac tumors occur in children:
  - Fibromas
  - Hamartomas
  - Hemangiomas
  - Rhabdomyomas
- Symptoms and signs are determined by tumor location rather than histology

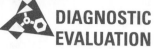 **CLINICAL PRESENTATION**

SYMPTOMS AND SIGNS

- Symptoms of heart failure, such as dyspnea
- Palpitation due to arrhythmias
- Constitutional symptoms:
  - Weight loss
  - Fatigue
  - Fever
- Chest pain
- Asymptomatic with incidental finding on an imaging study

PHYSICAL EXAM FINDINGS

- Elevated jugular venous pressure with right heart tumors
- Signs of congestive heart failure

DIFFERENTIAL DIAGNOSIS

- Metastatic tumors
- Thrombus
- Nonbacterial thrombolic endocarditis
- Vegetations from infective endocarditis
- Flail or prolapsing valve leaflets
- Giant aneurysm of the coronary artery
- Pericardial cyst
- Diaphragmatic hernia
- Lipomatous cardiac infiltration
- Normal anatomic variants:
  - Chiari network
  - Eustachian valve
  - Septum spurium
  - Thebesian valve
  - Left superior pulmonary vein
  - Atrial septal aneurysm

DIAGNOSTIC EVALUATION

LABORATORY TESTS

- CBC: anemia, leukocytosis
- Elevated erythrocyte sedimentation rate

ELECTROCARDIOGRAPHY

- Conduction abnormalities
- Arrhythmias

IMAGING STUDIES

- Echocardiography:
  - Excellent for endocardial tumors
  - Good for myocardial tumors
  - Poor for pericardial tumors
- CT and MRI:
  - Excellent for paracardiac tumors and can often distinguish tissue type, such as lipoma

DIAGNOSTIC PROCEDURES

- Coronary angiography may be indicated before surgery
- Cardiac biopsy via catheter or limited surgery may be required

TREATMENT

CARDIOLOGY REFERRAL

- Suspected cardiac tumor
- Heart failure
- Chest pain
- Arrhythmias

HOSPITALIZATION CRITERIA

- Heart failure
- Hemodynamic compromise
- Need for procedure or surgery

MEDICATIONS

- Pharmacologic therapy is adjunctive for specific tumors

THERAPEUTIC PROCEDURES

- Radiation therapy is adjunctive for specific situations

SURGERY

- Surgery can be curative or can be used to reduce symptoms
- Cardiac transplantation is an alternative for unresectable tumors

MONITORING

- ECG monitoring in hospital as appropriate

ONGOING MANAGEMENT

HOSPITAL DISCHARGE CRITERIA

- Resolution of problem
- After recovery from surgery

FOLLOW-UP

- Depends on tumor and treatment

COMPLICATIONS

- Sudden death
- Heart failure
- Syncope

PROGNOSIS

- Excellent prognosis for benign primary tumors after successful surgical removal
- Grim prognosis for malignant cardiac tumors without transplantation

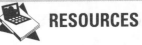

RESOURCES

REFERENCE

- Vaughan CJ et al: Tumors and the heart: molecular genetic advances. Curr Opin Cardiol 2001;16:195.

WEB SITE

- www.emedicine.com/med/topic280.htm

Variant or Prinzmetal Angina

 ## KEY FEATURES

ESSENTIALS OF DIAGNOSIS

- Chest pain at rest, which does not occur with exercise or emotional stress
- Transient ST-segment elevation on ECG
- Resolution of pain and ECG changes spontaneously or after nitroglycerin administration
- Focal arterial spasm may be demonstrated on coronary angiography

GENERAL CONSIDERATIONS

- Much more common in Japan than in the United States
- Has become less common in North America possibly because of widespread use of calcium channel blockers or nitrates
- On coronary angiography, sites of vasospasm have at least minimal atherosclerosis as detected by intravascular ultrasound
- Precise mechanism is not clear, although the following is known:
  - Reduced production of nitric oxide
  - An imbalance of endothelium-derived vasoconstrictor versus dilators
- Cigarette smoking is an important risk factor
- Patients with this disorder are younger than patients with angina secondary to atherosclerosis
- Myocardial infarction (MI) and sudden cardiac death may occur
- Rare cases may develop this disorder after coronary artery bypass surgery (CABG)
- It may occur in association with aspirin-induced asthma
- Alcohol withdrawal may provoke an attack
- Chemotherapy may provoke variant angina (5-fluorouracil and cyclophosphamide)

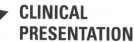 ## CLINICAL PRESENTATION

SYMPTOMS AND SIGNS

- Severe chest pain unlike angina
- Syncope
- Clustering of chest pain between midnight and 8 AM
- Normal exercise capacity and rarely, if any, chest pain on exertion

PHYSICAL EXAM FINDINGS

- Usually normal between episodes
  - Previous MI may change clinical examination
- During chest pain an S_4 may be heard

DIFFERENTIAL DIAGNOSIS

- Unstable chronic ischemic heart disease
- MI
- Pericarditis
- Other conditions mimicked on ECG, such as early repolarization

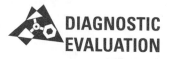 ## DIAGNOSTIC EVALUATION

LABORATORY TESTS

- CBC, metabolic panel
- Cardiac biomarkers during acute episodes

ELECTROCARDIOGRAPHY

- ECG shows transient ST elevation suggestive of acute MI during pain
- Holter monitoring may reveal asymptomatic ST elevation

IMAGING STUDIES

- Echocardiography may demonstrate left ventricular wall motion abnormalities during pain

DIAGNOSTIC PROCEDURES

- Coronary angiogram
- Fixed stenosis of a proximal vessel may be seen in the majority of patients
- Diagnostic of the condition are:
  - Normal coronary angiogram in the absence of ischemia
  - Focal coronary spasm during ischemia
- Right coronary artery spasm is more common than left
- Spasm at different sites or sequential involvement of different sites may be noted
- Acetylcholine provocation test may be helpful
- Ergonovine provocation is not recommended

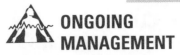

 TREATMENT

CARDIOLOGY REFERRAL

- All patients should be referred to a cardiologist

HOSPITALIZATION CRITERIA

- Hospitalization during acute episodes

MEDICATIONS

- Sublingual nitroglycerin for acute attacks
- Long-acting nitrates
- Calcium channel blockers
- Avoidance of beta blockers unless required for concomitant coronary atherosclerosis
- Percutaneous or surgical revascularization is rarely successful
- Aspirin increases severity of ischemic episodes

THERAPEUTIC PROCEDURES

- Percutaneous coronary intervention and occasionally CABG may be helpful if there are associated discrete, fixed, proximal lesions

SURGERY

- CABG generally not required except in associated fixed, proximal lesions

MONITORING

- Holter monitoring for effectiveness of medications

DIET AND ACTIVITY

- General healthy life style
- Cessation of smoking

ONGOING MANAGEMENT

HOSPITAL DISCHARGE CRITERIA

- Once symptom free
- After an MI (72 hours)

FOLLOW-UP

- Two weeks after hospital discharge
- Thereafter depends on symptoms but annual reassessment indicated

COMPLICATIONS

- Acute MI
- Resultant left ventricular dysfunction
- Sudden cardiac death rare

PROGNOSIS

- Long-term survival is excellent (95% at 5 years)
- Often an active phase is followed by a long period of quiescence
- Serious ventricular arrhythmias during acute episodes are associated with high risk for sudden cardiac death

PREVENTION

- Cessation of smoking
- Calcium channel blockers and nitrates may prevent further episodes

RESOURCES

PRACTICE GUIDELINES

- Coronary arteriography in patients with spontaneous episodes of chest pain and ST-segment elevation that resolves with vasodilators (nitroglycerin and/or calcium antagonists)
- Treatment with vasodilators (nitrates and calcium antagonists) in patients whose coronary arteriogram is normal or shows only nonobstructive lesions

REFERENCES

- Sueda S et al: Limitations of medical therapy in patients with pure coronary spastic angina. Chest 2003;123:380.
- Tanabe Y et al: Limited role of coronary angioplasty and stenting in coronary spastic angina with organic stenosis. J Am Coll Cardiol 2002;39:1120.

INFORMATION FOR PATIENTS

- www.nhlbi.nih.gov/health/dci/Diseases/Angina/Angina_WhatIs.html

WEB SITE

- www.americanheart.org

Venous Insufficiency

KEY FEATURES

ESSENTIALS OF DIAGNOSIS

- Pain and swelling of the leg with prolonged standing
- Dilated superficial veins (venous stars, varicose veins)
- Increased skin pigmentation, lipodermatosclerosis
- Ulcerations, usually on the medial aspect of the lower leg
- Duplex ultrasound useful to detect and locate refluxing segments

GENERAL CONSIDERATIONS

- Chronic venous insufficiency is a common problem that occurs more frequently in the legs than the arms
- Venous insufficiency is caused by incompetent venous valves
- With varicose veins alone, the incompetent valves are in the superficial veins
- Deep venous thrombosis damages deep vein valves leading to the postphlebitic syndrome, which is characterized by:
  - Chronic swelling and pain of the leg
  - Varicose veins
  - Hyperpigmentation (stasis dermatitis)
  - Ulcerations

CLINICAL PRESENTATION

SYMPTOMS AND SIGNS

- Leg swelling and pain that are exacerbated by prolonged sitting, standing, or vigorous exercise

PHYSICAL EXAM FINDINGS

- Stasis dermatitis of the affected leg
- Venous stars and varicosities
- Edema
- Ulcerations

DIFFERENTIAL DIAGNOSIS

- Deep venous thrombosis
- Phlegmasia cerulea dolens
- Localized lymphedema
- Enlarged inguinal lymph nodes obstructing flow
- Heart failure

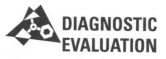 DIAGNOSTIC EVALUATION

IMAGING STUDIES

- Doppler ultrasonography with imaging: can localize the refluxing venous segments

DIAGNOSTIC PROCEDURES

- Photoplethysmography: uses color change to assess reflow rates in small skin veins after exercise which are reduced in patients with venous insufficiency
- Direct venous pressure measurements: typically elevated

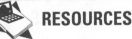

 ## TREATMENT

CARDIOLOGY REFERRAL

- When heart failure is suspected

HOSPITALIZATION CRITERIA

- For surgery
- For complications

MEDICATIONS

- Graduated compression stockings, leg elevation
- Local wound care for ulcerations

THERAPEUTIC PROCEDURES

- Isolated superficial venous insufficiency can be treated with sclerosis or vein stripping

SURGERY

- Deep vein insufficiency can be treated surgically in selected patients

MONITORING

- Leg circumference during therapy

DIET AND ACTIVITY

- Low-sodium diet
- Restricted activity

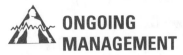 ## ONGOING MANAGEMENT

HOSPITAL DISCHARGE CRITERIA

- After successful surgery
- After resolution of complications

FOLLOW-UP

- Depends on the severity of the problem

COMPLICATIONS

- Cellulitis
- Pulmonary embolus

PROGNOSIS

- About 20% of patients with deep venous thrombosis of the leg develop postphlebitic syndrome

PREVENTION

- Prevention of venous thrombosis is key to preventing venous insufficiency, although some cases are hereditary

RESOURCES

PRACTICE GUIDELINES

- Venous insufficiency usually responds well to conservative therapy
- Surgical approaches, especially for deep vein insufficiency, have been disappointing

REFERENCES

- Barwell JR et al: Comparison of surgery and compression alone in chronic venous ulceration (ESCHAR study): randomized controlled trial. Lancet 2004;363:1854.
- Carpentier PH et al: Prevalence, risk factors, and clinical patterns of chronic venous disorders of lower limbs: a population-based study in France. J Vasc Surg 2004;40:650.
- Prandoni P et al: Below-knee elastic compression stockings to prevent the post-thrombotic syndrome: a randomized, controlled trial. Ann Intern Med 2004;141:249.

INFORMATION FOR PATIENTS

- www.drpen.com/459.81

WEB SITE

- www.emedicine.com/med/topic2760.htm

Ventricular Arrhythmia, Idiopathic

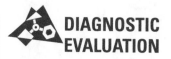 KEY FEATURES

ESSENTIALS OF DIAGNOSIS

- Ventricular tachycardia occurs with no evidence of structural heart disease
- Lack of structural heart disease is defined by normal findings on ECG, echocardiogram, and coronary angiography

GENERAL CONSIDERATIONS

- Tachycardia may be caused by triggered activity (right ventricular outflow tract tachycardia) or reentry (left ventricular tachycardia)
- Triggered outflow tract tachycardias are dependent on cyclic adenosine monophosphate and respond to IV adenosine
- MRI may be abnormal and show ventricular fatty deposits or frank right ventricular dysplasia
- The most common is right ventricular outflow tract tachycardia (90%) and is recognized as a left bundle branch block (LBBB) pattern with inferior axis during ventricular tachycardia
- The idiopathic left ventricular tachycardia is more often induced by atrial pacing and is sensitive to verapamil
- Sudden death is rare, and implantable cardioverter defibrillator (ICD) is not required
- Overall, the arrhythmia carries a benign prognosis
- These tachycardias are generally monomorphic

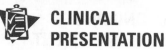 CLINICAL PRESENTATION

SYMPTOMS AND SIGNS

- Palpitations
- Syncope
- Presyncope

PHYSICAL EXAM FINDINGS

- Normal physical exam findings

DIFFERENTIAL DIAGNOSIS

- Intramyocardial reentrant ventricular tachycardia
- Arrhythmogenic right ventricular dysplasia (ARVD)
- Mahaim tachycardia
- Tachycardia following repair of tetralogy of Fallot

DIAGNOSTIC EVALUATION

LABORATORY TESTS

- Thyroid-stimulating hormone
- Comprehensive metabolic panel

ELECTROCARDIOGRAPHY

- ECG to assess morphology
- LBBB, inferior axis suggests right ventricular outflow tract (RVOT) origin
- Right bundle branch block (RBBB), left or superior axis suggests left posterior fascicle in origin
- RBBB, right inferior axis suggests left anterior fascicle in origin
- Exercise stress test may be used to initiate tachycardia
- Signal-averaged ECG may be helpful (unremarkable in RVOT and ventricular tachycardia, and abnormal in ARVD)

IMAGING STUDIES

- MRI of the heart to exclude right ventricular dysplasia

DIAGNOSTIC PROCEDURES

- Electrophysiology study to establish mechanism and determine suitability for ablation

TREATMENT

CARDIOLOGY REFERRAL

- All patients require evaluation by a cardiac electrophysiologist

HOSPITALIZATION CRITERIA

- Following syncope

MEDICATIONS

- Beta blockers, metoprolol 50 mg PO twice daily to a maximum usual dosage of 200 mg/day; or verapamil, start 180 mg/day, next dose 360 mg/day
- Class IA, IC, or III antiarrhythmic agents
- In acute conditions, in the emergency room adenosine can be used to terminate ventricular tachycardia

THERAPEUTIC PROCEDURES

- Radiofrequency ablation in appropriate cases

SURGERY

- Generally not required

MONITORING

- ECG monitoring in hospital

DIET AND ACTIVITY

- General healthy life style

ONGOING MANAGEMENT

HOSPITAL DISCHARGE CRITERIA

- After initiation of medication or radiofrequency ablation

FOLLOW-UP

- Two weeks after ablation or medication initiation
- Thereafter, follow-up every 6 months to assess lack of recurrence

COMPLICATIONS

- Trauma from syncope
- Sudden death extremely rare

PROGNOSIS

- Very good in the long term

RESOURCES

PRACTICE GUIDELINES

- Structurally normal heart includes ECG, echocardiogram, and coronary angiogram being collectively normal
- RVOT tachycardia is the most common tachycardia
- Radiofrequency ablation is very effective in the treatment of this condition
- ICD implantation is not required

REFERENCES

- Wall TS, Freedman RA: Ventricular tachycardia in structurally normal hearts. Curr Cardiol Rep 2002;4:388.
- Wever EF, Robles de Medina EO: Sudden death in patients without structural heart disease. J Am Coll Cardiol 2004;43:1137.

INFORMATION FOR PATIENTS

- www.nlm.nih.gov/medlineplus/arrhythmia.html

WEB SITE

- www.hrsonline.org

Ventricular Septal Defect

KEY FEATURES

ESSENTIALS OF DIAGNOSIS

- History of murmur appearing shortly after birth
- Pansystolic murmur at left sternal border, radiating rightward
- Echocardiographic findings of left atrial and left ventricular or biventricular enlargement; Doppler evidence of flow across the interventricular septum; increased pulmonary Doppler flow velocities

GENERAL CONSIDERATIONS

- Many ventricular septal defects (VSDs) close spontaneously in childhood
- Large defects often cause heart failure and are usually diagnosed early in childhood
- Most defects diagnosed in adulthood are small and not hemodynamically significant
- Persistent, large defects in adulthood are usually associated with Eisenmenger syndrome
- VSDs are most commonly classified according to anatomic location:
  - Perimembranous (also called infracristal, subaortic, or conoventricular), the most common, located below the aortic valve in the left ventricular (LV) outflow tract
  - Supracristal (also called subpulmonary, outlet, infundibular, conoseptal, or doubly committed subarteria) are also defects involving the membranous septum
  - The muscular VSDs, often multiple, may be located in the inlet or outlet regions or located within the trabecular septum
  - Posterior (also called inlet, canal-type, endocardial cushion-type, atrioventricular septum type) occur posterior to the septal leaflet of the tricuspid valve

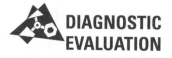 CLINICAL PRESENTATION

SYMPTOMS AND SIGNS

- Small shunts rarely cause symptoms, and the patient's history is usually that of a murmur present from early childhood
- Exertional dyspnea is present in patients > age 30 with moderate-sized defects
- Patients with large defects and Eisenmenger syndrome are the most disabled
- Hemoptysis may occur in patients with Eisenmenger syndrome

PHYSICAL EXAM FINDINGS

- Findings depend on the size of the defect and the relative resistance of the systemic and pulmonary circulations
- The patient with uncomplicated VSD is acyanotic with a laterally displaced, hyperdynamic LV apical impulse
- Pansystolic murmur, with or without an associated thrill, is loudest in the left fourth or fifth intercostal space radiating to the right
- Accentuated pulmonic component of S_2
- Narrowly split or single S_2 in the presence of a moderate-to-large VSD
- An S_3 gallop and diastolic rumble
- Patients with large defects have:
  - Cyanosis
  - Digital clubbing
  - Prominent right ventricular (RV) lift
  - A soft, short systolic murmur due to rapid equilibration of LV and RV pressures

DIFFERENTIAL DIAGNOSIS

- Other causes of exertional dyspnea
- Other causes of pulmonary hypertension
- Tricuspid regurgitation
- Mitral regurgitation

DIAGNOSTIC EVALUATION

LABORATORY TESTS

- Erythrocytosis in patients with Eisenmenger syndrome

ELECTROCARDIOGRAPHY

- Left atrial enlargement
- LV hypertrophy
- RV hypertrophy and strain in Eisenmenger patients

IMAGING STUDIES

- Chest x-ray: heart size and pulmonary vascularity vary from normal to increased depending on the size of the VSD; patients with Eisenmenger syndrome have normal heart size with prominent pulmonary arteries
- Two-dimensional and Doppler echocardiography usually defines the location and size of the VSD. Other findings include left atrial and LV dilatation, dilated main pulmonary artery, RV hypertrophy and enlargement (usually suggests pulmonary hypertension)
- MRI: useful but not usually performed unless echocardiography is not feasible or nondiagnostic

DIAGNOSTIC PROCEDURES

- Transesophageal echocardiography: used occasionally to better visualize the location of the VSD and the magnitude of shunting
- Cardiac catheterization (not necessary in all cases, except when surgical repair is contemplated):
  - Right heart catheterization findings include an oxygen saturation step-up within right ventricle
  - Calculation of the QP/QS ratio can be made in addition to the determination of the pulmonary artery pressure and pulmonary vascular resistance

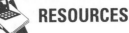

 ## TREATMENT

CARDIOLOGY REFERRAL

- Any patient with a suspected or confirmed VSD
- Congestive heart failure
- Pulmonary hypertension

HOSPITALIZATION CRITERIA

- Congestive heart failure
- Syncope
- Symptomatic severe pulmonary hypertension
- Hemoptysis
- Endocarditis or brain abscess

MEDICATIONS

- Appropriate therapy for congestive heart failure
- Pulmonary vasodilator therapy in patients with elevated pulmonary vascular resistance

THERAPEUTIC PROCEDURES

- Catheter-based closure of the VSD may be considered, depending on the location and anatomy of the defect and the surrounding structures

SURGERY

- Surgical repair is indicated in asymptomatic children and adults with normal pulmonary pressure if the pulmonary to systemic flow ratio is greater than 2:1
- Early repair may prevent progression of aortic insufficiency
- Closure of the VSD is contraindicated in patients with established severe pulmonary vascular disease

MONITORING

- ECG monitoring during hospitalization
- Fluid balance

DIET AND ACTIVITY

- Low-sodium diet, fluid-restricted diet for patients with congestive heart failure
- Avoidance of strenuous activity in patients with moderate-to-large VSDs

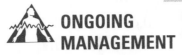 ## ONGOING MANAGEMENT

HOSPITAL DISCHARGE CRITERIA

- Stable cardiac rhythm and vital signs
- After successful closure of the VSD

FOLLOW-UP

- Visit with cardiologist within 2 weeks of hospital discharge
- Follow-up echocardiography and further visits to be determined by the severity of disease and symptoms

COMPLICATIONS

- Residual VSD
- Right bundle branch block
- Heart block requiring permanent pacemaker implantation
- Residual LV dysfunction
- Ventricular arrhythmia
- Progressive aortic insufficiency
- Eisenmenger complex
- Infective endocarditis
- RV outflow tract obstruction

PROGNOSIS

- Surgical mortality rate of 3–5% for VSD repair
- Patients with small VSDs who are asymptomatic have excellent long-term prognoses
- Prognosis of patients with moderate-to-large VSDs depends on the size of the defect, development of pulmonary vascular disease, RV outflow tract hypertrophy and obstruction, heart failure, and aortic insufficiency or endocarditis
- Patients with Eisenmenger syndrome have reduced survival and may be considered for heart-lung transplantation

PREVENTION

- Endocarditis prophylaxis is recommended

RESOURCES

PRACTICE GUIDELINES

- Patients with moderate- to large sized defects with pulmonary to systemic shunt magnitudes ≥ 2:1 should be considered for closure of the defect
- If feasible, percutaneous closure may be considered
- Patients with severe pulmonary vascular disease and evidence of Eisenmenger physiology should not undergo VSD closure
  - In these cases, treatment with pulmonary vasodilator therapy and/or heart-lung transplantation should be considered

REFERENCES

- Ammash NM: Ventricular septal defects in adults. Ann Intern Med 2001;135(9):812.
- Knauth AL: Transcatheter device closure of congenital and postoperative residual ventricular septal defects. Circulation 2004;110(5):501.

INFORMATION FOR PATIENTS

- http://www.nlm.nih.gov/medlineplus/ency/article/001099.htm
- http://www.americanheart.org/presenter.jhtml?identifier=11066

WEB SITE

- http://www.emedicine.com/ped/topic2402.htm

Ventricular Septal Rupture, Acute

 KEY FEATURES

ESSENTIALS OF DIAGNOSIS

- New holosystolic murmur days after an acute myocardial infarction
- Sudden hypotension or heart failure after myocardial infarction
- Echocardiographic evidence of a ventricular septal defect

GENERAL CONSIDERATIONS

- Occurs in up to 0.2%% of acute myocardial infarction (MI) in the thrombolytic era
- Half of the ventricular septal defects (VSD) occur in anterior wall MI
- This often occurs in the setting of first acute MI for the patient
- Peak incidence is between 3 and 7 days
- Acute mitral regurgitation secondary to acute MI has similar clinical presentation
- Increased risk of rupture occurs with old age and hypertension
- The apical septum is affected in anterior MI and the basal septum in inferior MI
- Complete heart block, atrial fibrillation and bundle branch block are not infrequent in VSD

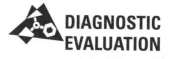 **CLINICAL PRESENTATION**

SYMPTOMS AND SIGNS

- Shortness of breath
- Cardiogenic shock

PHYSICAL EXAM FINDINGS

- Hypotension
- New harsh, holosystolic murmur with a thrill
- Elevated jugular venous pressure

DIFFERENTIAL DIAGNOSIS

- Hypotension or heart failure with acute MI for other reasons
- Acute mitral regurgitation due to papillary muscle rupture or dysfunction
- Cardiac rupture with pseudoaneurysm formation

DIAGNOSTIC EVALUATION

LABORATORY TESTS

- CBC
- Basal metabolic panel including serum creatinine (typically creatinine increases in shock secondary to poor renal blood flow)
- Cardiac biomarkers

ELECTROCARDIOGRAPHY

- ECG typically shows a transmural infarct

IMAGING STUDIES

- Echocardiogram may visualize the defect, but often it is difficult to see because it takes a circuitous course through the muscular interventricular septum
- Echo shows the septal wall motion abnormality and may show an enlarged right ventricle owing to the left-to-right shunt
- Color Doppler is best for identifying the leak across the septum
- Pulsed or continuous-wave Doppler can quantify the gradient and estimate right ventricular pressure

DIAGNOSTIC PROCEDURES

- Right heart catheterization identifies the oxygen step up in the right ventricle
- Coronary arteriography to identify the extent of the coronary artery disease (CAD)

TREATMENT

CARDIOLOGY REFERRAL

• All patients with suspected VSD after MI should be seen by a cardiologist

HOSPITALIZATION CRITERIA

• All patients should be hospitalized to the cardiac intensive care unit

MEDICATIONS

• Diuresis for heart failure
• Pressor support for hypotension
• IV sodium nitroprusside if blood pressure allows

THERAPEUTIC PROCEDURES

• Percutaneous transcatheter devices can be used to close ventricular defects, but experience is limited in the acute MI setting

SURGERY

• Emergent corrective surgery with coronary artery bypass graft (CABG) as needed

MONITORING

• Invasive hemodynamic monitoring
• ECG monitoring

DIET AND ACTIVITY

• After the patient recovers, diet and life style similar to what is recommended for CAD patients

ONGOING MANAGEMENT

HOSPITAL DISCHARGE CRITERIA

• Ambulating, symptom-free, and hemodynamically stable after the corrective procedure

FOLLOW-UP

• Two weeks after discharge from the hospital and thereafter depending on symptoms
• Annual stress tests may be performed on follow up

COMPLICATIONS

• High risk of mortality from the event
• Possible residual heart failure in survivors

PROGNOSIS

• Mortality rate of 74%
• Worse prognosis in inferior MI patients

PREVENTION

• Prompt revascularization at onset of MI

RESOURCES

PRACTICE GUIDELINES

• Management: emergent cardiac surgery unless further care is considered futile
• CABG at the time surgery
• Intra aortic balloon bump recommended for almost every patient considered for surgery

REFERENCE

• Birnbaum Y, Fishbein MC, Blanche C et al: Ventricular septal rupture after acute myocardial infarction. N Engl J Med 2002;347:1426.

INFORMATION FOR PATIENTS

• www.nhlbi.nih.gov/health/dci/Diseases/Cad/CAD_WhatIs.html

WEB SITE

• www.americanheart.org

Ventricular Tachycardia

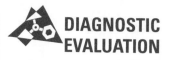 KEY FEATURES

ESSENTIALS OF DIAGNOSIS

- Monomorphic ventricular tachycardia (VT)
- Nonsustained: three or more consecutive QRS complexes of uniform configuration and of ventricular origin at a rate of more than 100 bpm
- Sustained: lasts more than 30 seconds or requires intervention for termination
- Polymorphic: beat-to-beat variation in QRS configuration

GENERAL CONSIDERATIONS

- VT along with ventricular fibrillation causes 400,000 sudden cardiac deaths (SCD) in the United States
- Most common with ischemic substrate and depressed left ventricular function
- Idiopathic dilated cardiomyopathy is also a frequent cause
- Bundle branch reentry occurs most often with idiopathic dilated cardiomyopathy
- VT rarely occurs with a structurally normal heart
- Myocardial infarction (MI)–induced scar plays an integral role in reentry that facilitates monomorphic VT
- Acute ischemia facilitates polymorphic VT
- Wide QRS tachycardia is mostly secondary to VT
- Aberrant conduction as a cause of wide QRS tachycardia is rare
- In patients with a history of MI, wide QRS tachycardia is almost always secondary
- Hemodynamic stability does not exclude VT
- Sustained versus nonsustained VT does not imply clinical significance

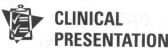 CLINICAL PRESENTATION

SYMPTOMS AND SIGNS

- SCD
- Syncope
- Near syncope
- Palpitations
- Lightheadedness
- Can be asymptomatic

PHYSICAL EXAM FINDINGS

- Cannon *a* waves
- Hypotension if there is hemodynamic disturbance

DIFFERENTIAL DIAGNOSIS

- Supraventricular tachycardia with aberrancy
- Wolff-Parkinson-White syndrome with antidromic tachycardia

DIAGNOSTIC EVALUATION

LABORATORY TESTS

- CBC, basal metabolic panel
- Serum magnesium
- Cardiac biomarkers
- Arterial blood gases if patient is hypoxic

ELECTROCARDIOGRAPHY

- ECG with rhythm strip to confirm VT
  - Atrioventricular dissociation, presence of fusion beats, and duration of R wave to nadir of S wave > 65 ms (left bundle branch block type) and > 100 ms (right bundle branch block type) in chest leads help to differentiate VT from supraventricular tachycardia with aberrancy
- Holter monitoring to identify VT

IMAGING STUDIES

- Echocardiogram to evaluate left ventricular function and hypertrophic cardiomyopathy (apical variety may associated with monomorphic VT)

DIAGNOSTIC PROCEDURES

- Coronary arteriography to identify and quantify coronary artery disease along with ventriculogram and hemodynamic assessment
- Electrophysiology study to establish diagnosis and determine suitability for ablation

TREATMENT

CARDIOLOGY REFERRAL

- All patients should be seen by a consulting cardiologist and possibly a cardiac electrophysiologist

HOSPITALIZATION CRITERIA

- All symptomatic patients must be hospitalized initially in an intensive care unit

MEDICATIONS

- Medication for stable patients:
  - Amiodarone (150 mg IV over 10 min, then 1 mg/min IV for 6 hours, then 0.5 mg/min for 18 hours) *or*
  - Lidocaine (100 mg IV bolus followed by 1–4 mg/min IV)

THERAPEUTIC PROCEDURES

- Unstable patients (hypotension, congestive heart failure, or chest pain) need immediate synchronized cardioversion
- For patients with recurrent sustained VT and survivors of sudden death, implantable cardioverter-defibrillator (ICD) is indicated
  - Amiodarone may be needed to reduce frequency of shocks
- For recurrent nonsustained VT in the presence of ischemic left ventricular dysfunction, consider electrophysiologic studies or ICD for primary prevention
- VT ablation may be successful in selected patients

SURGERY

- Epicardial ICD if there is no venous access
- Left ventricular aneurysmectomy in selected patients
- Intraoperative VT ablation rarely done today

MONITORING

- ECG monitoring in the hospital

DIET AND ACTIVITY

- Restrictions based on underlying heart disease

ONGOING MANAGEMENT

HOSPITAL DISCHARGE CRITERIA

- After ICD implantation or adequate amiodarone load (or other pharmacologic therapy) or definitive procedure

FOLLOW-UP

- After ICD implantation, follow-up in 1 week, then every 3 months and every time the ICD discharges
- Follow-up for treatment of systolic dysfunction

COMPLICATIONS

- SCD
- ICD complications including long-term complications of infection and frequent shocks—either appropriate or inappropriate

PROGNOSIS

- Depends on underlying left ventricular function
- Worse for patients with an ischemic etiology, poor left ventricular function, and presentation as SCD

PREVENTION

- Similar to that for coronary arery disease

RESOURCES

PRACTICE GUIDELINES

- Indications for ICD implantation:
  - Secondary prevention of cardiac arrest
  - Primary prevention in both ischemic and nonischemic substrate with ejection fraction < 0.35 and QRS duration > 120 ms
- Hemodynamically significant VT with structural heart disease warrants ICD placement

REFERENCES

- Saliba WI, Natale A: Ventricular tachycardia syndromes. Med Clin North Am 2001;85:267.
- Talwar KK, Naik N: Etiology and management of sustained ventricular tachycardia. Am J Cardiovasc Drugs 2001;1:179.

INFORMATION FOR PATIENTS

- www.drpen.com/427.5

WEB SITES

- www.hrsonline.org
- www.acc.org
- www.americanheart.org

Wandering Atrial Pacemaker

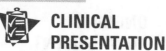

KEY FEATURES

ESSENTIALS OF DIAGNOSIS

- Progressive cyclic variation in P-wave morphology
- Heart rate 60–100 bpm
- Variation of P-wave morphology, P-P interval, and P-R interval

GENERAL CONSIDERATIONS

- This rhythm is benign
- This rhythm and multifocal atrial tachycardia are similar except for heart rate
- The other possible explanation is that there is significant respiratory sinus arrhythmia, with uncovering of latent foci of pacemaker activity
- Usually, it is associated with underlying lung disease
- In the elderly, it may be a manifestation of sick sinus syndrome
- In the young and athletic heart, it may represent enhanced vagal tone

CLINICAL PRESENTATION

SYMPTOMS AND SIGNS

- Usually causes no symptoms and is incidentally discovered
- Occasional patient may feel skipped beats

PHYSICAL EXAM FINDINGS

- Variable S_1

DIFFERENTIAL DIAGNOSIS

- Multifocal atrial tachycardia (heart rate > 100 bpm)

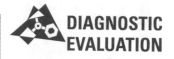

DIAGNOSTIC EVALUATION

LABORATORY TESTS

- None specific

ELECTROCARDIOGRAPHY

- ECG to document rhythm

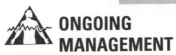

TREATMENT

CARDIOLOGY REFERRAL

• Not required

MEDICATIONS

• No specific treatment
• Monitor and treat the underlying cause, such as sick sinus syndrome or lung disease

DIET AND ACTIVITY

• No restrictions
• General healthy life style

ONGOING MANAGEMENT

FOLLOW-UP

• Once a year if sinus node abnormality is suspected; otherwise when symptoms arise

COMPLICATIONS

• May progress to sick sinus syndrome

PROGNOSIS

• This condition by itself is benign

RESOURCES

PRACTICE GUIDELINES

• Indications for pacemaker:
  – If part of sick sinus syndrome
  – Is associated with documented symptomatic bradycardia

REFERENCE

• Sergio FC, Steinberg JS: Supraventricular tachyarrhythmias involving the sinus node: clinical and electrophysiologic characteristics. Prog Cardiovasc Dis 1998;41:51.

INFORMATION FOR PATIENTS

• www.nlm.nih.gov/medlineplus/arrhythmia.html

WEB SITE

• www.hrsonline.org

Index